Applied Theatre: Performing Health and Wellbeing

The **Applied Theatre** series is a major innovation in applied theatre scholarship, bringing together leading international scholars that engage with and advance the field of applied theatre. Each book presents new ways of seeing and critically reflecting on this dynamic and vibrant field. Volumes offer a theoretical framework and introductory survey of the field addressed, combined with a range of case studies illustrating and critically engaging with practice.

Series Editors

Michael Balfour (Griffith University, Australia)
Sheila Preston (University of East London, UK)

Applied Theatre: Development
Tim Prentki
ISBN 978-1-4725-0986-4

Applied Theatre: Resettlement
Drama, Refugees and Resilience
Michael Balfour, Bruce Burton, Penny Bundy,
Julie Dunn and Nina Woodrow
ISBN 978-1-4725-3379-1

Applied Theatre: Research
Radical Departures
Peter O'Connor and Michael Anderson
ISBN 978-1-4725-0961-1

Applied Theatre: Aesthetics
Gareth White
ISBN 978-1-4725-1355-7

Applied Theatre: Performing Health and Wellbeing
Veronica Baxter and Katharine E. Low
ISBN 978-1-4725-8457-1

Applied Theatre: Facilitation
Sheila Preston
ISBN 978-1-4725-7693-4

Applied Theatre: Performing Health and Wellbeing

Veronica Baxter and Katharine E. Low

Series Editors
Michael Balfour and Sheila Preston

Bloomsbury Methuen Drama
An imprint of Bloomsbury Publishing Plc

B L O O M S B U R Y
LONDON • OXFORD • NEW YORK • NEW DELHI • SYDNEY

Bloomsbury Methuen Drama
An imprint of Bloomsbury Publishing Plc

Imprint previously known as Methuen Drama

50 Bedford Square	1385 Broadway
London	New York
WC1B 3DP	NY 10018
UK	USA

www.bloomsbury.com

BLOOMSBURY, METHUEN DRAMA and the Diana logo are trademarks of Bloomsbury Publishing Plc

First published 2017

© Veronica Baxter and Katharine E. Low, 2017

Veronica Baxter and Katharine E. Low have asserted their right under the Copyright, Designs and Patents Act, 1988, to be identified as editors of this work.

All rights reserved. No part of this publication may be reproduced or transmitted in any form or by any means, electronic or mechanical, including photocopying, recording, or any information storage or retrieval system, without prior permission in writing from the publishers.

No responsibility for loss caused to any individual or organization acting on or refraining from action as a result of the material in this publication can be accepted by Bloomsbury or the authors.

British Library Cataloguing-in-Publication Data
A catalogue record for this book is available from the British Library.

ISBN: HB: 978-1-4725-8456-4
PB: 978-1-4725-8457-1
ePDF: 978-1-4725-8459-5
ePub: 978-1-4-725-8458-8

Library of Congress Cataloging-in-Publication Data
A catalog record for this book is available from the Library of Congress.

Series: Applied Theatre

Cover design: Louise Dugdale
Cover image © Shutterstock

Typeset by Fakenham Prepress Solutions, Fakenham, Norfolk, NR21 8NN

Contents

List of Illustrations ix
Acknowledgements xi
Notes on Contributors xiii

Part 1

Introduction *Katharine Low* 3

1 Understanding Health, Wellbeing, the Millennium Development Goals and Health Inequities *Katharine Low* 11

2 Aesthetics, Instrumentalism and Ethics in Health and Wellbeing *Veronica Baxter* 41

Part 2

3 Ageing: Dementia Care, Death and Dying (the UK and North America) 75
   3.1 Introduction *Katharine Low* 75
   3.2 Essay – Participatory theatre and dementia *Nicola Hatton* 77
   3.3 Interview – A discussion about death? 'I feel more alive now' *Sue Mayo in conversation with Liz Rothschild, Director of* Kicking the Bucket: A Festival of Living and Dying 89

4 Communicable Diseases: Tuberculosis (South Africa), Malaria (Malawi) and Dengue Fever (Brazil) 97
   4.1 Introduction *Katharine Low* 97
   4.2 Essay – Tuberculosis: The forgotten plague *Veronica Baxter and Michele Tameris* 99

4.3	Snapshot – Dialogical theatre: Reconsidering the role of Theatre for Development for malaria prevention in Malawi *Zindaba Dunduzu Chisiza*	111
4.4	Interview – *Public Enemy No. 1*: Dengue fever in the *favelas* of Brazil *Johayne Hildefonso is interviewed by Jan Onoszko*	114

5 Non-Communicable Diseases: Lifestyle and Post-Colonial Stress Disorder (Canada), Nutrition and Health Eating (Denmark), Diabetes (UK)   121
   5.1 Introduction   *Katharine Low*   121
   5.2 Essay – 'Acting Out' our health: Assisting youth in making healthy lifestyle choices through linking Indigenous perspectives about wellbeing with Applied Theatre   *Julian Robbins, Warren Linds, Linda Goulet, Jo-Ann Episkenew and Karen Schmidt*   123
   5.3 Snapshot – Health theatre for children   *Dan Grabowski and Jens Aagaard-Hansen*   135
   5.4 Snapshot – Creativity and change in the lifestyles of South Asian communities in Yorkshire   *Geetha Upadhyaya*   142

6 Sexual Health: Practice from South Africa and the Asia–Pacific Region   145
   6.1 Introduction   *Veronica Baxter*   145
   6.2 Essay – 'It's difficult to talk about sex in a positive way': Creating a space to breathe   *Katharine Low*   146
   6.3 Snapshot – Performing the solution: Cautions and possibilities when using theatre conventions within HIV prevention programmes   *Helen Cahill*   162

7 Cancer: Research from the UK, USA and Australia   167
   7.1 Introduction   *Katharine Low*   167
   7.2 Essay – Proud disclosures and awkward receptions: Between bodies with cancer and their audiences   *Brian Lobel*   168

    7.3 Snapshot – *Alive and Out There*: Theatre addressing stigma around cancer in diverse communities in Sydney, Australia   *Astrid Perry and Lynne Baker*   180

8 Women's Health and Gender Inequity: Experiences from India, Malawi and the Solomon Islands   185
    8.1 Introduction   *Veronica Baxter*   185
    8.2 Essay – The ambiguities of *Shakti*: Performing women's well-being in India   *Nandita Dinesh*   186
    8.3 Snapshot – Women's drama group in Malawi targets mothers and children for burns prevention   *Effie Makepeace*   199
    8.4 Snapshot – *Stages of Change*: Using theatre to address domestic violence in the Solomon Islands   *Kiara Worth*   201

9 Mental Health: Perspectives from South Africa, the UK and Brazil   205
    9.1 Introduction   *Veronica Baxter*   205
    9.2 Essay – Between the 'traditional' and the theatrical: Forms and performances of healing depression in South Africa   *Sinethemba Makanya*   206
    9.3 Snapshot – *Mad Gyms and Kitchens*, Bobby Baker and Daily Life Ltd   *Caoimhe McAvinchey*   217
    9.4 Interview – Dionysus and ritual ecstasy: Madness and medicine   *Vitor Pordeus is interviewed by Katharine Low*   223

10 Snapshots of Practice: Environmental Health, Medical Dramaturgy, Addiction and Ebola   229
    10.1 Introduction   *Veronica Baxter*   229
    10.2 Snapshot – Ecological health in Violeta Luna's *NK603: Action for Performer & e-Maiz*   *Lisa Woynarski*   230
    10.3 Snapshot – Storying climate change adaptation: Theatre as a research tool in an Ecohealth research process in the Eastern Cape, South Africa   *Nicholas Hamer and Alexandra Sutherland*   234

10.4 Snapshot – Generating a medical dramaturgy: Live intersections between intermediality and health   *Deirdre McLaughlin and Joanne Scott*   238

10.5 Snapshot – 'Dance lifts us up in the world': Socially engaged theatre with people in recovery from addiction   *Zoe Zontou*   241

10.6 Snapshot – The performance of Ebola: A critical analysis of *Ebola Doctors*   *Gloria Ernest-Samuel*   245

Afterword   *Veronica Baxter and Katharine Low*   249
Notes   253
Index   307

List of Illustrations

Figure 1 Sara Cocker and a Storybox participant. Photo © Roshana Rubin-Mayhew for Small Things Creative Projects. 83

Figure 2 Pop Art image from *Carina's Choice* advises coughing into your elbow (not hands) to prevent the spread of tuberculosis. Photo © Veronica Baxter. 105

Figure 3 An *Aedes aegypti* mosquito looking satisfied at causing dengue fever, *Public Enemy No. 1*, 2009. Photo © AfroReggae. 118

Figure 4 *Husbands for Ma Lindi*. Photo © Patrick Selemani 160

Figure 5 Darpana's creation–performance–feedback loop in *Acting Healthy* & *Shakti*. 194

Figure 6 Women performing in *Stages of Change*, a theatre piece discussing domestic violence in the Solomon Islands. Photo © Kiara Worth. 201

Figure 7 *Mad Gyms and Kitchens*, Bobby Baker. Photo © Tim Smith 2012. 220

Figure 8 Violeta Luna – *NK603: Action for Performer & e-Maiz*. Photo © Greg Craig. 232

Figure 9 *Letting It Go*, Recipe for Life, West Yorkshire Playhouse. Photo © Kevin Hickson, Space2, http://www.space2.org.uk. 244

Acknowledgements

Katharine Low

It is impossible to thank everyone as fully as they deserve in print, but I will make up for that in person. My sincere and grateful thanks to Veronica Baxter, a kind and fantastic co-editor, and to all of our contributors to this book – your work has made this book and we are so excited to see it in print.

I also express my deep thanks both to my colleagues at the Royal Central School of Speech and Drama and to my colleagues, locally and further afield, all of whom epitomize collegiality and are excellent critical friends: Gilli Bush-Bailey, Steve Farrier, Gareth White, Amanda Stuart-Fisher, Selina Busby, Ben Buratta, Nicky Abraham, Lisa Woynarski, Joe Parslow and Tanya Zybutz; and to Sylvan Baker, Sue Mayo, Kerstin Mercer, Caoimhe McAvinchey, Ali Jeffers, Dave Calvert, Clara Vaughan and all those in the TaPRA Applied and Social Theatre Working Group. Many thanks also to both the Research Office and Theatre Applied: Centre for Research in Performance and Social Practice at Central for supporting my sabbatical, awarding research funding for some of the research in this book and for research assistance funding.

Thank you to my wonderful extended family and 'framily' in the UK and South Africa: my mum for being outspoken and always there, my dad for helping me celebrate all the small things in life, my brother for his generosity of spirit, and to Steve, without whose friendship and love, the world would be very boring. My last thanks are for all the women in my life who celebrate and jubilate each other's successes and stand shoulder to shoulder through the harder times. Thank you all.

Veronica Baxter

I gratefully acknowledge that in part, this research was made possible by a teaching relief grant from the University of Cape Town, and research travel funding from the National Research Foundation, South Africa. In addition, I thank Michele Tameris from SATVI for our collaboration, and the Wellcome Trust for funding our anti-tuberculosis community engagements. I am grateful to Jeremy David and Kerstin Mercer for their invaluable editing.

Kat Low has been a constant pleasure to work with – she has a rare generosity of spirit and her optimism has been unwavering. She and our co-authors have my gratitude and respect for their work.

I thank my colleagues at the University of Cape Town, in particular Nandita Dinesh and Pedzisai Maedza. My students remain an inspiration, reminding me that there is life in this old bird. I would also like to thank Nomazizi Msenge, whose support makes my focus on research work possible.

I stand on the shoulders of those who have gone before me, and thank them. My sisters, family and my heart's child, Georgia, have my eternal gratitude.

Notes on Contributors

Jens Aagaard-Hansen (MD, anthropologist, MPH, DTM, specialist in general medicine) has a double training background as medical doctor and social anthropologist. He has worked with anthropology in Europe, Africa and Asia for the past twenty-four years, focusing on children, health promotion, orphanhood, schooling, food security and medical anthropology. Much of the research has been conducted in close collaboration with local anthropologists as part of long-term projects, and dozens of anthropological Masters and PhD students have been trained. Over the years Jens has published on a wide range of topics, including health promotion and issues in relation to cross-disciplinarity.

Lynne Baker practices within the paradigm of process-oriented psychology. Using awareness, film and dramatic techniques, she opens up conversations. Some examples of her work include *Death, Dying and Ecstasy*, and *Article 3*, which addresses fundamental principles of human rights. She explores the diversity of marginalized people and lived experience. Her focus ranges from individuals to groups and socio-political concerns and crosses countries, cultures and hemispheres. Her qualifications include an MBA, a Diploma in Process Oriented Psychology and a Diploma in Screen. Lynne is a consultant psychologist, psychotherapist and film-maker.

Veronica Baxter is programme convener for Applied Theatre Masters, Honours and doctoral degrees at the University of Cape Town, South Africa. Her research and practice is mainly concerned with applied/social theatre, process drama and arts-based research working in health, education and social justice contexts. Veronica also conducts research and supervises postgraduate studies in South African and African theatre and performance. Drawing on extensive theatre practice in youth development, land restitution and HIV/AIDS work, she has partnered with health professionals around theatre approaches to the tuberculosis epidemic in the Western Cape region. Her most recent publications are chapters in *Applied Theatre: Development*, the *Methuen Drama Guide to South African Theatre* and *New Territories: Reconfiguring Theatre and Drama in Post-Apartheid South Africa*.

Helen Cahill is Associate Professor in student wellbeing and deputy-director of the Youth Research Centre, Graduate School of Education, University of Melbourne, Australia. She leads research, development and teaching in the fields of youth participation and wellbeing, specializing in the use of drama as critical pedagogy. She has developed a number of Australian and international health education programmes addressing issues related to drugs and mental health. Helen has led a number of prevention projects within developing countries in the Asia–Pacific region addressing life skills, reproductive health, HIV prevention and the reduction of gender-based violence.

Nandita Dinesh holds a PhD in Drama from the University of Cape Town, and an MA in Performance Studies from the Tisch School of the Arts at New York University. Her practice and research are centred on the potential and challenges of using theatre in response to conflict. With this focus, Nandita has conducted community-based theatre projects in India (Ahmedabad, Nagaland, Jammu and Kashmir), the United States (New Mexico), Mexico, Costa Rica, Guatemala, Rwanda, Uganda, Kenya and Zimbabwe.

Zindaba Dunduzu Chisiza is currently a PhD candidate at the University of Leeds. His research examines the effectiveness of a range of Theatre for Development practices as a dialogical tool for engaging young Malawian men in exploring identity and HIV/AIDS. He received his MA in Performance Research from the universities of Amsterdam and Warwick. His research interests are Theatre for Development, masculinities and gender politics in HIV/AIDS. Since

2012, Zindaba has worked as a lecturer in Drama at the University of Malawi, Chancellor College, and has been involved in devising theatre interventions with communities on human trafficking, cancer and agro-ecology.

Jo-Ann Episkenew was Director of the Indigenous Peoples' Health Research Centre and Professor of English at the First Nations University of Canada. An active researcher, her interests include Aboriginal youth health, applied literatures and trauma studies. Jo-Ann is author of *Taking Back Our Spirits: Indigenous Literatures, Public Policy, and Healing* (2009), winner of two Saskatchewan Book Awards. In 2015 the YWCA Regina recognized her with their Women of Distinction Lifetime Achievement Award.

Gloria Ernest-Samuel, a lecturer at the Department of Theatre Arts, Imo State University, Owerri, Nigeria, holds a Master of Arts degree in Media and Communication from the University of Calabar, Calabar, Nigeria. She is currently a PhD candidate at the University of the Witwatersrand, Johannesburg. Gloria has a special interest in Nollywood, and thus focuses on media, communication and cultural studies. She has published many academic articles in many local and international journals.

Linda Goulet is Professor of Indigenous Education at First Nations University of Canada, where she teaches Indigenous pedagogies and health and arts education. Her research with First Nations youth using the arts to explore social issues of health grew out of her interest in exploring effective teaching with Indigenous youth. In addition to other publications, Linda recently co-authored *Teaching Each Other: Nehinuw Concepts and Indigenous Pedagogies* (2015).

Dan Grabowski has a background in educational sociology and a PhD from the University of Southern Denmark in health education and health promotion. He works as a researcher at the Steno Diabetes

Center in Copenhagen and has published extensively on the topic of school children's health identities and health behaviour. Currently Dan's main research interest is family health promotion, with a particular interest in how to generate mutual involvement in families faced with problems pertaining to obesity and/or type 2 diabetes – thereby preventing the inter-familial spread of lifestyle diseases and negative health behaviour.

Nicholas Hamer works as a research associate at the Department of Environmental Science and the Institute for Water Research at Rhodes University, where he manages a project focusing on Climate Change Adaptation. His research interests include understanding how scientific knowledge can effectively be shared within a research process in rural communities, with a study on the effectiveness of a drama process to share knowledge relating to Climate Change Adaptation. At the Institute for Water Research, Nicholas leads a case study that collaborates with citizen-researchers to understand and respond to water resources challenges in Grahamstown, South Africa.

Nicola Hatton is a theatre practitioner and a lecturer in Drama at the University of Winchester. Her current research explores the creative role of artists in care settings, with a focus on how they engage with the sensory and aesthetic qualities of care homes. Nicola's recent publications include 'Re-imagining the care home: a spatially-responsive approach to arts practice in residential care', published in *RiDE, The Journal of Applied Theatre and Performance*.

Johayne Hildefonso is AfroReggae's Artistic Director as well as being the co-ordinator of their Wally Salomão Cultural Centre in Vigário Geral, Rio de Janeiro. He is also a theatre and improvisation teacher at Rio's renowned O Tablado Theatre. Johayne has worked as an actor, director and choreographer in film and theatre for more than 20 years, as well as directing international shows for AfroReggae, including their *Favela to the World* show at London's Barbican Theatre in 2007.

Warren Linds is Associate Professor in the Department of Applied Human Sciences at Concordia University, Montreal, Canada. His area of expertise is in exploring arts-based research as social intervention and applying forum theatre techniques to address issues of social justice. Warren is co-editor, with Elinor Vettraino, of *Playing in a House of Mirrors: Applied Theatre as Reflective Practice* (2015).

Brian Lobel is a Wellcome Trust Public Engagement Fellow and Senior Lecturer in Theatre at the University of Chichester. His publications include *BALL & Other Funny Stories About Cancer* (2012) and *CANCER CANCER CANCER CANCER CANCER* (2012), articles in *PAJ*, *CTR* and *Performance Research* and chapters in many collections. Brian writes primarily on the patient narrative and illness discourses, and works to introduce social models of disability to understanding cancer and chronic illness. His performance works include *An Appreciation*, *Purge*, *Carpe Minuta Prima*, *Cruising for Art* and *Fun with Cancer Patients*, all of which have toured internationally.

Katharine Low is a practitioner and researcher in socially engaged theatre practice, specializing in sexual and reproductive health (SRH), and is a lecturer in Applied Theatre and Community Performance at the Royal Central School of Speech and Drama. Since 2003, she has been researching and developing social theatre practices as an approach to SRH communication. As a practitioner, Katharine has developed applied theatre practices as ways of engaging young adults and women living with HIV in discussions around SRH in South Africa, Tanzania and the UK. Her current research interests lie in the fields of arts and health, sexual health communication, women and theatre, prison theatre and South African theatre. She has published her research in a number of journals and is currently writing a monograph on her applied practice in South Africa for Palgrave Macmillan. Katharine has also co-authored forthcoming chapters on theatre with women in the criminal justice system and theatre-making with HIV+ women. Between 2012 and 2016, she was a co-convenor of the Theatre and Performance Research Association's Applied and Social Theatre Working Group, and she is a trustee of the London Arts and Health Forum.

Sinethemba Makanya is a PhD candidate at the University of the Witwatersrand (WITS) Institute for Social and Economic Research (WISER) in Medical Humanities. She is a drama therapist trained at New York University (2012) and an initiate in the tradition of Indigenous healing. Sinethemba is the first of two black drama therapists in South Africa and is using her research to think through how drama therapy can integrate with Indigenous knowledge to offer integrated theories of personhood. She teaches at the University of Pretoria, and Drama for Life at the University of the Witwatersrand.

Effie Makepeace is a community theatre practitioner. She graduated from her Masters in Participation, Power and Social Change at the Institute of Development Studies in 2014. She has worked with community groups in the UK and internationally for eight years, using theatre to explore issues relevant to the communities she is working with. Effie is currently working at Cardboard Citizens in London and continues to explore theatre as a research tool, with particular focus on the area of sexualities.

Sue Mayo is a theatre-maker and academic who specializes in intergenerational arts practice. She has worked extensively with arts charity Magic Me, for whom she led the innovative Women's Library Project – eleven years of intergenerational women's projects. Sue teaches at Goldsmiths, University of London, where she is Convenor of the MA in Applied Theatre: Drama in Educational, Social, and Community Settings. Her research interests include creativity and dementia, the role of the artist in participatory work, and the semiotics of participation. Recent writing includes *A Marvellous Experiment* and the *Artist in Collaboration* and chapters in *Performance and Community: Commentary and Case Studies* (2013).

Caoimhe McAvinchey is a senior lecturer in Drama, Theatre and Performance at Queen Mary University of London. Throughout her research in socially engaged arts practice, she has collaborated with artists and arts organizations working in prisons (Clean Break), intergenerational arts practice (Magic Me), participatory arts with young people (Phakama) and arts and mental health (Bobby Baker and Daily Life Ltd). Caoimhe's publications include *Theatre and Prison* (2011) and *Performance and Community: Case Studies and Commentary* (2013) and she is currently preparing the forthcoming publications: *Applied Theatre: Women and the Criminal Justice System*, *Phakama: Participatory Performance in the Making* (co-edited with Lucy Richardson and Fabio Santos) and a monograph about Clean Break theatre company.

Deirdre McLaughlin is the Director of MA Acting at Arts Educational Schools in London. She has worked professionally as an actor, director and dramaturg in the US and UK at venues including Shakespeare's Globe, the National Theatre Studio, The Place, Williamstown Theatre Festival and New York Stage & Film. She is a PhD candidate at the Royal Central School of Speech and Drama. Deirdre is a founding member of the Embodied Cognition, Acting and Performance working group at the Society for the Study of Artificial Intelligence and the Simulation of Behaviour.

Jan Onoszko is a British journalist living in Rio de Janeiro. He started his career at BBC Radio Leeds before spending more than nine years at ITV as a reporter, presenter and documentary maker. In 2009 he moved to Rio, where he works as a freelance journalist, translator and producer.

Astrid Perry is the manager of the Multicultural Health Service, South Eastern Sydney Local Health District and convenor of the state-wide Multicultural Health Services network. She holds a PhD in Sociology from the University of Western Sydney. Astrid has a particular interest in research, health promotion, training and models of care to improve access to culturally appropriate health care and health services. Her recent publications include 'eSimulation: a novel approach to enhancing cultural competence within a health care organization' in *Nursing Education in Practice* (2014) and 'Love stories, understanding the caring journey of aged Greek-Australian carers' in *Health and Social Care in the Community* (2015).

Vitor Pordeus is a theatre-maker, transcultural psychiatrist and co-creator of the Hotel and Spa of Madness (at the Nise da Silveira Mental Health Institute in Rio de Janeiro). He trained in theatre under Amir Haddad, Ray Lima and Junio Santos. Vitor is also the founding director of the Centre for Culture, Science and Health of the Public Health Office of Rio de Janeiro City, and co-founder of the People's University for Art and Science, and has authored many papers ranging in topic from immunology to psychiatry.

Julian Robbins is mixed race with Mi'kmaq ancestry. He is currently employed as a post-doctoral fellow at the Indigenous Peoples' Health Research Centre in Saskatchewan, where he is helping to organize health and wellness research (that uses culture and the arts) around the general area of suicide prevention for Aboriginal youth of the File Hills Qu'Appelle Tribal Council (FHQTC), situated in southern Saskatchewan. Julian completed his PhD dissertation in Indigenous Studies at Trent University in 2014.

Liz Rothschild is a writer, director and actor who trained at the Bristol Old Vic Theatre School in the UK, before pursuing a busy and active career, embracing mainstream and socially engaged theatre. Alongside this, Liz has developed *Kicking the Bucket, a Festival of Living and Dying*, which is held bi-annually in Oxford, UK.

Karen Schmidt is of Cree and German descent and is a member of Cowessess First Nation in Saskatchewan. She has resided in the Fort

Qu'Appelle area for most of her life and has served as Health Educator for File Hills Qu'Appelle Tribal Council for ten years. In that role, Karen has acted as liaison between the *Acting Out in a Good Way* research project, the community and the tribal council.

Jo Scott is a live media practitioner-researcher and lecturer in performance at the University of Salford. Her research explores the creation, activation and experience of events created through live media modes of practice. Jo has presented her practice-as-research at various events and symposia, including recently a contribution to the 'Networked Bodies' symposium at Watermans Art Centre in Brentford and a live set for the 2015 Sonic Fusion Festival at MediaCityUK, Salford

Alexandra Sutherland is Associate Professor in Drama Studies at Rhodes University, South Africa, where she heads the Applied Theatre programmes for undergraduate and postgraduate students. Her teaching and research activities focus broadly on the creation of play and performance spaces within institutional settings as a way to generate alternative physical, social, emotional and political modes of representation. This has included a theatre project with young people in a street children's shelter, and the uses of performance to interrogate race and class within higher education. Alexandra's current research involves the social and aesthetic meanings of performance in forensic institutions.

Michele Tameris is a medical practitioner and has been a clinical research officer at the South Africa Vaccine Initiative (SATVI) in Worcester, South Africa, since 2003. She has served as Principal Investigator on several vaccine trials. Michele is well acquainted with the participant community because she has been closely involved in developing material for SATVI community projects, including the comic and performances of *Carina's Choice*. Michele has been a driving force in SATVI's efforts for community involvement, by active facilitation of SATVI's Community Advisory Board.

Geetha Upadhyaya is an NHS Consultant in the field of medical pathology, metabolic medicine and endocrinology. She also has a postgraduate degree in classical Indian dance/music and has worked in India and Malaysia with children with learning disabilities and autism. She co-founded, and is the Artistic Director of, Kala Sangam, a South Asian arts and culture and heritage company. In addition, Geetha has founded charities for people with autism in Bradford and south India. She has received the Beacon of Cultural Diversity award from the Asian Business Network and an honorary doctorate from Bradford University.

Kiara Worth is a writer, photographer, development consultant, social activist and world traveller. With a background in community development, she has a particular interest in using the creative arts as a communication tool and has worked as a development consultant internationally. Kiara has led a range of civil society groups focused on community development and sustainability, and currently works as a photographer documenting multilateral negotiations on the environment and development. She spent five years working in Papua New Guinea as a writer and photographer, with a unique opportunity to experience the diverse and colourful cultures of the Pacific.

Lisa Woynarski is Lecturer of Theatre in the Department of Film, Theatre and Television at the University of Reading. She works at the intersection of performance and ecology, specializing in urban ecology and contemporary performance practices. Lisa received her PhD from Royal Central School of Speech and Drama for her research articulating an ecological performance aesthetic. As a performance-maker and ecodramaturg, she makes research-engaged performances exploring climate change resilience and urban ecology. Lisa's work has been published in *Contemporary Theatre Review*, *RiDE*, *Performance Research* and the Centre for Sustainable Practice in *The Quarterly*. She was recently a postdoctoral researcher on Tonic Theatre's Advance project on gender equality in the UK performing arts. Lisa is co-convener of the Culture and Ecology Network (London).

Zoe Zontou is Lecturer in Drama at Liverpool Hope University. Her principal research interests lie in the field of socially engaged theatre with people in recovery from substance misuse. Her research covers a wide range of topics, including autobiography in performance, addiction studies and cultural policy, which are examined through their relationship with socially engaged theatre. Zoe has worked as a practitioner and researcher in a number of organizations and has published in the area of socially engaged theatre research and practice. Her most recent publication, co-edited with James Reynolds, is the book *Addiction and Performance* (2014).

Part One

Introduction

Katharine Low

The biggest challenge facing our global community today is health. Both health inequities and poor health, coupled with limited access to universal health care, has resulted in a situation in which the global burden of disease is significant for many countries. However, the crisis rests predominantly in the Global South and low-income countries. Richard Horton, editor of *The Lancet*, a British medical journal, summarizes the state of the world's health, based on the findings of the 2010 Global Burden of Disease study (GBD):

> Tuberculosis and malaria are estimated to have killed around 1.2 million people each in 2010. 8 million people died from cancer in 2010, over a third more deaths than 20 years ago. One in four deaths was from heart disease or stroke. 1.3 million deaths were due to diabetes. Deaths from road traffic injuries increased by almost half. Blood pressure is the biggest global risk factor for disease, followed by tobacco, alcohol, and poor diet. And young adults are emerging as a new and neglected priority in global health: GBD 2010 finds that young adults, especially men, are dying in far higher numbers than previously appreciated. But the most afflicted continent remains Africa. Here, maternal, newborn, and child mortality, along with a broad array of vaccine-preventable and other communicable diseases, remain urgent concerns.[1]

Indeed, while the burden of infectious diseases (such as HIV) begins to plateau, we are living longer: life expectancy has increased globally from 65.3 years in 1990 to 71.5 years in 2013,[2] which in turn has an impact on our health. We see this in the rise of age-related illnesses, such as Alzheimer's disease and other dementias, and the rising death rates from non-communicable diseases (NCD) and injury.[3] However, it is the impact of poverty on health that remains one of our biggest challenges. For example, over 95 per cent of tuberculosis-related deaths occur in the developing world, and 80 per cent of NCDs are found in low- to middle-income countries.[4] Furthermore, low- to middle-income countries often 'face a heavy triple burden of infections, NCDs, and injuries'.[5]

The current state of the world's health has led to a call to action by the Commission on Social Determinants of Health to both governments and NGOs, as well as to civil society.[6] There is clearly a role to play for the arts in this setting. In a recent article, Peter Bazalgette, chair of the English Arts Council, noted the following:

> As it happens, quietly and with increasing effectiveness, medics and carers, health authorities and local councils alike are turning to the arts as one way to help boost the wellbeing of the nation. This is about prevention rather than cure. And, as ever with the arts and culture, it's about enriching lives, too.[7]

However, while there is an increasing recognition of the importance of the arts in health (see for example the 2014 launch of the All Party Parliamentary Group for Arts, Health and Wellbeing in the UK Parliament),[8] there remains caution as to how the arts are perceived to 'function'. For example, John Ashton, President of the British Faculty of Public Health, warns:

> If the arts are to play their full part in health, we must make their contribution explicit throughout the human life cycle, from birth and health through adolescence and adult life to decline, death and mourning. Arts and culture are a part of every human's makeup and potential, assets that should be explored and developed – not commodities that can be separated from the essence of the person and exploited.[9]

It is here that theatre, performance and art-making can make a powerful impact. Theatre-making in response to particular health situations, and as part of a creative human process as a human right, has been long-standing. This book brings together practice and practitioners who work in the field to oversee a wealth of practice occurring across the world, contrasting work taking place in the Global South with that of the Global North. We bring these examples of work to this book to challenge, critique and celebrate innovative practice in the field of Applied Theatre and performance.

Broadly, we define Applied Theatre and performance as theatre-making with, for and by particular groups of people and in locations that are not traditionally associated with theatre. The origins of the term Applied Theatre have been vigorously debated elsewhere;[10,11,12] however, there is a general consensus that Applied Theatre practice, in its most pared down form, involves theatre-making with and/or for a particular group of people. The settings in which the theatre-making takes place are varied, from conflict zones to inter-generational work, focusing on literacy or health. As health is the focus of *Performing Health and Wellbeing*, the following chapters contain a range of research essays, brief snapshots and accounts of projects and interviews in order to examine and discuss particular understandings of theatre-making in specific health contexts. It is useful here to frame how we are examining theatre-making in a health context. When considering the field of Applied Theatre and performance around health, two strands, 'arts in health' and 'arts for health', emerge. In the arts in health category we see the art-making to be the primary intent of the arts activity, with any health benefits or education emerging as a welcome outcome. In the arts for health strand, the arts are viewed as the medium of engagement with the health issue with direct pedagogical intentions. However, as will become evident in the practice discussed in this book, these two categories are very broad; often practice is not as easily or simply categorized as one or the other, which we believe is a good thing since art-making should transcend categorization. We must also be wary of the instinct to categorize, as in that categorization we are potentially medicalizing the arts.

As authors, we understand that the differentiation between these two categories lies in the intentions of the practice as well its context. The work in this book therefore clusters around four broad categories: educational work around health issues (with specific pedagogic and interventionist approaches); art-making/making art in response to specific health issues; addressing health through creativity/artistry/art-making (wellbeing); and finally performance research, which involves researching people's health through participatory arts (or arts-based research)[13] methodologies. Again, that is not to say that the practices examined in this book fall neatly into these categories – on the contrary, we are fully conscious of the problematics of viewing the theatre-making in such binary terms. Rather, we feel it is a useful way of framing some of the analysis which allows for more in-depth discussion. As co-editors, we do have differing views on approaches to practice, particularly around questions of intention, instrumentalism and aesthetics, and in Chapter 2 Veronica Baxter argues that this is contextualized by perspectives from the Global South and the Global North. In this book, we will distinguish between academic scholarship and practice, namely acknowledging the importance of the scholarship, for example from medical anthropologists, in terms of contextualizing and grounding the practice within broader health discourses.

Essentially, we consider creativity and the aesthetic as fundamental elements to all practice and view with *dis-ease* approaches to practice which reduce the experience of theatre-making to solely reaching a particular need. We are also conscious of a neoliberal agenda whereby arts practice is being employed as a salve or plaster for widespread and complex social ills.

In their recent book *Art as Therapy*, Alain de Botton and John Armstrong critique the view that art should be for art's sake, arguing that they find the art world's negative responses to attempts to determine the purpose of art somewhat reductionist.[14] Rather, they suggest that if we consider art as therapy – taking the notion of the therapeutic as broadly enhancing our lives – art becomes a means of this improvement. In short, they believe that art has a latent therapeutic potential and that the goal of art should be self-improvement. While in essence de Botton and Armstrong are discussing visual arts, the arguments that they make do have resonances for performance-based practices. However, when viewed from a health perspective we challenge de Botton and Armstrong's reductionist view of the purpose and impact of art-making. Defining the aetiology of art's purpose in this context is not particularly useful – there are so many other possibilities for this form of art-making. Furthermore, asking such a question sets up an unhelpful false binary of 'art without purpose' versus 'art with a purpose'. The question should not be 'is art for self-improvement or not?' Rather, we should explore if art does lead to improvements in health, if a number of other factors are at play. For art to have 'improvement' qualities it needs to succeed as art in of and as itself; fundamentally it requires 'success' in terms of aesthetic qualities, amongst others. We take heed of Emma Brodzinski's warning against theatre-making that neglects artistry in favour of the intentions of the work.[15] Additionally, we are informed by François Matarasso's view of art: 'Art may be defined as a means through which we can examine our experience of ourselves, the world around us, and the relationship between the two, and share the results with other people in a form that gives free rein to our intellectual, physical, emotional and spiritual qualities.'[16] Thus, in this book the reader will encounter practice that is innovative, challenging and extraordinary, but above all, the practice will contain a strong aesthetic, and creativity will be integral to its process and form. We believe that without a creative, aesthetic focus, arts and health practice can be commodified, whereby the art is serving the goals of the health message, public health provider or funders. However, where instrumentalist practice is discussed in this book, its aesthetics are rigorously critiqued.

We have divided the book into examining work from both the Global South and the Global North, with a view to comparing and analysing practice from both regions. An initial categorization of countries as either Global North or Global South is a development from the Cold War-era categories of First World, Second World and Third

World. Predominantly based on the United Nations Development Programme's Human Development Index (HDI), a division between countries into either category is linked to the global political economy. Traditionally richer and 'more developed' countries, often located in the North, are defined as Global North. These include the UK, North America, numerous European countries and developed parts of Asia and Oceania, such as Australia and New Zealand. Countries that have medium to low HDI ratings[17] (such as Tonga and the Gambia) are described as belonging to the Global South, a categorization that broadly includes most developing countries and many countries that are geographically located in the southern hemisphere. While the current categorizations of Global South and Global North are being challenged, in that they are reductive and do not take into account the growing economies of countries in the Global South,[18] we have maintained the existing classification because of the way in which inequities around the economy, gender, societal and structural factors impact on the health of the people in the Global South. For example, while HIV is significantly important as a health crisis in sub-Saharan Africa in terms of numbers, infection in the UK is relatively low, and other growing health issues, such as dementia, are important. In addition to the burden of disease as experienced differently in North and South, the Gini-coefficient shows that, generally, developed nations have lower inequality between citizens, with Global South countries amongst the highest. A Gini index of 0 represents perfect equality, while an index of 100 implies perfect inequality. For example, the World Bank places Norway at 25, the UK at 33 and Germany at 30.1. Peru is scored at 44.7, the USA at 41.1 and South Africa at 63.5.[19]

The contributors to this book are practitioners, academic researchers, medical doctors and sociologists. They work across a range of fields within different contexts and they represent new and sometimes unheard voices from areas of the world that are underrepresented in discussions of arts and health practices. We hope that the breadth of work presented in this book is as exciting for the reader to engage with as it as has been for us to work with. The book is divided into two parts: the first part offers, in Chapter 1, introductions to the fields of health, wellbeing and health inequities and, in Chapter 2, the history of Applied Theatre and performance in the field of health. The second part of the book considers eight specific health areas, namely the ageing population and death and dying; communicable diseases; non-communicable diseases; sexual health; cancer; women's health and gender inequity; mental health; and emerging health concerns. For each of these areas, we have gathered two or three contributions from differing countries and contexts and have provided brief introductions to the topics in question. In closing, returning to the Commission on Social Determinants of Health's call to action mentioned at the start of this Introduction, the practice discussed and analysed in this book demonstrates ways of exploring and challenging health issues throughout 'the human life cycle'. We hope that readers will find inspiration and provocation alike in the work discussed as we work alongside each other creating and making art in and for health.

1

Understanding Health, Wellbeing, the Millennium Development Goals and Health Inequities

Katharine Low

In this chapter, I explore understandings and perceptions of health and wellbeing[1] and consider how these terms are employed in the field of healthcare and arts in health. Health and wellbeing are terms that are sometimes used interchangeably; however, that is not the case in this book. In brief, we define health as as an individual's emotional, spiritual and physical condition. We engage with the notion of social health and wellbeing, and we define wellbeing as a social construct that intersects with individuals' and communities' perceptions of their own health. The subtleties of these definitions will be critiqued in the chapter that follows. Alongside this, I offer an introduction to the impetus and need for health promotion, framing this against an analysis of the Millennium Development Goals and existing global health inequities in order to provide a context and an explanation for the importance of theatre and performance-based responses to health concerns globally.

Health

The complexity of identifying the meaning of health is illustrated by the Ancient Greeks' way of treating the ill in temples dedicated to Apollo's son, Asclepius, the god of health and medicine. Called 'asclepia', these temples were established as healing sanctuaries to which pilgrims travelled for care.[2] These temples, as Edwin Heathcote explains, followed the notion of 'holos' or holistic understanding of treatment, whereby the whole person was cared for, mind and body: '[T]he cure was cultural, spiritual, topographical and medicinal.'[3] Remains of asclepia can be found across Greece and Turkey; however, what is fascinating is that they were not only comprised of temples: rather, each asclepion would often include a theatre (an odeion), a temple dedicated to Asclepius, baths, gymnasiums and sleep lodges (abatons). During the patients' 'stay', the pilgrims would watch rituals enacted by the attendants before sleeping in the lodges and discussing their resulting dreams with the priests.[4,5] Heathcote notes that '[t]heatre, the ultimate cathartic entertainment, was central to the experience, a purging of emotion'.[6] While the Greeks could be perceived as prescribing art as medicine, such an understanding of the wholeness of a person's needs and health can be seen in other cultures over time. Indeed, as Eleonora Belfiore notes, the arts in health have a long history 'which extends beyond the Western intellectual tradition'.[7] Drawing on Rafael Campo's research, Belfiore points to practices of incantations and rituals using poetry as healing practices found in Native American cultures and within Egypt at the time of the Pharaohs.[8]

Yet, over time the wholeness or *holos* understanding of health seems to have disappeared and a normalizing understanding has appeared in its place. Susan Sontag most notably draws attention to this in her two essays, *Illness as Metaphor and AIDS Its Metaphors*, as she considers how ill-health and disease are constructed and described in American society in the 1970s and 1980s.[9] Commenting on Sontag's essays, Marilyn Bordwell points to how Sontag illustrates that the perception of disease 'is not merely a value-neutral biological malfunction, of interest only to the patient and the physician. Rather, "feelings about evil are projected onto a disease. And the disease (so enriched with meanings) is projected onto the world." '[10] Indeed, the concept of health is historically difficult to capture and definitions of the meaning of health are regularly debated. In *The Gay Science*, first published in 1882, Friedrich Nietzsche argued:

For there is no health as such, and all attempts to define a thing that way have been wretched failures. Even the determination of what is healthy for your *body* depends on your goal, your horizon, your energies, your impulses, your errors, and above all on the ideals and phantasms of your soul.[11]

More recently, François Matarasso has noted that it is 'fruitless' to attempt a definition of health, pointing out that 'a general definition of good health is impossible since health is always experienced and the value each of us sets on different aspects will vary'.[12] Thus, understandings of health are complex; while Matarasso draws attention to the individuality of health and the way in which we experience it, Kenneth Boyd points to the numerous obstacles in defining health. In his analysis of health concepts, Boyd draws on Nietzsche's view that attempting to define health as the absence of disease or infirmity leads to complications as, for example, some people may have symptoms of illness such as nausea but have no obvious disorder, and secondly, Boyd notes that these terms are often 'rooted in metaphor' and embody specific value judgements.[13] Indeed, as Boyd proceeds to argue, the definitions of health, healing and wholeness will continue to remain elusive until the 'arguments which reduce first-person experience to third-person psychological, sociological or evolutionary explanations' are countered.[14] This remains the crux of the problem: definitions of health usually refer to notions of wholeness, absence of disease or ability to recover. For example, the medical historiographer George Canguilhem proposes the following: 'To be in good health, means being able to fall sick and recover.'[15] That is to say, a healthy body is one that does not have a chronic disease or illness, or is able to recuperate. Malcolm MacLachlan argues that such views of health are 'encouraged by a purely disease (or medical) conception of health and illness', which seems to indicate that if you have a broken arm, genetic disease or form of cancer 'you are in an undesirable state and therefore ill'.[16] Furthermore, as Boyd points out, such definitions remain ambiguous, intangible and do not capture the whole picture. Both Boyd and

MacLachlan separately argue that these definitions are problematic because they suggest a normative aim whereby the person suffering from disease is not 'whole'. MacLachlan problematizes such a view by pointing out that if health is defined by lack of illness, how do you define a person's health if they have, for example, previously suffered from hallucinations but no longer have them or if a person is HIV positive but is not displaying any symptoms?

Yet, it remains difficult to define or name health other than through the absence of illness or disease, a fact to which Alan Blum draws attention in his book, *The Grey Zone of Health and Illness* (2011). Blum argues that 'it always seems as if health can only be determined by disease, existing as nothing more than the time spent thinking about not being ill or in following regimes designed to fortify itself against such a disturbance'.[17] Furthermore, MacLachlan argues that people and their health are more complicated than a binary between healthy or unhealthy, noting that 'we can at once be relatively healthy in some aspects of life and relatively unhealthy in other aspects of it'.[18] In a similar vein, Blum develops this argument further by commenting on the difficulty of 'justifying the "good feeling" assumed to come from healthfulness and well-being in-itself'.[19] He argues that without having the possibility of using any disturbances (or 'feeling bad') to describe one's health, we appear to fall into a trap where our descriptions of our health 'seem rhapsodic or at least every bit as vacuous or incommunicable as describing one's pain'.[20] Blum suggests that one of the reasons for this is due to the way in which our bodies and our minds communicate, indicating that such communication may not be straightforward. He suggests that 'the body "records" influences from the environment in a way that the mind might not grasp', explaining further: 'The body, then, is much like an interlocutor to the mind, which "replies" to it as if a representative of the unknown environment, recording its influences in a way that could question any action.' [21] While Blum draws attention to the difficulty of communicating with another one's pain or experiences of ill health, the focus on alternative ways of communicating understandings of health is exciting as it encourages the possibility of recognizing other means of sharing understandings and experiences of health, pain and wellbeing, not simply verbally but rather through performance, movement and art.

Alongside the difficulty of defining health vs ill-health, there exists a normative or normalizing view around health, where certain health behaviours are promoted in order to help improve their community's or individual's health situation. As Marian Pitts and Keith Phillips have argued, there exists

> [...] a common-sense notion that a relationship exists between good health and personal habits. Plato said, 'where temperance is, there health is speedily imparted'. Many groups have codified 'good' living habits into their religions and there is strong evidence of the outcome of healthy living and abstinence in such communities: Mormons in Utah have a 30 per cent lower incidence of most cancers than the general population of the USA (Matarazzo, 1983)[22]

While the matter of what constitutes 'good' health and the normalizing emphasis on 'good' 'views' will be discussed in more detail when considering notions of wellbeing below, it remains that ideas of health are frequently normative and prescriptive; indeed, as a result of religious doctrines or frameworks of morality, certain behaviours are condemned by society, religious leaders or public officials as placing a person's health at 'risk'.

There are several critiques of the definition of health: not appreciating the extent of the health experience and the wholeness of a person, the complexities of how diverse communities define health and the lack of a holistic understanding of health, which I turn to now. Considering the World Health Organization's (WHO's) definition of health – 'Health is a state of complete physical, mental and social wellbeing and not merely the absence of disease or infirmity'[23] – an initial reading does appear to acknowledge that to be in good health means more than the absence of disorder in the body. However, the notion of 'complete' is problematic as some people may feel that they are healthy, despite suffering from chronic pain. Additionally, critics have argued that it is not a practical definition:[24] it is too utopian and, crucially, tends to equate health with happiness, which, as Rodolfo Saracci argues, is the equivalent of equating two distinct experiences with little relationship between each other.[25] The equation of health with happiness is again part of a normative approach to health, whereby individuals are guided to follow a particular interpretation of health depending on where they happen to live. Currently, there appears to be a push for a definition of health as being all-encompassing in nature, drawing together a range of possibilities so as to work for everyone. For example, the South African Department of Health states that its mission is to 'improve health status through the prevention of illnesses and the promotion of healthy lifestyles and to consistently improve the healthcare delivery system by focusing on access, equity, efficiency, quality and sustainability' in order to achieve its vision of 'a long and healthy life for all South Africans'.[26] The Department of Health in Papua New Guinea notes that its vision for health is 'A healthy and prosperous nation that upholds human rights and our Christian and traditional values'[27] and the Ministry of Health in Singapore states its vision as 'Championing a healthy nation with our people – To live well, live long & with peace of mind.'[28] Yet, as with the WHO definition, such ideals are both utopian and highly problematic in that it is not possible to agree a global definition of health given differences in cultural understandings, structures of feelings and access to health care and material conditions. Rather, I believe it is important to examine more diverse and holistic understandings of health; for example, Saracci suggests that we consider using a more helpful descriptor of health and offers the following: 'Health is a condition of well-being free of disease or infirmity and a basic and universal human right',[29] which sets up an interesting and timely parallel between health and human rights.

Alternatively, Niyi Awofeso points to the Australian Aboriginal people's definition of health which incorporates both community health and spiritual and wellbeing as core features of their definition, a decision that he argues would help to 'enrich' the WHO's existing definition of health.[30] In full, Aboriginal health is defined by the

National Aboriginal Community Controlled Health Organization (NACCHO) as follows:

> 'Aboriginal health' means not just the physical well-being of an individual but refers to the social, emotional and cultural well-being of the whole Community in which each individual is able to achieve their full potential as a human being thereby bringing about the total well-being of their Community. It is a whole of life view and includes the cyclical concept of life–death–life.[31]

Here a more holistic and life-cycle view of health is apparent and there exists an acknowledgement of the subtleties of health and experiences of health as being continually emerging. For example, Mike White, discussing the notion of health within the field of arts in health, and particularly in participatory arts, offers a linking of dignity with health. Considering how self-esteem is often used as an indicator of a successful arts in health project, White draws on Richard Horton's argument that '[i]njuries to individual or community dignity may represent a hitherto unrecognised pathogenic force with the destructive capacity towards physical, mental and social well-being at least equal to that of viruses and bacteria'[32] in order to suggest that a more appropriate measurement might be the dignity of those involved. White argues that '[d]ignity might be measurable too in that we all have an instinctive understanding of when our own has been violated'.[33] There is clearly a push towards a more holistic understanding of health across diverse fields, as is evident in a recent report on global health from the WHO's mandated Commission on Social Determinants of Health, which was established by the WHO in 2005 as an independent commission to promote health equity by analysing and gathering evidence and data to help encourage global action. The Commission noted that 'the success of societies must be measured not only in terms of economic growth but also in terms of sustainability and the increased well-being and quality of life of citizens. Health is a key contributor to this wide range of societal goals.'[34] Such a statement, to me, illustrates a clear view of the holistic and all-encompassing nature of health, in which health is not seen in an individualistic or normative manner, but a view which is responsive to both societal input and individual desires and intentions. A more holistic and encompassing view of health is fundamental as it is impossible to agree one definition that fits or suits a global population; rather, I believe that it is important to carefully consider the implications and needs for each country and its citizens. This chapter contributes to the overarching ambition of this book: to give insight into different examples and ways of creating work that may help to inform and contextualize practice occurring elsewhere and offer a resounding argument for the role of the arts in health. Alongside this, discussions of health are often closely linked to descriptors of wellbeing or achieving a certain aspect of wellbeing, which, considering the slipperiness of the term 'wellbeing' and how the term is employed, calls for an attentive analysis of the concept.

Wellbeing

The notion of 'wellbeing' is controversial. Politicians and policymakers frequently refer to notions of wellbeing, but the goals and understandings of the term are quite different, as are their uses of the concept. For example, before being elected as British Prime Minister in 2010, David Cameron argued for the need to measure the nation's happiness, suggesting:

> It's time we admitted that there's more to life than money, and it's time we focused not just on GDP, but on GWB – general well-being. Well-being can't be measured by money or traded in markets. It's about the beauty of our surroundings, the quality of our culture and, above all, the strength of our relationships. Improving our society's sense of well-being is, I believe, the central political challenge of our times.[35]

While Cameron was clearly attempting to gain support for his notion of a 'big society' and increased civic action to gather evidence to justify public service cuts,[36] there has been a worrying shift in thinking whereby 'participation in social activities is seen as a powerful determinant of health and happiness'.[37] For example, Marc Pilkington notes how the World Happiness Report and the *Journal of Happiness Studies* are making a case for measuring levels of happiness as an indicator of subjective wellbeing, which can then be potentially employed as a measure of economic progress.[38] Similarly, in his analysis of indicators of neoliberalism, William Davies observes how indicators of wellbeing growth are being employed to measure and compare market growth, noting that '[r]eports from [the World Economic Forum's] Davos meeting suggested that concern with wellbeing (mental and bodily) may now even have trumpeted competitiveness (Greenhill, 2014)'.[39] To us, as editors, this rise in a neoliberal use of wellbeing as an achievable 'indicator' of a country's success is deeply troubling. Considering wellbeing as an indicator of economic progress is also highly problematic as it suggests that it is possible to quantify an individual's sense of wellbeing or happiness and that it is possible to compare these indicators with others, without acknowledging the myriad other factors that may influence an individual's sense of happiness, for example links to a community, culture and economic status. Rather, I suggest that notions of wellbeing should be perceived in the holistic, all-encompassing sense whereby, like health, many other factors are acknowledged, thus allowing for greater diversity of experiences and broader understandings of wellbeing.

In another example of how the term 'wellbeing' is employed, surgeon and public health researcher Atul Gawande considered the idea of wellbeing in his final 2014 Reith Lecture, focusing on the provision of health care. With a particular interest in mortality and longevity, the medical advances of the past century and the care we provide our elders, Gawande argued that 'the advancement of human well-being requires understanding how to build and sustain such institutions [heath care providers] effectively. And we are only in the infancy of that knowledge.'[40] Specifically, Gawande posited that basic primary care, encompassing ease of access and continuity with a medical professional for emergencies, management of chronic conditions and prevention, is fundamental to human wellbeing. Here Gawande's argument is firmly placed within the medical sector and provision where the focus is on providing for the individual's physical and psychological needs. While Gawande is making a forceful argument for equal access to basic primary care, such definitions of wellbeing can also be interpreted too narrowly.

While notions of wellbeing are clearly being employed as part of neoliberal agendas globally, the term is also closely associated with understandings of culture (in an artistic sense), a person's social structures and traditions as well as with social capital. Beginning with the notion of social connectedness, considerations of wellbeing have been closely associated with feelings of safety and connections within a particular society. A study of the increasing levels of anxiety found in adolescents in the US in the late 1980s, compared with data from the 1950s, suggested that young people's anxiety was linked to feelings of social isolation, concern over a perceived increase in environmental dangers and the breakdown of the 'safe society'. The study's author, Jean M. Twenge, concluded that, 'Until people feel both safe and connected to others, anxiety is likely to remain high.'[41] Wellbeing then is often implicitly connected with an individual's sense of community or social connections. Ray Pahl, a British sociologist, has expressed concern with such an implicit link, arguing that, 'We have to explore precisely which kinds of social connectedness, encompassing which kinds of quantitative needs and functions relate to which kinds of health outcomes.'[42] Nonetheless, most researchers are in agreement that culture is intrinsically connected to a person's or a community's understanding of wellbeing. For example, in his analysis of cultural trends found in modern Western culture, such as 'consumerism', 'individualism' and 'secularism', Richard Eckersley argues that despite the benefits that these 'isms' have produced (for example he suggests that feminism 'has enhanced the status of women and given them more control over their lives'),[43] they do have the potential to negatively impact on people's sense of wellbeing and their health. Specifically, he points to the increase in antisocial values or 'the tension generated between cultural ideals and social realities'.[44] However, while some feminisms can be seen to have advantaged women, the response has also included vilifications and, now, social media gives vent to 'trolls' set upon exerting new controls to quell the current rising of feminist sensibility. Here, Eckersley makes an argument about the impact that culture, and the influences that surround a particular culture, can have on a person's subjective wellbeing. In his analysis, he offers a summary of the research into the different influences on subjective wellbeing and suggests that there are three aspects that implement a person's wellbeing: 'a cognitive aspect; life satisfaction; and pleasant and unpleasant affect (moods and emotions)'.[45] However problematic I might find his discussion of the influence of the 'isms' on Western societies' sense of wellbeing, Eckersley makes a convincing case about the intrinsic relationship between cultural structures and social traditions and a community's or an individual's sense of wellbeing. This argument, in my view, continues to underline the need to acknowledge the importance of working holistically and to do so within the arts and health.

The evaluators of the Arts Council England's Be Creative Be Well programme[46] used the following definition of wellbeing to analyse the success of their project: 'Wellbeing is more than happiness or the absence of illness. It is fundamentally about how people experience their own lives, whether they feel able to achieve things and have a sense of purpose. It's also about a sense of belonging and being part of the social fabric, connected to other people and supportive local networks.'[47] This definition of wellbeing is interesting as once again the notion of social connectedness and an individual's wellbeing are linked. The Be Creative Be Well programme specifically targeted London boroughs that were impoverished or had a long histor of social housing and found that by increasing access to artistic and cultural practices, the participants noted improved wellbeing at the end of the project. This builds on a similar understanding of wellbeing developed by the British New Economics Foundation (NEF) in 2008.

The NEF reviewed over 400 studies which examined different aspects of health and wellbeing in order to develop an understanding of 'everyday well-being' and identified five actions that could be taken to improve individuals' wellbeing, in the following areas: 'social relationships, physical activity, awareness, learning, and giving'.[48] Again, the emphasis is on the social and the potential importance of increasing relationships and an emerging sense of connectedness for a person's understanding of their own wellbeing. The individual is placed more carefully in the locus of this description of wellbeing. Yet the potential use of this understanding of wellbeing by politicians or policymakers in a neoliberal manner is not acknowledged. I believe wellbeing often remains a term imposed on a population or group rather than one negotiated with them.

This is not a view found solely in Britain, however. For example, as will be discussed further in their essay in Chapter 5, Julian Robbins and his colleagues offer another interpretation of what health means for Indigenous people. Discussing their theatre-based workshops focusing on decolonization with First Nations youth in Canada and the possible effects of post-colonial stress disorder in an earlier article, Felice Yuen and colleagues discuss how young people might determine what attributes they feel belong to a healthy community.[49] In their analysis, the researchers propose that a community's health can be defined through its young people's ongoing development and understanding of what wellbeing could be for their community. What is interesting about the work of Yuen and her colleagues is that they make a clear link between a group's culture and their sense of wellbeing, and the impact that this has on the community's health. Similarly, MacLachlan associates community health with a community being healthy, connected and demonstrating a sense of belonging.[50] He argues that different cultures have different concepts of health and wellbeing:

> One feature of encountering a different culture may be having to understand a different perspective on the factors responsible for health and illness. Within most western societies the biomedical

model predominates, which attributes health and illness to changes in our biochemical and physiological substrate, changes that often occur at such a microscopic level that belief in them is, for most people, an act of faith. On a worldwide scale, faith in other causal mechanisms, such as the intervention of displeased spirits or the use of witchcraft, is probably more widespread.[51]

Acknowledging these diverse viewpoints, it is apparent that culture (in terms of people's traditions and artistic engagement) does have a bearing on people's sense of wellbeing, which is an understanding that underlines the practice discussed in this book. It is fundamental to remember that we are dealing with cultural atmospheres and structures of feelings; wellbeing is subjective, but the arts can respond to and work with subjective understandings, creating practice that illuminates and celebrates diverse understandings. That said, however, we need to be cautious of an instrumentalist use of the arts being employed or applied in order to 'improve' wellbeing and to increase the development of a population's social capital because the government believes it is vital to improving market values. In her book *Theatre in Health and Care*, Emma Brodzinski cautions against how the fields of arts and health work with each other, noting that '[i]t seems, particularly within arts in health, that the arts aspect may be viewed as a means to achieve a health goal (i.e. an instrument) rather than exploring the qualities of the arts activity in itself … In terms of the two cultures speaking to each other it seems important that they should maintain equal status rather than one purely serving the other.'[52] Similarly, commenting on the British field of arts and health, White warns against seeking 'cultural value in cultural well-being'.[53] In particular, White draws attention to the dangerous path where arts in health projects have been encouraged or pushed 'to identify instrumental therapeutic effects', a trend that ignores the projects' common focus on social interaction.[54] White further argues that '[i]n evaluation studies to date, arts in health projects have frequently been required to demonstrate physiological and mental health benefits whilst neglecting the potential of the arts to help to shape people's world view, influencing their choices, autonomy and social engagement'.[55] Here, White draws attention to what is missing from the instrumentalist focus on employing cultural values as an impact indicator of wellbeing, despite the existing difficulties of evaluating and determining such indicators. Furthermore, such an approach tends to fail to notice the participatory nature of arts in health projects, which can encourage collective creativity, understanding of quality and artistry, and social inclusion, all of which may also impact on an individual's sense of wellbeing – though this remains difficult to quantify.[56] Indeed, in medicine there exists a 'hierarchy of evidence'[57] where randomized-controlled trials and detailed quantitative reviews are perceived as solid evidence. These methodological approaches are impossible for arts in health projects to reproduce (in terms of cost and scale) and are also reductive in that these methods would not 'capture' the subtle and detailed shifts that may occur for individuals. Indeed, Belfiore draws attention to this disparity in the arts evidencing impact, noting that '[t]he question of evidence also poses obvious problems of justification and legitimacy, especially where arts and health practice is publically funded. Particularly during times of austerity and contracting budgets for the provision of public health services, developing robust evidence of the kind that scientists consider reliable and credible will remain a priority for the arts and health community.'[58] Yet again, the focus here remains on the field of arts and health 'proving' impact, and this is an argument that we, as practitioners, need to hold more completely in our own hands. We must continue to boldly determine and name our own values of our work and find ways of avoiding situations where – as Deirdre Heddon, speaking at a 2015 TaPRA Applied and Social Theatre research event on impact and value, has warned – the arts can often be employed as the medium through which to disseminate research or 'as tools to engage, mediate, knowledge transfer, to be catalyst and … a means of garnering impact', but not used as research.[59]

Reviewing the history of the social impact of the arts, Belfiore and Oliver Bennett considered the theories that argued that arts can be used as an indicator of personal wellbeing. They concluded that views on the impact the arts can have on health and wellbeing fall into two categories: '*pleasure-giving* as the central function of the aesthetic experience' and the 'therapeutic role of both artistic production and consumption of everyday life as well as in the medical setting'.[60] Belfiore and Bennett argue that while the current specific focus on the relation between the arts and health and wellbeing has been generated by discussion around quality of life, they emphasize that this debate is one that has a long history and 'is ultimately related to the Aristotelian notion of tragic catharsis'.[61] The point that they are arguing is that an instrumental use of the arts is not a new approach; rather, it is an approach that has arguably existed for over 2,500 years[62] and that it remains vital for us as a field to be wary of such uses. In essence, in our practice we need to be cautious of an instrumental view and approach to arts practice whereby the artistic practice is linked with wellbeing in order to resolve a health situation; it is not as simple as 'applying' arts to a situation. While it remains important to actively acknowledge and appreciate that cultural effects have an impact on a person's sense of wellbeing, the arts are not a panacea. We have, as artists, a thorough belief in the impact the arts may have, but we also need to acknowledge the wider influences that affect a person's health. Yet, as Karen Taylor, the programme manager for the Be Creative Be Well project, has argued, 'I have no problem with what people call "instrumentalism". So what if artists want to change the world through their practice? What's so terrible about that?'[63]

Health promotion and education

While instrumentalism can be viewed with suspicion, and there will always be 'risks' attached to the potential moral frameworks held by groups or individuals who determine boundaries of acceptable behaviours, there remains an urgent need to do something in the face of the burden of disease and inequality faced by the global population. Health promotion and education is an important part of this. As Peter Baelz notes, 'Health education is never simply the imparting information by one who knows to one who does not know. It is communication of insights, shared exploration of shared humanity, *a venture of persons in the making*'.[64] Health promotion is an underlying aspect of significant amounts of arts in health work; sometimes when we are discussing the health benefits of a project there is some form of health promotion or education implicit within it. While clearly there are specific issues around health promotion, particularly around power dynamics and who chooses the 'issue' in question, there remains a commitment to share ideas and views in order to achieve a form of equitable health for all. Analysing Baelz's idea, White describes the intent of health promotion as 'a quality relationship around the communication of health',[65] which is in essence what I would argue is the role of the WHO.

The idea of an organization that focuses on global health was discussed in 1945 during the establishment of the United Nations, and the WHO was formally established on 7 April 1948. The WHO is seen primarily as having a public health role: leading on global health concerns, deciding and maintaining global standards, informing and engaging with research, and providing technical assistance to countries. It asserts that 'in the 21st century, health is a shared responsibility, involving equitable access to essential care and collective defence against transnational threats'.[66] However, an outward facing view of health and responsibility is a relatively new concept. Health promotion, which is an integral aspect of the WHO's work, came to the fore in 1978 following the Alma Ata Declaration whereby an agreement was made to address and combat the gross inequalities in health status between countries. In essence, the Alma Ata Declaration upheld the understanding that good primary health care is the way to attain 'Health for All'. The Declaration emphasized the need to support health promotion in developing countries by including the population in the development of health care practices. The Declaration initiated a global process of thinking more broadly about health and what impacts on people's health. MacLachlan has argued that what is interesting about the 1978 Declaration is that it is the first time that culture is not viewed as being distinct from community;[67] however, this shift in thinking around the importance of inequalities actually began earlier – in 1847, with Rudolf Virchow's work.

Virchow was a major proponent of social medicine, arguing that there is no distinction 'between being a health professional and a political activist'.[68] Virchow rejected the notion of 'humoral pathology' in medicine, arguing that disease is linked to cellular pathology and social conditions.[69] In 1847, as a government-employed doctor, Virchow was sent to discover the source of the typhoid epidemic in Upper Silesia. In his report, he argued that disease has two causes: pathological and political, and that the outbreak could not be contained solely by drugs or treatment programmes; rather, societal changes were required, including economic freedom, education and better welfare. Virchow argued that while typhoid is linked to hygiene, the fact that the workers lacked the means to adequately care for themselves (they had limited access to water and proper food, and were living in extreme poverty) coupled with their harsh working conditions meant there existed a social cause to the outbreak, which, in effect, was a capitalist-led inequality.[70,71] He argued that social conditions foster disease and concluded that '[e]very individual has the right of existence and health, and the State is responsible for ensuring this'.[72] Virchow began a way of thinking in which disease and health were being reconnected to culture and society, echoing the calls to wholeness known to us though Ancient Greece's understanding of health. Furthermore, principles that recognize and seek to observe wider social and economic impacts on health now inform the WHO's planning and strategy. Currently, the WHO has identified six priority areas in which they take leadership in resolving, namely universal health care coverage; developing and sustaining International Health Regulations across countries; increasing access to medical products; determining and better understanding the social, economic and environmental determinants of health; an increased focus on non-communicable diseases as a rising cause of major health consequences around the world; and focusing on the health-related Millennium Development Goals (MDGs).[73] Before discussing health inequities, a consideration of the MDGs is necessary because they inform the context behind the need for facilitating and funding arts-based practice, particularly in the Global South, as they identify specific areas in crisis.

Millennium Development Goals

The Millennium Development Goals were developed following the Millennium Summit in September 2000 at the United Nations' New York headquarters. Initiated as the world's first anti-poverty drive and global partnership, the United Nations' Millennium Declaration committed all 189 United Nations member states to reaching a series of international development targets by 2015.[74] Predominately focusing on poverty eradication across the globe, eight MDGs were agreed. These comprised a commitment to (1) eradicate extreme poverty and hunger; (2) achieve universal and primary education; (3) promote gender equality and empower women; (4) reduce child mortality; (5) improve maternal health; (6) combat HIV AIDS, malaria and other diseases; (7) ensure environmental stability; and (8) develop a global partnership for development.[75] In the establishment of the MDGs, significant emphasis was placed on the role of poverty as being the epicentre of most inequality found across the globe, and strong links were made between poverty reduction and increased global security for all countries. Indeed, the focus on inequalities that arise through poverty forms the fundamental basis of the MDGs. As Jeffrey Sachs, the Special Adviser to the Secretary-General on the MDGs, stated:

> Extreme poverty can be defined as 'poverty that kills', depriving individuals of the means to stay alive in the face of hunger, disease, and environmental hazards. When individuals suffer from extreme poverty and lack the meagre income needed even to cover basic needs, a single episode of disease, or drought, or a pest that destroys a harvest can be the difference between life and death.[76]

Emphasis was also placed on the ethos of the goals in terms of achieving global justice, ensuring human rights for all and reducing the need to resort to violent conflict as a result of resource scarcity.[77] Although these were not the world's first development targets, as Matthew Clarke and Simon Feeny observe, the MDGs received 'unprecedented support' globally and, crucially, in agreeing to the targets, world leaders, particularly those from developing countries, and international donors 'had made themselves more accountable to taxpayers and voters'.[78]

Specifically, the MDGs focused on improving human wellbeing in developing countries and it is for this reason that I consider them in this chapter, acknowledging the multiple factors that impact on a person's health. The focus of many MDGs is on health crises and situations predominantly found in Global South countries, and it is important to understand the international drive to attain the MGD targets in these countries. Specifically, the practice examined in this book focuses on some of the issues addressed in the MDGs, namely gender equality and empowering woman, child and woman health, and infectious diseases such as TB, HIV and malaria. However, throughout the fifteen-year target period, concerns were noted about the feasibility of achieving the MDG targets.[79] A 2013 British Department for International Development (DfID) report noted that although some progress had been made in reducing child mortality, particularly in North Africa and most of Asia, in sub-Saharan Africa and Oceania child mortality remained a concern.[80] It also determined that overall global progress in achieving this MDG was 'lagging'. Similarly, improving maternal health was also described as 'lagging', with low to moderate reductions in maternal mortality overall (only 57 per cent of all births in sub-Saharan Africa and Asia are attended by skilled personnel) and slow progress in providing universal access to reproductive health (apart from East Asia). Finally, MDG 6, which aimed to reverse the spread of HIV and achieve universal access to treatment for HIV/AIDS, has also not been met globally, despite some significant progresses in particular regions such as sub-Saharan Africa, where the epidemic has begun to stabilize. Significantly, of the 15 million people who need treatment, as of 2011 only 8 million were accessing treatment globally. However, it is the lack of focus on TB that is particularly worrying, as TB is the main cause of death for HIV+ people; further research and action is needed in this area[81] – a concern that Veronica Baxter and Michele Tameris address in their essay in Chapter 4.

While there have been a number of critiques of the attainability of the MDGs, these are generally clustered around four areas: countries lacking the technical and infrastructural abilities necessary; more limited financial resources and fiscal mobility; particular policies or institutional capacity; and societal and cultural values.[82,83] The major stumbling block, however, has been that the MDGs were seen as targets aligned to individual countries rather than global targets. In his critique of the MDGs, Jan Vandermoortele has argued that it is difficult to judge each nation on the level to which, individually, they have achieved the eight MDGs, as each country set their own developmental targets.[84] Vandermoortele furthers this analysis, noting that trying to compare one nation's progress against the global MDG achievement map and benchmark list can 'distort the real picture of progress at the country level' and that '[i]t has tragic consequences because countries that start from low levels of human development are frequently presented as failures, even though they achieve respectable progress.'[85]

What Vandermoortele is arguing against here is fundamental, as assumptions can be made when reading these world maps. Seeing countries coloured in red or amber on a world map or described in a targets list as 'failing' or 'lagging' can result in a particular narrative being prescribed, one that often does not take into account the specifics of the history of a particular nation. The narratives that should be considered, but often are not, include the high rates of global debt and the historical impacts of colonialism and, more currently, capitalism. While we are careful not to spread and uphold these narratives in this book, it still remains pertinent to consider world tables in order to bring an understanding of the numbers of people involved and, in some cases, the dire need for some form of external assistance. Furthermore, these analyses of targets often do not consider the impact that conflict has had on a nation reaching its targets. The aforementioned DfID report, having examined data from all of the developing countries, concluded that 'no low income, fragile or conflict affected state has yet achieved a single MDG'. Indeed, of the thirty-four countries who were struggling to meet the MDGs, twenty-two were currently in or emerging from diverse conflicts.[86]

Additionally, Malcolm Langford, Andy Sumner and Alicia Ely Yamin propose that the MDGs have been reformulated as a particular ideal or norm by which certain behaviours and actions are expected. Acknowledging that although the MDGs have quantitative targets, as the editors of *Millennium Development Goals and Human Rights* (2013), they suggest that they also include a particular ethical and moral imperative. Drawing from Sakiko Fukuda-Parr and David Hulme's (2000) research on the development of the 'poverty norm', Langford and colleagues suggest that the MDGs' 'indicator framework was and continues to be embedded within attempts to legitimise certain ideas on norms and incentivise particular actions'.[87] This idea of establishing a particular norm, which in turn leads to the development of particular encouraged behaviours, demonstrates how the MDGs can be used as a means of pressurizing countries into adopting specific targets. While this could be viewed as a global call to action to reduce poverty, my reading of this 'legitimization' of certain actions is that it is a neoliberal drive towards normative behaviour. Obviously equality and health equity across the world is key, but there is a fine line between telling people what to do and encouraging governments and populations to decide what is right for their country and themselves.

Yet the situation remains that a significant number of people are still at risk from infectious diseases and have difficulties in accessing health services and understanding their health needs. As this critique of the MDGs has shown, inequities remain major determinants of the world's health and it is these inequalities that need to be addressed. While performance and theatre cannot address some of these inequities directly, they can potentially question, challenge and pressurize for change, which can be seen in the examples of practice in the chapters that follow. For example, in Chapter 8, Effie Makepeace and Kiara Worth discuss women's health and gender inequity; and in Chapter 10, Lisa Woynarski, Nicholas Hamer and Alexandra Sutherland consider ecological health arising from different inequities. However, it is important to understand the different influences that inform health inequities. While a major part of the MDGs' focus was to address to health inequities, it has been argued that this has not been successful, owing to overfocusing on target numbers rather than better understanding the reasons for the existing health inequities. It is for this reason that I now turn to discuss health inequities in order to better understand the contexts and performative-based responses to health inequalities that the contributors to this book address in the analyses that follow.

Health inequities and inequalities

Health inequities or health inequalities are terms used across health care, social care, cultural policy and politics. They are determined with reference to the socioeconomic spectrum of a country or region in order to understand the impact of globalization on the health of a particular society. In essence, these terms are primarily employed by a range of organizations, researchers and governments as a comparative tool to gain an understanding of where a particular population is placed in terms of their health situation in comparison with another region or country. However, the terms are also used as a political call to action: by identifying different types of inequity in health, the different causes or determinants (societal, structural and economic) can be explored and challenged, particularly through theatre and performance forms. Inequities in health are described by the WHO as '*avoidable* inequalities in health between groups of people within countries and between countries',[88] and it is generally understood, as Michael Marmot argues, that 'the more favoured people are, socially and economically, the better their health'.[89] In essence, the determinants of health inequities fall into three broad categories: structural and cultural; location and locality; and trade and economy.

In his book *Pathologies of Power: Health, Human Rights, and the New War on the Poor*, Paul Farmer draws attention to how power imbalances lead to inequalities, which have wide-ranging effects on people's health and ways of life. Described as 'a kind of quiet brutality', Farmer argues that an asymmetry of power and the resulting inequalities results in ongoing structural violence for those who are without power.[90] Drawing from Johan Galtung's conceptualization of structural violence, Farmer further defines it as 'a host of offensives against human dignity' which includes all forms of inequality such as gender and social inequality, human rights abuses and extreme and relative poverty.[91] Locating the examples for his theories in Haiti (a country where he has worked as a doctor and an anthropologist for over twenty years), Farmer describes how people who live in extreme and relative poverty are victims of structural violence, because their suffering has originated through both historical and economic causes (such as colonialism or trade agreements). Farmer illustrates how structural violence is a social determinant of health: a health inequity. He makes a powerful argument that people's decisions or ability to act, or 'their agency', will be 'limited by racism, sexism, political violence, *and* grinding poverty'.[92] Specifically, Farmer makes a link between poverty and health:

> Today, the world's poor are the chief victims of structural violence – violence that has thus far defied the analysis of many who seek to understand the nature and distribution of extreme suffering. Why might this be so? One answer is that the poor are not only more likely to suffer; they are also less likely to have their suffering noticed.[93]

In this statement, Farmer is arguing that in order to understand suffering you need to reveal the individual suffering and then 'one must embed individual biography in the larger matrix of culture, history, and political economy'.[94] The need to take the time to consider an individual's experience is made explicit by Farmer's analysis and this need and intention is a fundamental argument of this book: to create a space to share moments of practice created with groups that are not often reached within traditional public health interventions. So, for example, Astrid Perry and Lynne Baker describe theatre projects reaching diverse audiences in Australia in Chapter 7. It is important to gain a wider understanding of how diverse groups and populations experience health and wellbeing, since a greater understanding of this, as Farmer argues, will help to develop and strengthen our practice.

Farmer's research into inequities has had far-reaching impact. For example, the WHO's Commission on Social Determinants of Health,[95] drawing from both Amartya Sen's and Farmer's research, argues that:

> Social inequity manifests across various intersecting social categories such as class, education, gender, age, ethnicity, disability, and geography. It signals not simply difference but hierarchy, and reflects deep inequities in the wealth, power, and prestige of different people and communities. People who are already disenfranchised are further disadvantaged with respect to their health – having the freedom to participate in economic, social, political, and cultural relationships has intrinsic value. (Sen, 1999)[96]

In its analysis, the Commission pointed to the clear indicators of the impact that social inequality, power and locality of a person has on that person's health and the health equity available to them. The 2008 report was a forceful and strongly worded call to attention to the social justice disaster unfolding, and identified the global shared responsibility to respond to this disaster. The Commission advocated that '[c]hanges in power relationships can take place at various levels, from the "micro" level of individuals, households, or communities to the "macro" sphere of structural relations among economic, social, and political actors and institutions', and drew attention to the state's responsibility in alleviating health inequities as well as the importance of the promotion of civil society action on health inequities.[97]

In contrast, Brazilian arts-based company AfroReggae is addressing health inequities and issues in a way that encourages civil society action through their work in the *favelas* surrounding Rio de Janeiro (please see the snapshot interview in Chapter 4). Writing about the long-standing and ongoing practice of AfroReggae, Paul Heritage and Silvia Ramos draw attention to the 'age, colour and place for death in Brazilian cities', whereby it is the poor, young, black population who live on the periphery of the cities that have the highest death toll.[98] In their analysis, Heritage and Ramos argue that the structural violence – what they refer to as 'intentional lethal violence' surrounding these communities – is a public health problem. They consider how the artistic directors of AfroReggae view the changes that have occurred in their communities to be the result of the artistic practices and their focus on the 'bodies' of the young people they work with by emphasizing the links between health and aesthetics. Heritage and Ramos conclude that:

> AfroReggae has developed their own unique form of protecting communities from the life-threatening conditions that decimate and degrade them. It understands, as the pioneers of public health knew at the beginning of the twentieth century, that defence and protection is more effective than the attempt to 'cure' and that improving the health of individuals is intrinsically linked to reforming the city itself.[99]

In this example of AfroReggae's work, an understanding of structural inequality forms part of the artistic practice that has led to changes and positive outcomes for many of those young people involved. Similarly, an engagement with and challenging of the societal and gender inequalities that Nandita Dinesh addresses in her analysis of gender inequity in India in Chapter 8 is another example of the importance of understanding the breadth of impact inequity can have on a population's health.

Inequality is not something that is confined to developing countries; it originates from divisions within society, from wealth disparities, trade disparities, different cultural and social norms and existing structural violence. These divisions, as Daniel Dorling argues, 'are everywhere; they are the stuff of geography. They are found along country lanes in Lincolnshire, between regions in Europe and between countries worldwide.[100] There is clear evidence that the location where people live directly impacts on their health and employment, predominantly owing to the health equity available to them.[101] For example, the 2010 Global Burden of Disease study (GBD),[102] which is the world's largest investigation into the global causes and occurrence of health risks, diseases and injury, concluded that while some improvements are being made, such as rising life expectancy for both men and women and a decrease in the burden from malaria and HIV, there still exist significant discrepancies between nations. While the GBD concluded that the results of the 2010 study demonstrated a 'hopeful picture', the authors warned that 'huge gaps remain in progress for some regions of the world'.[103] Richard Horton draws attention to the fact that much of the burden of disease is still located in the Global South, and particularly in Africa. Part of the success of the GBD is that through the results of the study there is now a clearer understanding of the cause and effects of certain diseases and of these global trends. Horton argues that it is now possible to 'independently (and dispassionately)' discuss and address the health priorities certain countries face.[104] Indeed what is so interesting about the recent results of the GBD study is how the different disease burdens have shifted in the past ten years. It is now evident that since the last study in 1990, there has been an increase in non-communicable diseases, including heart disease, lower respiratory infections and strokes, which has a significant impact on the populations' disability-adjusted life years (DALYs).[105] So, for example, in 1990, 47 per cent of DALYs worldwide were linked to communicable and nutritional disorders/diseases, 43 per cent of DALYs to non-communicable diseases, and 10 per cent to injury. This has now changed, in 2010, to non-communicable diseases representing 54 per cent of DALYs worldwide and communicable and nutritional diseases dropping to 35 per cent.[106] This finding is echoed by Christopher Murray and colleagues, who note that '[s]ubstantial heterogeneity exists in rankings of leading causes of disease burden among regions',[107] which is to say that most of the burden remains in the Global South, specifically in Africa. In particular, Murray and colleagues draw attention to the largely unidentified burden of mental illness and the pressing need for 'practical strategies for managing these disorders in low-income and middle-income countries'.[108] The difficulty with addressing mental health is discussed by Sinethemba Makanya in her essay in Chapter 9.

Finally, while gross inequalities exist between Global North and Global South countries, within individual countries, irrespective of global status, wealth inequalities have a major impact on the population's health. For example, despite an overall global decline in child mortality, the UK child death rate per 1000 births is 4.9, which is almost double the rate of other European countries such as Sweden (2.7) or Iceland (2.4).[109] Researchers from two different reports (the *Global Burden of Diseases, Injuries, and Risk Factors Study 2013* and *Why Children Die: Death in Infants, Children and Young People in the UK*) independently concluded that '[s]ocial and economic inequalities are matters of life and death for children',[110] pointing to the role of poverty and deprivation, including the ruling government's cuts to welfare funding, which 'were directly linked to the deaths of the youngest children'.[111] However, for Global South countries, much of the issue lies in the existence of wealth deprivation. Dorling offers an interesting analysis of the international divides in health inequality between the Global South and the Global North. Specifically, he argues that there is a direct and indirect connection between geographical locations, in terms of both trade policies and cultural policies resulting from colonization. Using the Democratic Republic of the Congo (DRC), Belgium and Norway as examples, Dorling draws attention to the marked difference in health care provision where the European countries have some of the best health in the world compared with one of the worst in the DRC. He suggests that this is partly due to trade agreements where the Western countries require specific commodities (such as diamonds or minerals) that come from the Congo but do not pay well for them, which helps to maintain the divide.[112] He acknowledges that while direct connections between poverty and wealth between nations can be difficult to determine, there are some links to be found. Drawing on Matthew Connolly's argument that from the late nineteenth century onwards, the longevity and health of Europeans, North Americans and the Japanese began to improve 'partly *because* people in other parts of the world [were] suffering deprivation and dying young',[113] Dorling points to the devastating effects of Belgium's control of the Congo under King Leopold II (1885–1909) as an example of the consequences of material exploitation and genocidal policies that continue to have striking repercussions on the health of the Congolese today.[114]

Yet while the impact of income poverty on health is significant, we must remain conscious of other potential impacts, including social exclusion. For example, Marmot argues that the existing 20-year gap in life expectancy between Aboriginal and Torres Strait Islander peoples and the average Australian is not solely linked to income poverty, and instead we need to consider more broadly the different causes, including the impacts of social exclusion in a community/country.[115] Marmot concludes that '[i]f the major determinants of health are social, so must be the remedies',[116] which offers a strong argument for the use of performance and theatre-based responses which have a keen focus on communication and inclusion. However, while this chapter has attempted to provide a dispassionate overview of the burden of disease on the world, in this very analysis, there is still a tendency towards a taxonomical, and pathologized, approach rather than interrogating analyses of the causes of inequalities. While data and trends are vital knowledge with which to respond to and challenge certain health burdens, what is needed is a more in-depth analysis of the social determinants of health, along with an understanding of how wealth inequities and cultural differences have an impact on a person's health. Part of this research has been undertaken by the WHO's Commission on Social Determinants of Health. Specifically, as the Marmot Review notes, 'a major thrust of the Commission is turning public-health knowledge into political action'.[117] The tone and framing of this Commission is interesting in that it is a highly political call to action which has been initiated and supported by the WHO, an organization that sometimes is perceived as being quite reserved or slow to react.[118] Some of the Commission's statements are politically sensitive as it brings together the agendas of health equity and climate change and acknowledges the impacts that environmental change can have on a population's health. The language used in the Commission's brief is also challenging: they describe themselves as taking 'a holistic view of social determinants of health' and draw attention to the fact that the clear health inequalities seen globally arise from 'the unequal distribution of power, income, goods, and services, globally and nationally'. Arguing that this 'consequent unfairness' for the poor, when coupled with the 'toxic combination of poor social policies and programmes, unfair economic arrangements, and bad politics' and people's daily living conditions, leads to clear health inequalities around the world.[119] Despite this comprehensive push to understand and resolve global health inequalities, it is apparent that in 2015 minimal progress has been made. With specific reference to the MDGs, Vandermoortele points to the limited societal or economic improvements for the poorest globally, arguing that '[t]he main reason why the world is not on track for meeting the 2015 targets is because the bottom 30%–40% of the population in most countries have not benefited much from social progress and economic growth'.[120] The continuing and growing wealth inequity between the poor and the rich remains a major factor in the continuing health inequities across the world.

Part of the reason for the limited degree of change may be a lack of real understanding of what poverty is for many people. Thomas Pogge, Professor of Philosophy and International Affairs at Yale University, challenges the idea that poverty and inequity can be resolved.[121] Discussing the global jubilation and fanfare that followed the World Bank's 2012 declaration that global poverty had reduced despite the global economic crisis, Pogge argues that there is a misunderstanding of what living on less than $2 actually means for the 2471 million people who do so daily. He contends that people are surviving, not living. Pogge's suggestion about the misunderstanding of the depth of poverty is coupled with the lack of political attention that health inequities often receive. Usually governments respond at crisis points, and there are often few long-term structures put in place to resolve certain issues. For example, David Buck, a Senior Fellow on Public Health and Inequalities at the King's Fund, questions the lack of attention health inequalities receive in the UK. In particular, he draws attention to how little is actually done in terms of counteracting health inequalities, noting that there has been no sustained response from the British government.[122]

Indeed, as Gabriel Scally, an Associate Fellow at the Institute for Public Policy Research in the UK, has argued, 'Health inequalities have ceased to be fashionable. From a position where the goal to reduce inequalities was a core objective of the health system – with national targets to reduce them by 10 per cent – we have seen it steadily marginalised.'[123] Although Scally is referring to the UK, and more specifically England, he is making a crucial point that despite the WHO Commission's forceful statements, globally little has happened, even in rich countries. However, returning to Marmot's notion of the need for social remedies alongside state-based responses, here lies a strong argument for the importance of both better understanding the more fluid and subtle social determinants of health and responding to these inequities in diverse ways. It is here that the creative arts have a key role to play and the examples of practice discussed in this book offer different ways of responding to and understanding health issues globally, thereby building a more detailed picture of the existing research and practice in this field. This chapter has considered understandings of health and wellbeing, the emergence of health promotion and the complex field of health inequities to establish a clear context for the analysis of practice that follows. In the next chapter, Baxter considers the ways in which the creative arts, particularly performance-based approaches, have historically addressed health issues.

2

Aesthetics, Instrumentalism and Ethics in Health and Wellbeing

Veronica Baxter

This chapter will predominantly focus on analysing the 'application' of theatre and performance to health and wellbeing – in particular where artistic practices intentionally work as pedagogy and intervention towards effective and affective outcomes. Through the presentation of case studies selected to foreground Applied Theatre in health from Global South contexts, the discussion will explore the relationship between the urgency of health education and the aesthetic choices made in theatre. In the Global South, the term most often used to describe Applied Theatre practices is Theatre for Development (TfD),[1] resulting in some synergies in this chapter with Tim Prentki's *Applied Theatre: Development*, a volume in this series.[2] In particular, TfD practitioners often view their work through a socio-political frame, specifically intending to address issues of social justice. As Katharine Low has indicated in Chapter 1, health care provision is an issue of social justice. The overlap with Prentki's work is therefore an ideological one, interpreting the nature and form of Applied Theatre in health from a socio-cultural standpoint. However, this analysis (and the chapters that follow) will illustrate praxis in 'developing' nations by engaging with programmes that respond or engage with the specific focus of health.

Many of the examples that follow illustrate the relevance of addressing alcohol abuse and its socioeconomic and health impact on communities. The World Health Organization (WHO) reports that 3.3 million deaths each year are attributable to the harmful use of alcohol, and that overall the global burden of disease – measured in Disability-Adjusted Life Years (DALYs) – is 5.1 per cent.[3] Alcohol is directly attributable to over 200 different disease and injury conditions, and causal relationships are established between alcohol consumption and gender violence, tuberculosis and HIV/AIDS.[4]

This chapter will also investigate arts practices where health and wellbeing are potentially enhanced by participation in art-making. This will address the contested terrain of 'art for art's sake', questioning what an 'un-applied' theatre would look like, and the aesthetic considerations for practice across diverse contexts. In analysis of 'wellbeing', the crucial component of resilience will be viewed through discussion of 'community arts', the 'positive psychology' movement and the selected research evidence that is emerging.

Much of the writing will attempt to provide new perspectives on the debates around the impact of, inter alia, participatory and non-formal learning in community contexts, 'effect', 'affect', pedagogical and interventionist theatre, socio-cultural aspects of health and wellbeing, the role of poverty in health and wellbeing, and a discussion of relativism in aesthetic taste. The examples will also investigate the relationship between the psychologically-based approaches to learning and the evaluation of impact in community health projects.

Last, the chapter will discuss research into the arts, health and wellbeing, and some of the gaps in current work. For further analysis of research into, and through, Applied Theatre, see Peter O'Connor and Michael Anderson's book in this series.[5] The research method, arts-based research, or what O'Connor and Anderson refer to as 'applied theatre as research' (ATAR), is a developing area of Applied Theatre in health.

'Effects' and 'affects'

One of the chief reasons put forward in favour of Applied Theatre and performance practices is that they engage participants cognitively and emotionally. TfD emerged with a focus on people's education and social justice, with a mix of political idealism and advocacy of the theatre's capacity to intervene in community contexts. Prentki, along with other scholars in the field, discusses the nuances of the various forms that TfD took over the years on theatre's interventions to educate, inform, empower, reconcile and revolutionize.[6,7,8] For the purposes of this discussion and to summarise, it would be true to say that these approaches emphasized the cognitive potential of theatre, rather than its affective properties. To some extent this has remained the case in TfD approaches. However, more recently, practitioners have argued that only focusing on 'effects' divests theatre of the intrinsic value of affective responses. There has been a surge of interest in 'affect' in Applied Theatre and performance, which is presented as counter to the utilitarian purposes that drama[9] and theatre has fulfilled in a number of settings.[10] The relationship between form and function is being re-evaluated, and there is also a marked reappraisal of aesthetics.[11] Some of this interest has been generated by James Thompson, who suggests that Applied Theatre 'is limited if it concentrates solely on effects – identifiable social outcomes, messages or impacts – and forgets the radical potential of the freedom to enjoy beautiful radiant things'.[12] Thompson along with subsequent writers draw on Jacques Rancière's idea of an emancipated spectator, where it is argued that:

> … artists do not wish to instruct the spectator. Today they deny using the stage to dictate a lesson or convey a message. They simply wish to produce a form of consciousness, and intensity of feeling, an energy for action. But they always assume that what will be perceived, felt, understood is what they have put into their dramatic art or performance.[13]

It is the last sentence that speaks directly to the dilemma faced by all theatre and performance, that is, the multiplicity and instability of meanings generated, which makes both *effects* and *affects* on audiences and participants difficult to assess. However, simplifying applied approaches to focus on feeling has several unintended consequences, not least the impact of privileging feeling over cognition, ascribing personal 'taste' to aesthetic judgement, and setting up a binary between emotion and cognition.

Many of these arguments around aesthetics appear to deny the diversity or context of what is considered art, and subsequently its affective responses. The measure of art, despite postmodernity, is still often associated with hierarchies of venue or purpose – greater value is placed on art that is formal, urban or site specific, like a museum or theatre. Art practised on the side of the road, in the case of sculpture, is called 'craft'. Morris dancing is referred to as 'folk' dance, or *ngoma* as 'traditional'. Performances in clinics, on farms, in a clearing or on the street become 'popular' or 'people's' theatre – often perceived as inferior art. By this measure, pedagogical and interventionist art for health is seen as lesser, invoking the infamous adage from George Bernard Shaw, 'He who can, does. He who cannot, teaches.'[14]

The expected emotional response to art is influenced by culture, performance styles and their purpose and meaning. However, many arguments around *affect*, when broken down, simply seem to apply Kant's advocacy of art for art's sake – which Brad Haseman and Joe Winston criticize as 'creat[ing] a hierarchy of taste, with the refined and cultivated being seen as able to enjoy the best art purely for its aesthetic qualities, as distinct from the popular or "agreeable" pleasures of everyday cultural activities that need no special education for us to learn how to appreciate them'.[15] Citing Rancière and Helen Freshwater, they reject Boal's assertion that the spectator is passive. Rather, they argue that practitioners must re-evaluate the role of the spectator of the event, 'and by implication the role of the aesthetic in these acts of watching, interpretation and transformation'.[16]

Negative impact of emotional engagement

A research project on undergraduate students' perceptions of date rape is an example of the instability of meaning and the unintended consequences of dramatization. In European theatre theory Brecht's *Verfremdungseffekt* has suggested that aesthetic distance (or critical distance) is desirable for learning to take place.[17] Robert Landy suggests that under-distancing in theatre results in too great an emotional response, blurring cognition. Over-distancing means that the spectator (or participant) does not engage emotionally with the character or content of the theatre, and it is therefore pointless as either art or education.[18] He argues that there is an optimal distance between under-and over-distancing that is the aesthetic distance.

A psychology study conducted with undergraduate students in South Africa problematized this relationship between cognition and emotion, by investigating patterns of 'blaming' the victim in heterosexual date rape.[19] The project sought to compare participants' responses to three dramatized video scenes or written vignettes. The detailed written vignette was exactly the same as the enactment of the scenes in the video, moment by moment. The video scenes and written vignettes depicted three possible scenarios specific to date rape, which research has showed to be significant factors, i.e. alcohol, flirtation and 'being owed'. Therefore, in one scenario the 'victim' was drunk; in the second, the 'victim' was flirtatious or 'leading on'; and in the third, the 'rapist' had bought dinner and a movie for the 'victim' and therefore felt he was 'owed' sex.

The results of the dramatized scenes demonstrated both positive and negative consequences for using written vignettes versus dramatization. Participants who read the written vignette were more likely to blame the victim for being drunk, and far fewer identified this vignette as a case of date rape. The report suggests that this is due to the instability of meaning in the written vignette – due to the participants filling the gaps with imaginative and personal associations with alcohol and rape, possibly imagining the drunken behaviour as worse than it appears in the video. Also the emotional consequences of the rape on the woman were not revealed through reading a neutral, distanced account.[20] However the video of the woman's flirtatious 'leading on' resulted in a marked increase in blaming of the woman.

The report suggests that the participants' emotional responses to the enacted scenes were significant, arguably because no details were left to the imagination, and the 'rapist' was seen as a real person, not an imagined monster. Fewer respondents identified the 'leading on' scene as date rape.

The implications for theatre and performance are a mixed blessing – theatre elicits a great deal of emotional engagement. However, heightened emotion can affect the stability of meaning in and interpretation of theatre and performance. When there is an urgent need to engage an audience, there is considerable skill to balancing the emotional and cognitive potential of theatre, and a pendulum swing towards one or the other is not helpful.

Debates around participation

Prentki shows that the changes in TfD were developed out of the criticism of the travelling or popular theatre model, which were largely non-participatory.[21] This analysis will not be repeated here, other than in discussion of two health-related projects that illustrate the relationship between participation and what Zakes Mda[22] calls 'optimal intervention'. The examples are old, and while Applied Theatre practices may have moved on from this description, the roots of practice speak to contemporary challenges. In this analysis Mda describes the way in which the models of TfD were changed to conquer 'the culture of silence'.[23] In this study of Lesotho's Marotholi Travelling Theatre, he shows how community participants become increasingly active, assuming control over the processes of structural change, as the outside catalyst's role reduced. Some of the complexity in these struggles resulted from the class and race positions of catalyst-facilitators of the development communication, now often referred to as Social and Behaviour Communication (SBCC).[24] Mda discusses what he calls Community-generated (Comgen) theatre where high participation is achieved by the community, contrasting this with what he calls Participatory Agit-Prop, where a catalyst theatre piece that brings new information to the community is made and performed with limited participation. Mda's examples of Lesotho's Maratholi Travelling Theatre's *Alcohol Play* (1989) and the *Rural Sanitation Play* (1986) speak directly to the concerns with the TfD models at play in health during the 1980s and 1990s.

In the Participatory Agit-Prop model as shown in the *Rural Sanitation Play*, a loosely structured play was devised in collaboration with local health workers, and toured to community meetings in several villages. The play had strategic opportunities within its structure for dialogue between the actors and audience, and was performed by actors who were able to improvise the inclusion of local knowledge and conditions, as well as understanding the traditional format of a community meeting. The piece was unashamedly instrumental in its intentions – seeking to promote the building of pit latrines and hygiene – and this central aspect was constantly reinforced and encouraged. The campaign resulted in the building of latrines as a visible outcome of the theatre. As Mda points out, there was no opportunity to question the realities of structural oppression, the reasons why in the late twentieth century, villages in Lesotho still needed a play to encourage sanitation and hygiene and to stimulate the building of latrines.

In contrast, the TfD model used by Maratholi for the *Alcohol Play* was that of Comgen theatre, involving a few theatre practitioners from Maratholi living and working with the community of Tebellong for two weeks, collectively researching the community and creating a performance with community members using familiar performance forms. The theme of the play was decided upon through identifying community problems, most of which seemed rooted in excessive alcohol consumption. The eventual performance was well received and created a willingness to engage in further theatre work in order to engage in dialogue with community problems. A report from Tebellong hospital identified the form of theatre as being more accessible and entertaining than other communication methods. Mda is clear that Comgen theatre is more successful in generating participation than other models.[25] However, participation failed to engage the community in analysis of the socio-political reasons for the alcohol and associated problems in the community, creating despair, and leading to those involved blaming themselves for 'bad' behaviours.

> If only they could stop drinking, they say, they would defeat poverty. They are not aware of the political and economic structures both at local and national level that have kept them in the state of poverty ... The tendency to moralise, and to find the nearest scapegoat, in the naming of their problems is due to the fact that the peasants had not been equipped with the tools of critical analysis. They had been provided only with the technical tools of the theatre.[26]

Mda compares this with the much-quoted example from 1982, of the Kamariithu Cultural Centre in Limuru district, Kenya, where the broader community participated in the rehearsal of the play *Ngaahika Ndenda* (*I will marry when I want*), analysing the colonial and post-colonial land issues. The difference, he asserts, between the peasants of Tebellong and those of Limuru, Kenya, is that the latter theatrical process created socio-political critical awareness of the problems around landlessness, whereas the Tebellong community blamed themselves for alcoholism. In Tebellong it is more likely that this led to community paralysis on development issues, rather than action. Prentki harnesses arguments from Penina Mlama and David Kerr to emphasize the role of intervening facilitators, often university students, who do not have the socio-political understanding or experience to move the dialogue forward. Mda asserts that optimal intervention is the solution, but requires facilitators who 'have a higher level of social consciousness – and of critical awareness'.[27] This points towards the problem of training in TfD facilitation, with a theatrical toolbox that develops a deep analysis of the power structures in the community.

Antonio Gramsci spoke about the importance of nurturing 'organic intellectuals' in an oppressed community, 'whose task is to identify the social interests behind power; challenge traditional understandings of culture, power and politics; and share such knowledge as the basis for organising diverse forms of class struggle in order to create a socialist society'.²⁸ It is clear in Mda's analysis of both the Participatory Agit-Prop and the Community-generated models that neither delivered on conscientization or on developing organic intellectuals to take community development further. In these examples, arguably the problem was not the models used, but the overtly instrumentalist aims of the *Rural Sanitation Play*, and structural challenges to healthy behaviour in the *Alcohol Play*. One of the aspects of both performance projects in Lesotho is the limited duration of the interventions.

Kerr cites an example of a long-term health research project in Malawi (2003–4) on which he consulted as the theatre specialist.²⁹ He argues that the overtly didactic stance of TfD emerged from plays done by missionaries and colonial officers, and is based on a 'Mr Wise and Mr Foolish' formula, as does Zindaba Chisiza in Chapter 4. This formula leads to a simplistic set of messages that are far removed from the 'multi-layered performance techniques and motifs' and 'dilemma folktales' of indigenous performance. In working with Tukumbusyane Travelling Theatre, local to Lungwena, Kerr and his research assistant, Syned Muthathiwa, were able to complicate the use of 'Mr Wise and Mr Foolish' as stock characters, but at the same time encourage the use of two trickster figures trying to outwit each other, presenting dilemmas to the audiences. The research was collecting Knowledge, Attitudes, Practices (KAP) regarding polygyny, reasons for girls marrying at a young age, the impact of initiation ceremonies for boys and girls, reluctance to attend the clinic and use birth control, patterns of food consumption and attitudes to pit latrines. The Tukumbusyane actors worked effectively to construct a play and characters that effectively used indigenous performance traditions to provoke extensive debate between audience members, particularly between the men and women. Kerr suggests that one of the reasons this theatre company was effective was because it was a group of older, more experienced performers – 'unlike many similar groups in Southern Africa, these are not teenagers recently dropped out of school and looking for money or glory'.³⁰ In this sense they could be referred to as organic intellectuals of their communities, able to provide appropriate leadership on matters of social change.

TfD was originally based in progressive ideas about social justice, and in health, linked to, for example, the Universal Declaration of Human Rights, which advocates (in Article 25) that 'Everyone has the right to a standard of living adequate for the health and well-being of himself [sic] and of his family.'[31] Clearly theatre cannot provide the material 'standard of living' needed, and therefore Applied Theatre praxis often devolves to advocacy around accessing health resources, analysis of the obstacles to health, and education around personal and community development. In addition Applied Theatre has benefits for participants in relation to 'affect'.

There are studies of the impact of participation in arts activities (and theatre and performance specifically) that are useful to mention, in framing this analysis. One of the indicators of success often ignored in evaluation of Applied Theatre practices (and their aesthetic and pedagogical influence) is when that theatrical engagement fosters more theatre, creativity and learning. This was the case in a longitudinal pilot study conducted in Sri Lanka, with the objective of curbing excessive alcohol consumption.[32]

Two rural villages of similar size and scope were selected for the study, including their high prevalence of illicit distilleries and alcohol consumption. One was randomly selected as the control village, receiving no interventions. The other received an intervention including street dramas, poster campaigns, leaflets and individual and group discussions. The study was intended to monitor and influence the alcohol consumption patterns by males over the age of 18 in both villages, comparing these over a period of six months and then 24 months. For the sake of brevity, it is suffice to say that in the intervention village the excessive use of alcohol was significantly curbed, compared to an increase in the control village – alcohol dependency was reduced in the intervention village, but not in the control. These findings were borne out over the two-year longitudinal study, but significantly here, recall and influence of the street dramas was reported as follows:[33]

The recall of the intervention was very high for the baseline medical clinic (93%), street drama (85%) and poster (75%), whereas the leaflets (43%) and brief intervention (52%) were less well-recalled. The preferred intervention by the community was the street drama with 75% approval with the other interventions being 15%. This preference was reflected in that the villagers initiated two additional dramas during the intervention period (weeks 10 and 15), their own street drama was based around the original intervention themes.

Since alcohol is a leading health problem in Sri Lanka, the pilot study's findings are important for both the improved health and social wellbeing of the communities, and for the benefits of Applied Theatre, in this case, street dramas.

The street drama had both high-recall and the community preference. This was distinguished from other components of the intervention by high levels of community participation as an audience and then subsequently as participants. The early initiation of locally produced drama was a strong indication of the cultural acceptance of this intervention and is supported by the subsequent viewing of video by village members. Equally surprising and undoubtedly significant was the spontaneous formation of a community action group.[34]

The development of plays and formation of a community action group in the intervention village highlights two important points: the intervention was not a one-off campaign that fell into an organizational vacuum, and members of the community were involved in its success.

Moving away from the social

However, part of the neoliberal agenda in funding TfD often distances the work from its social justice roots. It is not in the interests of most funders to conscientize people into questioning the status quo. The work often privileges psychological analysis and 'affect' over the sociopolitical, and runs the risk of obfuscating the relationships of power that exist in any applied performance context. Along the way, it also privileges elitist and Western notions of aesthetics and art, using an unwritten code of 'good' and 'bad' theatre. Notions of 'bad' theatre also encompasses the difficulty in measuring impact or efficacy of 'arts for health' interventions and 'arts in health'. In contemporary scholarship, the fears of 'bad' (often equated with didactic) theatre has caused a pendulum swing from 'effect' to 'affect'; art with purpose to art 'without' purpose. Arguably such debates are most prevalent in Global North scholarship. Citing Sayre's Law,[35] an analysis of applied arts for health shows that overt instrumentalism is almost completely absent where health services are more developed and accessible (i.e. in the Global North), and this is where scholars regularly reject notions of effect. In other words, the 'arts in health' approach is more prevalent in the Global North, where the benefits to health and wellbeing are a by-product of arts engagement. In the Global South, health care services are often dysfunctional and education levels are lower, resulting in little understanding of primary health issues. There is a tangible sense of urgency to cope with the burden of disease – to intervene, educate and advocate – because the stakes are high.

The more pedagogical 'arts for health' approaches (often in Global South contexts) are to some extent endorsed by François Matarasso's research, in which he argues that 'artists are not pure beings, uninfluenced by the desires of patrons or publics, and all artistic policy is, consciously or not, partly instrumental'. He acknowledges that 'artistic policy is always a matter of contestation: at least in democracies that debate should be open. Art does not belong to anyone. Ideas of what it is and how it should operate are not owned by artists, professionals, academics, politicians or by any one of us.'[36]

Mike White and his co-researchers in Ireland, Australia, South Africa and northern England analyse their 'arts in health' work as being clearly linked to positive health outcomes.[37] Despite recounting successful community-based work with a broad range of communities, nationalities, cultures, socioeconomic contexts, and age, gender and race, White concludes by presenting the challenges to research the field effectively. He argues that many practitioners know by experience that their work helps participants' health and wellbeing, but proving this is more difficult. He suggests that there is a tension between the artistic and social aims of any project, but that the better approach is to focus on the artistry and its affect, and 'to understand the creative process better in order to generate better quality art', and to engage with the '"madness" of art and its making'.[38] Perhaps most importantly he invokes 'qualitative evidence from participants [that] repeatedly affirms the felt experience of art as a counter to the circumstances and symptoms of ill health or social exclusion'.[39] This 'felt experience of art' goes to the heart of the debates around aesthetics – and raises the question whether it is at all possible to sever the affect from the effect, the feeling from the thinking, the form from the content. Alain de Botton tweeted that, 'When we call a work of art "beautiful", we sense in it values to which we aspire but from which we have been exiled.'[40] In an ordinary person's practice or viewing of theatre and performance activities, the emotional response to the art evokes a movement towards reassessing the value of life. As White suggests above, the glimpses of beauty inspire all practitioners to 'generate better quality art'.

Eugene van Erven weighs in on the debate around aesthetics, in his discussion of community theatre, where he argues that:

> ... in the first place it privileges the artistic pleasure and sociocultural empowerment of its community participants. Its material and aesthetic forms always emerge directly (if not exclusively) from 'the' community, whose interests it tries to express.[41]

However, the move away from effect or social impact as primary is often motivated by fear that the theatrical or performance work is somehow deficient of an aesthetic, has no merits in form when judged against outsider criteria. In contexts where little exposure to the arts is possible, where there are fewer skills and cultural heritage has been eroded, it is too easy to dismiss the value of a 'rough' art, by using standards that derive from, for example, urban centres, other cultural traditions and other performance norms.

Claire Bishop cites Irit Rogoff in discussion of the dangers of neoliberal, instrumentalist appropriation of participatory and educational art-making, specifically that:

> there is a certain slippage between terms like 'education', 'self-organised pedagogies', 'research' and 'knowledge production', so that the radical strands of the intersection between art and pedagogy blur easily with the neoliberal impetus to render education a product or tool in the 'knowledge economy'.[42]

Rogoff discusses how the 'Academy' can respond against commodification of education and art, by viewing education as a space that can hold:

> the speculative tension between the question of what one needs to know and that of what one aspires to. Academies often focus on what it is that people need to know in order to start thinking and acting, but we choose to approach the academy as a space that generates vital principles and activities – activities and principles you can take with you and which can be applied beyond its walls to become a mode of life-long learning.[43]

Bishop takes up this discussion about pedagogic art projects in the social field (including Augusto Boal's technique of Invisible Theatre) which 'require us to examine our assumptions about both fields of operation, and to ponder the productive overlaps and incompatibilities that might arise from their experimental conjunction, with the consequence of perpetually reinventing both'.[44] This is as much an appeal against the stifling and formulaic use of Applied Theatre as it is to look at dissonance between practices and practitioners from different social contexts.

Contextual practices

One of Applied Theatre's perennial problems is that where interventions may employ excellent strategies in the field, structural oppression and poverty may result in little effect to the work. Where there is little local organization to support the work, it falls into an 'action' vacuum. For example, while Applied Theatre may advocate the use of antiretroviral therapy for HIV in the case of a decline in CD4 count (an indicator of immunity), the health service provision may not be adequate to meet the demand. The result is frustration on the part of the facilitator and participants or audiences, and in the process possibly discrediting the strategies rather than the health services.

Using TfD strategies as an attempt to educate a community about, for example, mosquito nets in malaria areas, may result in little uptake of the messages. This could be due to prevailing socioeconomic circumstances or cultural behaviour patterns specific to the region. In this case, because the uptake of mosquito nets is poor, practitioners may veer into examining the psycho-social reasons for the seeming intractability of the individuals and community, because of unchangeable socioeconomic and structural oppression. This may result in 'blaming' the community for its burden of malaria. A study in Tanzania reinforces this point:

> Studies that have over-privileged cultural factors have [been] challenged for failing to pay enough attention to the political and economic determinants of compliance to biomedical interventions (Garro, 1986; Dein, 2007). According to Farmer (1999), although those studies may provide some useful information, they tend to shift the blame onto the people by exaggerating their agency.[45]

One of the challenges of doing this work remains that as a result of its progressive roots, the participants have high hopes for better provision of health resources, development and social changes. This is particularly the case for 'outsider-in' interventions, possibly because the outsider is viewed as from the government, city or university, and therefore is viewed as being powerful. Faced with a community that expects the project to bridge changes in their immediate circumstances, when the theatre work fails to deliver on effect or social change, the methods/medium of analysis (i.e. theatre) are deemed ineffective. This is not because the community has *not* learnt from the engagement but because empowerment is not achieved in isolation, and theatre alone is not enough for sustainable development or education to take place. A better approach combines the theatre interventions with other organizations that can offer direct assistance in changing material circumstances.

Psychologism

Frustration with theatre's inability to change structural oppression has resulted in many practitioners moving towards what this research will call 'psychologism'. In short, 'psychologism' is the tendency to ascribe non-psychological socioeconomic and political conditions to a psychological explanation, the latter usually individualist in origin.[46] Applied theatre practitioners have experienced frustration with the failure to change social conditions, and therefore what feels like the 'rehearsal' (to appropriate Boal's term) not of revolution, but of defeat.[47,48] The 'defeat' turns the practitioner away from collective social analysis towards the individual.

James Thompson[49] identifies a version of 'psychologism' in his discussion of theatre approaches to trauma, arguing that a Western trope of telling individual 'stories' appears to have become rooted in Applied Theatre practices. He argues that the Western concept of how to deal with trauma has been to ask participants in a theatre workshop to tell their stories, witnessed by their fellow participants. He is dismissive of the culturallyinsensitive use of narrative and playback methods used in post-tsunami Sri Lanka that assume that sharing stories of trauma is the best approach to dealing with the situation. Arguing that this is a 'globalisation of a particular form of knowledge',[50] the methods ignore that culturally specific forms of addressing the situation are more appropriate.[51] These interventions are often more reliant on individualist approaches to healing or reconciliation and do not consider the interrelatedness of many cultural norms. Elsewhere James Thompson has argued that in traumatic or conflict situations the last thing people want to do is make theatre about the situation in hand – that in fact 'all they want to do is play'.[52]

Elektra Tselikas uses the term 'social theatre' to add to the debate around form and function, where she employs Bruno Latour's argument that the social or society is 'reassembled' through the act of making theatre, or 'to create spaces allowing for the "social" to emerge'.[53] She argues that applied or 'social' theatre practitioners often do not trust their artistic practices due to pressure to be psychologically effective, advancing her 'hypothesis that when theatre is blurred with psychology and counselling, it loses its artistic potential and transformational power for groups and individuals'. She continues that the term 'social' frees the theatre-making process to explore the subject matter, rather than focus on 'relational group dynamics',[54] whereas in therapeutic engagements, 'relationships are given primordial importance'. She argues that in the 'social' theatre, actors can set aside their own biographies and that of others, and focus on the 'new associations and "social" context' being made – distance that is reminiscent of Brecht's *verfremdungseffekt*.[55]

Social cognitive learning theory

Albert Bandura's social cognitive learning has had an impact in many Global South contexts through the development of what has been called entertainment-education.[56] The work of Bandura represents a move away from the social justice framework in the arts. 'Psychologism' is implicated in the Entertainment-Education (EE or edutainment) approaches to researching media and Information and Communication Technologies for Development (ITC4D). The discourses of EE have crept into TfD practices and are linked to servicing the goals of funding agencies:

> EE is the process of purposely designing and implementing a media message to both entertain and educate in order to increase audience members' knowledge about an educational issue, create favorable attitude, shift social norms, and change the overt behavior of individuals and communities.[57]

These approaches draw on, and arguably universalize, Bandura's[58] social cognitive learning theory. Bandura argues that human beings operate in social structures that affect them in their personal efficacy, but nevertheless stresses that the individual is an 'agent' in their own life. The focus of his work is the ability of symbolic communication (through theatre or the media) to influence the choices that the individual makes. Essentially he argues that there are two types of learning in these contexts: that which punishes and that which rewards. With this in mind, he introduces the concept of social modelling (by characters in a play, for example) in order to promote individual and social change – models that include 'the instructive, motivational, social prompting, and social construction functions'.[59]

> With regard to the instructive function, models serve as transmitters of knowledge, values, cognitive skills, and new styles of behavior. Observers also acquire emotional proclivities toward people, places, and objects through modeled emotional experiences. Observers learn to fear that which frightened or injured models, to dislike what repulsed them, and to like what gratified them. Self-debilitating fears and inhibitions can be eliminated by modeling that depicts effective coping strategies and instills a sense of coping efficacy.[60]

Key to this social cognitive learning theory is that the individual must have a strong sense of efficacy, that is, they should believe that they can effect change through their actions. This belief in efficacy is achieved, according to Bandura, through experiences where mastery is achieved. In addition to mastery, social modelling is the recognition of someone's similarity to yourself, for example, a character in a soap opera. If this character models efficacy and is rewarded, then these behaviours are something to emulate. A failure is deemed a punishment, from which the person learns not to emulate the behaviours that led to failure. In modelling, efficacy is what governs a person to strive, to overcome obstacles and work towards achievement. Bandura ties efficacy to the optimism and resilience of both the individual and the social group. In other words, if an individual or group is optimistic, this is likely to have emerged out of rewarded behaviours, and allows them to be more resilient to life's challenges. Bandura also rather neatly concludes that if people are not achieving efficacy, then they should make different choices, in this way overdetermining the extent to which ordinary people in difficult environments have choices.

Bandura's social cognitive theory has been used extensively in media campaigns using radio drama or television soap operas in mass communication of health messages. His refinement of the theories was done in collaboration with, for example, Miguel Sabido, South American telenovela pioneer. This theory, modelling in particular, along with enormous resources in dramatizing social and individual problems, has been applied to Entertainment-Education campaigns in health promotion and education all over the world, and, for example, in the HIV/AIDS education theatre campaigns of DramAidE in South Africa.[61,62,63]

Worldview as a factor in health and wellbeing

In many southern African contexts (although not exclusively), people may ascribe their social and health problems to external forces beyond their control. In its crudest form, a patient at a clinic may ascribe their illness to having been bewitched, rendering them disempowered. This prevailing explanation for individual or community misfortunes also releases the sufferer from taking responsibility for changing their behaviours. In hierarchical and patriarchal societies the individual or group may be required to navigate a complex set of externally located controls that block personal agency, simultaneously creating a 'learnt helplessness'.

In order to provide clarity on the behaviours of individuals who are faced with little or no control over life situations, Vatan and Lester[64] distinguish between the notions of 'hopelessness', 'helplessness' and 'haplessness' as follows: a) 'hopelessness is a cognitive attitude in which people are not optimistic and have lost motivation about their future'; b) 'helplessness is the belief that there is nothing the individuals can do to change their lives'; and c) 'haplessness is the belief that one's life is in the hands of fate or luck'.

Vatan and Lester's study shows that all three of these states of being are connected to both cognitive and affective responses to lived situations. Where a society is structured hierarchically, or people believe that they are helpless or their circumstances are unchangeable, perhaps overtly didactic, instrumental approaches are valid because people are *inured* to being told what to do. However, often instrumentalist approaches are used precisely because social and cultural changes are not in the best interests of those at the top of the hierarchy.

Genevieve Stander's study of Rotter's theory of Locus of Control[65] is instructive in this case. Locus of Control (LOC) is essentially based on an individual's perception of the agency (control) of their lives – the extent to which control is either externally located or internally located. Internal versus external control refers to the degree to which a person expects that a reinforcement or an outcome of their behaviour is contingent on their own behaviour or personal characteristics versus the degree to which persons expect that the reinforcement or outcome is a function of chance, luck, or fate, is under the control of powerful others, or is simply unpredictable.[66] It also has an impact on the type of emotional associations that a participant in an Applied Theatre process will make.

Stander tested LOC in South Africa, and corroborated her findings in India, in three surveys over a period of ten years; in 1995, 2001 and 2006. Her research is based on respondents' self-identifying themselves into social-class groups. Her study reveals that in lower- or working-class groups, there is a greater reliance on externalized LOC, whereas for the middle and upper classes, LOC is internalized. Since 1995 and South Africa's transformation from apartheid, overall there has been an increase in internalized LOC, related to increased social mobility and improved opportunities. However, LOC has great influence on those for whom an Applied Theatre project may work, in order to effect change in knowledge, attitudes and practices.

Developing agency amongst participants of Applied Theatre projects is crucial to the development of an internalized LOC. One of the ways of doing this, as Nick Hamer and Alex Sutherland point out in Chapter 10, is to involve members of the community as actors. This not only enables deeper knowledge to be shared in the longer term, but also ensures that intervention remains rooted in the social context and culture. In a study conducted in Mumbai, Pertti J. Pelto and Rajendra Singh,[67] members of the RISHTA project (Research and Intervention in Sexual Health: Theory to Action) cite the use of street theatre in health communication about alcohol consumption, sexual risk and male–female relationships in low-income, slum communities of Mumbai, India. Extensive qualitative research was conducted over 18 months, and used in the development of the plays. Using community actors sourced by an NGO, the Community of Resource Organizations (CORO), the street theatre played 150 times to audiences of between 100 and 300 people. The main focus came to be questioning the nature of masculinity as it related to alcohol consumption, relationships with wives and commercial sex workers, and the risks of sexually transmitted infections. Using the form of street theatre most prevalent in the area, the play was announced in each area by a figure known as 'Awaliyah or Fakir',[68] whose colourful costume, face painting and comic hat drew attention to the performance. This character also mediated the performance by telling jokes and engaging the audience in discussion. Two plays were performed with slightly different emphases, namely *Tota and Maina* (the names of the lead characters) and *Story of Destiny*. The latter was narrated by a nomadic minstrel, who proved to be an important figure in the audience's aesthetic appreciation of the work.

The performances were followed up by extensive surveys of 2,722 men who had watched the performances. Some 56 per cent of these men reported having seen the plays, or heard about the central information from someone who had seen them. Overall, 42 per cent of the men had seen more than one performance. Messages about excessive alcohol consumption were most remembered at 79 per cent, followed by sexual health at 57 per cent, and domestic violence at 54%. HIV/AIDS awareness was remembered by 49 per cent. Some 90 per cent of the men interviewed reported incorporating the messages into their lifestyles.

Pelto and Singh[69] suggest that a large degree of success in the street theatre campaign was due to the actors being from the communities they performed to; in other words, they became peer educators. The other aspect that led to the success of the street theatre was that the scripts were devised after extensive field research.

Concerning issues of alcohol use and abuse, the RISHTA project endline survey showed that it is possible to reduce men's alcohol use through aggressive awareness campaigns. The discussions after the street drama performances showed that men in the study communities are aware of the dangers of excessive alcohol use, and that interventions that dramatize problems and urge restraint can have a positive impact. Another lesson from the street plays and accompanying educational meetings is that the messages about alcohol abuse should be connected to other social issues, including health problems, risky sexual behaviours and domestic inter-spouse relations.[70]

Beth Osnes, working in Guatemala, focuses on increasing the participation of girls and women in effective sustainable development, arguing that Applied Theatre provides an imaginative, creative and dialogical space.[71] She argues that Applied Theatre works against the idea of a 'deficit' model of development, but rather that the techniques recognize that women are capable and that even without any interventions many do 'overcome the obstacles they face and rise up to become community organizers, attend university, or transgress other societal norms within their communities'.[72] In this way she echoes the 'capabilities approach' of Amartya Sen, as discussed by Nandita Dinesh in Chapter 8. Osnes' work with Guatemalan Mayan girls, developing Vocal Empowerment workshops for Starfish One by One,[73] was intended to allow each participant 'to have a physical experience of their public voices as strong and expressive', leading to their (cap)ability to 'communicate decisions they would make about their own lives, which related to empowerment'.[74] Using warm-ups, physical and vocal exercises and role plays, the girls were encouraged to first express themselves in a semi-public forum, with a community mentor who in future would track the girls' development. Their role-play tasks were increasingly difficult and moved from a community to a national platform, as well as identifying their obstacles to their 'occupational dreams'.[75]

Osnes recounts that the indicators that the goals had been met were universally located within an arts-based research approach: strength and development of voice, making eye contact and having confidence in their range of movement, and their willingness in a later part of the workshop to engage with improvised situations. Follow-up observation and interaction with the community mentor provided some feedback on the longer-term benefits of the workshop, including that the girls had used the exercises in their own meetings, and the skills in presentations at school. However, Osnes suggests that the recounted outcomes come 'from my own perspective but with an attempt to include multiple viewpoints'[76] and that a 'baseline set to measure what was important to us – vocal strength and expressive range – was our perception of the strength of the girls' voices and their expressive range at the beginning of the workshop'. She suggests that the workshop design would be altered for future use and that other ways of evaluating would be included. The descriptions of the participants' responses show that a great deal of affective appreciation was evident. Beth Osnes' example, however, shows that increasingly the practice of the arts is used to develop individualist self-efficacy and as an antidote or panacea for social alienation and its concomitant conditions.

Resilience

Regular practice of the arts is seen as beneficial to health and wellbeing, in particular in assisting the development of personal resilience.

Much of the research into resilience is in neuroscience and positive psychology, and in summary suggests that the development of resilience relies on the elements of 'compensating experiences outside the home, [and] self-esteem development'.[77] In addition, an 'outgoing temperament, maternal warmth, and stimulating activities promote resilience to socioeconomic adversity'.[78] The practice of theatre (and other arts activities) does promote a positive outlook, self-esteem and an outgoing temperament – perhaps even optimism. It also provides experiences outside the home that stimulate interpersonal bonds and provides opportunities to develop coping skills through facing adversity. Many children and young adults develop adaptive social strategies to cope with adversity, as well as positive internal self-beliefs that sustain them.

Shelley E. Taylor and Jonathon D. Brown[79] argue that there are three internal self-beliefs that are necessary to personal wellbeing and a sense of personal efficacy – these are 'positive illusions' that are necessary for wellbeing and not, in fact, a strictly realistic self-perception. One of these necessary positive self-beliefs is holding a high opinion of yourself, another is the idea that you can control things, and another is that you will get what you desire. The more these three positive illusions are held, the more likely you are to describe yourself as happy, and the greater your resilience. Martin Seligman has developed a 'Master of Resilience Training' or MRT that has been implemented and researched with UK teachers and the US Army.[80] The programme consists of three modules, building mental toughness, building strengths and building strong relationships. The programme leads the participants through various symbolically named strategies, revolving around a simple formula: C (emotional consequences) do not stem directly from A (adversity) but from B (your beliefs about the adversity). The process of learning mental toughness involves recognizing mental 'traps' in thinking, the 'iceberg' of fixed beliefs, catastrophizing, assessing personal strengths, gratitude and 'learned optimism'. The last of these is what Seligman's 'positive psychology' movement has theorized to counter what he terms 'learned helplessness'. Seligman shows that helplessness is learned when people have no way to influence change in their lives. As a result they score high on pessimism scales, and their resilience to negative life events is profoundly compromised. Seligman cites considerable evidence that suggests that optimism is a factor in protecting humans from cardiovascular disease, and referring to Sheldon Cohen's research, that 'people with high positive emotion before [receiving] the rhinovirus get fewer colds', the converse is also true – that people with a pessimistic outlook get more colds.[81] In suggesting these factors that contribute to health he suggests that a state of wellbeing includes doing something 'for its own sake' and refers to *ikigai*, the Japanese term loosely translated as 'having something to live for'.[82]

Participatory processes of theatre-making and performance fulfil some of the ways of developing a more positive affect, including doing something 'for its own sake' and 'compensating experiences outside the home'. In the process of developing a more positive affect, theatre-making gives participants an opportunity to examine various blocks to mental and physical resilience, and potentially a 'rehearsal' for 'learned optimism'. However, while the development of positive affect requires more than actualizing wishes and dreams, there are pitfalls similar to those of TfD practices mentioned before. The work may create false expectations of behaviour change in a participant, which, if not achieved, can be interpreted as a personal failure, hence 'blaming the victim'. The worldview of the individual or community may be based more on 'fate' than 'destiny', affecting the extent to which people accept their circumstances as unchangeable. Even if a participant experiences a profound shift during a workshop process, upon leaving that safe space there may be no facilities to support the participant further. For example, inmates in Cape Town's Pollsmoor prison in 2015 noted their changes of confidence, self-esteem, a decrease in drug use and development of a post-prison plan. However, upon parole, the inmates were released into the same socioeconomic conditions that initiated their criminal behaviour.[83] This points towards a major tension between positive affect or optimism, and the socioeconomic determinants of optimism, self-actualization. According to Abraham Maslow, the human spirit can move to self-actualization and self-transcendence only once the basic human needs of food, water, shelter, family and loving relationships are established.[84]

Researching wellbeing

Various research projects have evaluated the impact of the participation in the arts more generally on young and old people in various parts of the world. For example, the Sing For Your Life Silver Song Clubs in the UK[85] provide regular opportunities for older people to participate in community singing. According to Ann Skingley and Hilary Bungay, singing has several physical and mental benefits, including decreasing social isolation, increasing enjoyment, and improving breathing, mobility and mental acumen – in other words, improving resilience.[86] It is not surprising, therefore, that many of the poorest members of South African townships often spend entire days and nights singing and dancing in their churches, praying for release from their circumstances. Their results are endorsed for a range of arts-based interventions in two specifically developed, international journals, namely *Applied Arts in Health*[87] and *Arts in Health*.[88]

A recent UK Arts and Humanities Research Council (AHRC) report on the value of the arts acknowledges the use of 'community arts activities to engage people in thinking about their own health, and help individuals in disadvantaged areas (and with health problems) to build the capacity to address them'.[89] The authors assert that 'attention to social determinants, inequalities and globalisation locate the production of health and ill-health within complex relationships shaped across space and time'. Encouraging results for the benefit of arts in health came from Sweden: 'a randomly-selected cohort of 9,011 Swedish adults from the 1990–1 Swedish Survey of Living Conditions, followed up in 2003, showed that attendance at the cinema, theatre, art galleries, live music events and museums was associated with lower rates of cancer-related mortality'.[90] However, while most of the cases cited showed the benefits of arts engagement, the authors pointed to a lack of valid and reliable research. They also point to a conundrum in the research, in that it is difficult to tell whether those who benefit from engaging with the arts are also those who have a predisposition for the arts. Further research is needed in this regard.

No one would argue the point that in order to be effective, theatre needs to use a full range of artistic expression – creative expression that is shaped according to the context of its participants/audiences. An earlier study by Matarasso and his fellow UK-based researchers in 1997 focused on the social impact of participation in arts activities,[91] which was summarised as follows:

> Participation in arts activities brings social benefits; The experience of participation is unique and significant; Relationship is more significant than form; The social impacts of the arts are complex; Social impacts are inevitable but not necessarily positive; Participating in the arts brings risks and costs; Arts projects can provide cost-effective solutions; [and] Social impacts are demonstrable.[92]

Perhaps the move away from public funding of the arts has motivated a utilitarian approach and a feverish but flawed research process, in order to fulfil funding conditions by corporate donors who want measurable outcomes. With the global trend towards neoliberal policies (that promote self-interest and free-market principles), naïve altruism in Applied Theatre and performance practices has been replaced with some moral relativism, or at worst, opportunism. Most importantly, the pressure to account for effects has run counter to critical evaluation of Applied Theatre praxis, and a measured understanding of what impact is contextually appropriate. Matthew Jennings and Andrea Baldwin argue that:

> Evaluation has become a corporate chore, often contracted out to professional consultants, whereby boxes can be ticked and formulaic cases made for the justification of funding (Leeuw, 2009). Practitioners' and participants' experiences and backgrounds have been either ignored or reduced to quantitative indicators for the

fulfilment of socio-political objectives. There has been little space for the development of ongoing critical and reflective practice. In any case, practitioners have little motivation to assess their work critically, at least within the public sphere. Their continued employment has depended on positive (and positivist) individual project evaluations.[93]

What Jennings and Baldwin also point to is the absence of infrastructure to support the theatre practitioner in their work. Many theatre practitioners may lack the time and skills to fundraise, keep accounts or write comprehensive reports in addition to the theatre practice. However, often there is no money for support staff and so the work becomes unsustainable and under-researched. While the need for arts management in theatres is generally understood, very few arts administrators are trained to work specifically in the field of Applied Theatre, which arguably requires a different mind- and skill-set.

Facilitation and ethics

Christopher Odhiambo Joseph points to an important consideration in Applied Theatre practice – that the strength of the interventions rest to a large extent on the artistic skills and socio-political insight of facilitators. He points to ethical problems in the practices of Applied Theatre (in his study specifically related to TfD), citing his research into Kenyan practitioners and companies.[94] He ascertained from a questionnaire he administered in 2004 that 90% of practitioners had started to work in the field because of chasing donor money, not out of commitment to society. He also found that 70% of his questionnaire respondents did not know that there was 'a philosophy and ideology that defines and characterises the practice'.[95] This weakness in facilitators of TfD allows donors to exploit and dumb down the methods of TfD.

Additionally, donor agencies often disregard the research findings of the TfD processes, or use the theatre-facilitated dialogical process in the community as an avenue to impose their own pre-determined ideas. Lastly Odhiambo Joseph points towards the lack of adequate training in facilitators of TfD, with over 60% having received no training, and 40% having received some training through irregular workshops. While formal training as part of a degree programme was offered for the first time in 1997 at Moi University, Kenya, he argues that the 'ethos of commercialisation' is dominant.

Odhiambo Joseph's research raises questions about the TfD facilitator's ability to focus on the main dilemmas that may face a community, and effectively work to change them. In part this is due to the donor's agenda, which may be overtly didactic and not in keeping with the actual social needs of the area.

> In order to be seen, felt and finally succeed, many NGOs have perfected the art of dancing to a donor's tune. They come up with 'fashionable' causes and have learnt when to scream, when to push and when to act blind, deaf and dumb.[96]

The donor's objective may also ignore the structural problems in society in favour of an ameliorative approach to the problems. In other words, the limited efficacy of Applied Theatre in social justice contexts is potentially due to the problem of structural oppression and uninformed facilitation. Even if a local group or community could absorb the information and mobilize for social change, the organization or structures of society are not always aligned to the working-class benefit. This speaks to the importance of Odhiambo Joseph's call for the development of a code of ethics or charter that improves the training facilitators of Applied Theatre (or in Boal's terms, 'difficultators').[97]

The skill of facilitation rests on the ability to ask questions to probe the subject matter through a problem-posing performance, or literal questions in a participatory process. The art of questioning is an ancient one, documented by the classical Greek philosophers and the great teachers of Timbuktu. Socratic questioning has particular relevance to the facilitation of Applied Theatre, when questions are asked from a place of seeming ignorance. Peter Abbs suggests that Socratic questioning comes from a state of mind that is 'creative ignorance, inner perplexity and emotional unease that such perplexity created'.[98] This puts in mind Augusto Boal's Joker figure, who throughout the theatre interacts with the spect-actors in order to provoke deeper thinking and understanding of the social context, also congruent with Freire's 'dialogical'. Boal refers to the Joker as a 'midwife' of ideas and action, deliberately invoking Socrates' famous lines to his students.[99]

Organic intellectuals can appear in the form of *jongleurs* or *griots*, with a history in performance, according to Claudia Orenstein, where 'clowns from Western traditions … are usually antagonistic to social structures'.[100] It is the ability of the facilitator to be 'the fool [who] represents the free spirit, the unconventional thinker whose example encourages others to view the world in new and extraordinary ways'.[101] One of the important aspects of approaching health and wellbeing challenges through humour is the ability to laugh, providing a release from stressors and the development of optimism.[102]

However, in many instances of Applied Theatre in health it is necessary for the facilitator to be extremely skilled at theatre *and* to understand the subject matter in all its complexities. For a facilitator to run a workshop, for example on HIV/AIDS, and not have sufficient subject and contextual knowledge, runs the risk of undermining the objectives of the health intervention, putting people's lives at risk and bringing the theatrical approach into disrepute.

For example, South African Applied Theatre and performance practice is still haunted by the *Sarafina 2* debacle in the early 1990s, where a high-profile theatre director was commissioned to produce an 'AIDS musical' for local learning and entertainment. Not only did this musical cost upwards of R14 million (approximately £637,000 at the 2016 exchange rate), but it was deemed to be entirely misleading on the subject of HIV/AIDS, prevention, treatment and dying.[103]

Some health professionals argue that partnerships between an artist and medical specialist are ideal. However, the artist may have to make an improvisatory decision in the moment, without stopping the action for a consultation. In the Global South, health services are notoriously short-staffed and this may obviate partnerships in action.

Another key aspect to facilitation of Arts for Health and Arts in Health projects is to have extensive knowledge of theatrical and performance forms that are both local and global. If the mode of theatre and performance is used in developing health and wellbeing, then provision of the best possible experience is ideal. Clearly there are times when theatre is not the ideal medium for education or information giving, because a pamphlet, a 'lecture' or media could communicate better or just as effectively. There are other contexts in which 'live' performers or participants in physical contact with each other present too many risks, for example in the case of the Ebola virus outbreak (in 2014–15) in West African countries.

However, when specific objectives that are 'life and death' are delivered through theatre, the question of what is learned is ethically weighted. If a practitioner elicits (through theatrical processes) feedback from an audience, and the information therein is life-threateningly 'wrong', how does the facilitator resolve the situation without undermining indigenous, local knowledge and experience? If the theatre is a performance, and in the process of rendering it has created multiple readings, some of which are hazardous attitudes or practices, what are the ethical implications for the participants and/or audience and the reputation of Applied Theatre? Does an overtly instrumentalist performance fail to engage the participants because it created too little emotion? Can the affective responses overwhelm the cognitive potential in a performance or workshop? Part 2 of this book engages with extraordinarily varied ways in which practitioners negotiate the dialectical relationship between emotion and cognition, aesthetics and ethics. The diverse research processes in Applied Theatre and performance are well represented in Part 2, emerging from global challenges to health and wellbeing.

Part Two

3

Ageing: Dementia Care, Death and Dying (the UK and North America)

3.1 Introduction

Katharine Low

Across the world, in both low-income and high-income countries, life expectancy is rising due to better health care and significant reductions in childhood mortality and infectious diseases. In addition, there exists a growing ageing population, particularly in high-income countries, due to declining fertility rates worldwide.[1] However, with rises in life expectancy come increases in multiple health conditions which need a diversity of care, management and treatment. Furthermore, while dementia has previously been linked with developed countries, there has been a marked rise in cases of dementia in developing countries.[2] While increased interest in how to cope with ageing is being displayed in the Global South, there remains more focus on the issue in the Global North, which currently accounts for two-thirds of the world's ageing population. This is a trend that will soon change though, as the ageing population in the Global South is growing at faster rates.[3]

In the run-up to the 2015 British general election, significant debate arose over whose responsibility it was to reduce health inequalities and to 'ensure people age in better health'.[4] This drew attention to significant health inequalities, even in high-income countries like the UK, which are linked to location, ethnicity and poverty around life expectancy and care in old age.[5] Such debates are often closely associated with concerns over 'ageism' and views that older people or people with dementia are 'draining' the economy and are '"too far gone" to notice or care'[6] or contribute to society. The WHO's recent *World Report on Ageing and Health* notes, on the contrary, that the ageing population does not lead to greater dependency but rather celebrates the contributions elders bring to society.[7]

Similarly, Allan Kellehear, in his book 'A Social History of Dying', draws attention to how, through major improvements in medical technology, 'there is a widespread desire and optimism that the time of death can be controlled' in rich and wealthy parts of the world, while in poorer or more vulnerable communities there has been a rise in 'shameful deaths'.[8] He argues that 'shameful deaths' represent 'a moral and social failure to provide satisfactory models of social care for dying people at the economic margins of our world',[9] and calls for 'real products of social support, tolerance and courage to sit with the contagious or unrecognised dying'.[10]

Yet, death is often feared, ignored or hidden. Writing in 1973, Seymour Fisher argued 'It may not be a coincidence that the two things we keep most secret from our children are birth and death.' In Fisher's analysis of how children and ultimately adults view death, he considers how death is also kept from adults' view through the way the elderly are often institutionalized and severely ill people are isolated in ICU.[11] Clearly, death and dementia remain vitally important topics to discuss and acknowledge, both for individuals and more broadly as a society. In the essay and interview that follow, Nicola Hatton, Sue Mayo and Liz Rothschild draw attention to the role of art or the artist in setting up and engendering spaces through which topics such as death or people previously seen as being 'too far gone' can be celebrated and can have a place as artists. As you will see in their discussions, we are – thankfully – moving away from dismissive and suppressive attitudes. However, there remains much to be done in terms of combating reductive views of the elderly and facing death in a healthier way, and each contribution suggests exciting ways forward, placing the experiences of individuals at the centre of the process.

3.2 Essay – Participatory theatre and dementia
Nicola Hatton

This essay explores theatre practice with people who are living with dementia. Participatory arts with people with dementia have increased significantly in recent years, with projects taking place in arts venues, care homes, hospitals, day centres and a range of community settings.[12] However, despite a growing body of research about the arts in dementia care, there has been little investigation of theatre-based work. This essay investigates some of the different types of theatre practice that are taking place and considers the benefits and limitations of different approaches. My intention in exploring different types of theatre practice is not to endorse one approach over another but to question what theatre might offer in supporting people with dementia to be 'in the moment'. As such, I pay particular attention to improvisation, not just as a type of practice, but as a key aspect of *all* theatre practice with people who are living with dementia. Dramatic improvisation is based on the principle that a performance is created in the moment that it is performed. In order for an improvisation to be successful, performers must accept the line that is offered to them by another performer and add something new – a process commonly described as 'saying yes' or 'yes, and …'. People with dementia often improvise as part of their everyday lives, and the basic practice of 'saying yes' in dramatic improvisations is a strategy that can support their participation in theatre projects without fear of failure.

In an article about arts practices in care homes, the theatre scholar Caoimhe McAvinchey outlines the need to ask new questions about the value of the arts with older people: 'If we only ask questions about the social, economic and health value [of the work] … we continue to develop an evidence base that reiterates particular, already known, outcomes.'[13] McAvinchey suggests that 'examining the contexts, politics and processes' of performance practice with older people may lead to new understandings about 'innovations in form, artistic labour practices and cultural organisational capacity'.[14] This essay is informed by her argument and uses the principles of improvisation to draw attention to the artistic possibilities of theatre practice with people who are living with dementia.

Theatre and dementia work is developing at a time when dementia is particularly prominent in the public imagination. Global statistics on dementia can be difficult to track owing to poor levels of diagnosis. However, to give an indication of scale, there are an estimated 800,000 people living with a form of dementia in the UK, with Alzheimer's disease being the most prevalent type.[15] This figure is predicted to rise to 1.4 million in the next thirty years. In Europe as a whole, this figure is currently estimated to be 6 million,[16] and in the United States 5.3 million.[17] The predominant factor for this increase in diagnoses is the ageing population of the Global North, as the likelihood of having dementia increases exponentially with old age. With no cure and the number of patients increasing substantially each year, the economic challenge of managing the disease and providing high quality, affordable care has become a priority in many different parts of the world, perhaps particularly in the late capitalist economies of the West.

The increase in arts practices with people with dementia is largely attributable to a growing body of evidence that suggests that participation can have a positive impact on health and wellbeing.[18] As a result of this evidence, there has been an increase in projects that are funded by the health sector. However, there has also been an increased interest in the creative possibilities of the work, which is reflected in support from the arts and cultural sectors. In 2013, Arts Council England announced a £1 million grant to fund new projects in residential care homes. The aim of the grant was to 'support artistic excellence in residential care settings and stretch aspiration for the range of arts that residents can access and experience'.[19] This increase in capacity indicates a new commitment to develop artists' work, and echoes McAvinchey's argument that more attention be given to exploring the aesthetic value of arts practices in elder care settings.

Much of the theatre work that is taking place with people who have dementia has developed in response to this relatively recent demand for arts provision in care homes. However, the origins of participatory theatre with people who have dementia can be traced back much earlier to the Reminiscence Theatre movement of the 1970s and 1980s. In his book *Staging Ageing*, the theatre scholar Michael Mangan defines Reminiscence Theatre as 'a mode of documentary theatre-making which takes the memories and experiences of older people as a basis for a theatre script or performance'.[20] He traces the development of Reminiscence Theatre, describing the work of Devon-based theatre company Fair Old Times, who in the 1970s developed a set of documentary techniques in order to engage older people in their community. Baz Kershaw, who was co-director of the company at the time, describes the therapeutic intention behind the work, which was designed 'to improve the psychological and social health of the elderly'.[21] The result was a series of shows which interspersed rehearsed scenes with the live reminiscences of the older people in the audience.

While Fair Old Times' model of Reminiscence Theatre was built on the principles of drama therapy, the theatre director Pam Schweitzer was developing a different approach, which Mangan observes is now 'most firmly associated with reminiscence theatre'.[22] Schweitzer's model emerged from an intergenerational project in London involving school students and older people from their local community. The project involved students interviewing older participants about their experiences as young people and developing naturalistic scenes from their responses. Though the project was successful with the older participants, Schweitzer realized that it was limited by the fact that it had only been accessed by a small number of older people. This led her to form the Age Exchange Theatre Trust, a professional theatre company which dramatized the long-term memories of participants and toured them to older people in care homes and sheltered accommodation.

The development of Age Exchange's work for people living with dementia came when the company took their work into care homes. The company recognized that reminiscence may have therapeutic value for participants with dementia. However, Schweitzer observed that the naturalistic format of the reminiscence plays was not always appropriate for people with dementia, who may not be able to contribute verbally or make sense of a linear narrative. She realized that 'a more flexible approach was needed, geared more specifically to meet individual needs'.[23] Since then, Age Exchange have developed their reminiscence work for people with dementia, using a theme-based approach that includes improvisation, objects, sensory stimuli and one-to-one encounters.

A recent production was co-facilitated by Age Exchange and the Trinity Laban Conservatoire of Music and Dance. The performance featured people with dementia and their carers and was facilitated by the composer Natasha Lohan, choreographer Stella Howard and Age Exchange's Arts and Education Coordinator Malcolm Jones. The piece, which explored the participants' memories of going on seaside holidays in Britain, still contained a strong reminiscence component, but the story was told in a non-linear fashion through episodes of song, movement, dialogue and repeated words. This gave the performance an abstract quality and supports McAvinchey's suggestion that arts practices with older people, and particularly those with dementia, have the potential to demonstrate innovation in form. What was also different about the performance from other reminiscence productions I have seen was the opportunities it gave for unrehearsed contributions from the participants. When one of the participants began to sing in the middle of a movement sequence the rest of the company joined in, which took the performance in an unexpected direction. This moment highlighted the value of improvisation as a flexible form that supports the creative contributions of people with dementia in the way that they are expressed. Furthermore, it drew attention to the status of people with dementia as skilled improvisers who are accustomed to improvising in unfamiliar situations as part of everyday life.

This shift away from naturalistic storytelling has opened up a broader set of aesthetic possibilities for doing Reminiscence Theatre with people who have dementia. However, one of the limitations of reminiscence as a creative approach is that its focus on the long-term histories of the participants risks overlooking their creative responses to the present moment. Helen Nicholson suggests that theatre practice in care homes has the potential to draw attention to the creativity that is inherent in the everyday lives of people with dementia as they move 'between material and imagined worlds, between attention and inattention, between memories of the past and their creative responses to living in the here and now'.[24] Her suggestion indicates the need for theatre practitioners to balance an engagement with the past with an understanding of the creative contribution that people with dementia can make in the present. This is where the principle of improvisation can be particularly instructive, as it requires performers to be 'in the moment' in order for a dramatic encounter to take place.

One approach that has been highly successful in engaging people with dementia in the moment is Timeslips – an improvisational storytelling technique developed by the playwright Anne Davis Basting. Basting created Timeslips after working with people in the later stages of dementia. She was interested in developing a form of storytelling that captured 'the complexity of their worlds and our relationship to them ... complete with missing words, repeated sounds and hazy memories'.[25] Rather than encouraging participants to recall stories from the past, the purpose was to create new stories from imagination through a process of collaborative storytelling.

In 2013 I participated in a Timeslips workshop. Participants gathered in a circle in the lounge and were invited to choose an image from a selection of pictures. Realistic images were avoided so that participants did not associate them with an existing story that they may have had difficulty remembering. In this instance, the group chose a black and white photograph of a woman diving off a bridge into a river. The picture was distributed around the circle and the facilitator posed a series of questions about it. These would often focus on the sensory aspects of the picture ('What does the water feel like?'), or the imagined world outside the image ('Does the woman have a family?'). There was no 'wrong' answer and everything that was offered – sentences, words, sounds, questions – was recorded on a large sheet of paper and incorporated into the story. The story was then retold to the group word for word and given a title.

The philosophy behind Timeslips is that stories are created from imagination rather than the memories. Its emphasis on accepting every offer of the participants makes it a valuable technique for working with people at the later stages of the disease, for whom language and verbal communication may be challenging. Additionally, this process of 'saying yes' is a useful strategy for engaging with the diverse moods of participants. Basting explains that 'challenge answers' are an important aspect of the Timeslips process: 'When we asked a storyteller what we should call Ethel Rebecca's daughters, her reply was (very typically) "I don't know." The facilitator reassured her (also very typically) by saying "You can say anything you like." As if to say "oh yeah?" the storyteller smugly responded, "ABCDEFG." '[26] By weaving the answer 'ABCDEFG' into their story, Basting explains, the storytellers were assured that 'our promise to accept any answer was sincere'.[27] Additionally, by taking up the participants' suggestions in the way that they are offered, Timeslips stories are not restricted to a conventional narrative form. Instead, they are open to different forms of storytelling, which may include fragments, repetitions and sounds. Timeslips demonstrates the unique aesthetic contribution that can be made by people at the later stages of dementia, and the possibilities of improvisation in engaging with them on their own terms.

The Timeslips approach has been highly influential in the development of improvisational theatre projects for people with dementia in the US. Key projects include Elders Share the Arts, who run a story-based improvisation programme in New York, and The Memory Ensemble project in Chicago, which explores how improvisation can improve the quality of life for people who have recently received a diagnosis.[28] These programmes are based on the idea that improvisation's focus on the present moment, and its principle of 'saying yes' to everything that is offered, can allow people with dementia to contribute to a creative process without fear of getting it wrong. As

Clayton Drinko observes of the Memory Ensemble, 'Improvisation's focus on the present moment may make these participants who have dementia feel safer to play ... The "yes, and ..." rule reinforces this by not allowing failure.'[29] Practitioners from the Memory Ensemble suggest that improvisation is particularly successful with people at the earlier stages of the disease who still communicate verbally and for whom improvisation may 'challenge them to use their minds in a new way'.[30] However, I argue that improvisation is an important aspect of all theatre practice with people who are living with dementia, whatever the stage of the disease. As the Timeslips approach indicates, improvisation can support artists to engage people in the later stages of dementia as it enables them to respond to diverse contributions and different methods of communication. One project that is guided by this principle is the Storybox project in Manchester. I now turn to examining the Storybox process in order to reflect on the significance of improvisation when working in care home settings.

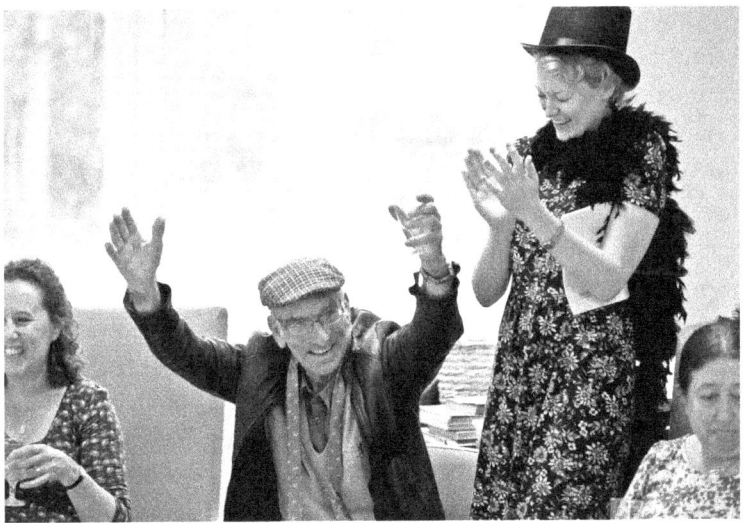

Figure 1: Sara Cocker and a Storybox participant. Photography © Roshana Rubin-Mayhew for Small Things Creative Projects.

Storybox is an improvisational storytelling programme for older people with a particular focus on those living with dementia. It was created by artists Liz Postlethwaite, Lowri Evans and Sara Cocker at the Library Theatre Company in Manchester and is now run by the Manchester-based company Small Things. Storybox takes place in care homes, day centres, hospitals and community centres over a ten-week period. Workshops are led by a Storybox practitioner and a visiting artist with a background in theatre or another art form. The programme encompasses different forms of performance and a typical workshop will involve props, costume, singing, role play, storytelling and movement which are brought together by a broad theme (see Figure 1). I spent a day with Storybox at a care home in Cheshire. The theme was the fairground. We arrived in a car crammed full of fairground-themed props including cock-a-hoop, coconuts, sparkly hats, 'goldfish' (carrot sticks in bags of water), balloons, inflatable balls and hook-a-ducks. It occurred to me as they were unpacked that some of these props may come across as patronizing to the residents, as they could be associated with children's play. This is an important consideration for theatre practitioners working in care homes, as the intention to introduce a theme into a care space quickly and simply may involve using objects that are bold and exaggerated. However, the seriousness with which Evans and Cocker engaged with the objects as props throughout the workshop seemed to foster a collective understanding of the theatrical intention behind them. Additionally, the artists were respectful in the way that they offered the props to participants, inviting them to select their own and accepting if someone did not want to take one.

The Storybox project evaluation suggests that improvisation is an integral aspect of the Storybox process, describing it as a 'bit of a journey where the destination is unknown'.[31] Although the artists plan each session carefully, the direction of the workshop is largely dictated by the residents themselves. This process is explained in the evaluation:

> Quite often if we do a game that involves holding hands in a circle an impromptu 'Auld Lang Syne' rendition starts up with the group. So we

just go along with it and everyone has an understanding that in that moment we are singing 'Auld Lang Syne' and have every right and reason to. We could then move on with the planned activity or accept the song and suggest, 'OK, so it's New Year's Eve then. Where are we having our party?' And so on.[32]

This balance between planning and improvisation is an important part of the Storybox process. It enables artists to take up the contributions of the participants while still maintaining a forward momentum to the workshops. This can lead to unexpected creative discoveries, such as a warm-up game turning into a New Year's Eve party. However, the artists acknowledge that the process of finding inventive ways of 'saying yes' to every contribution can be exhausting as they have to be continually thinking on their feet and responding to what is happening in the space at the time. In acknowledging the labour involved in this type of facilitation, Evans and Cocker stress the importance of having two facilitators:

> You need two people to deliver the session. It is important that one person can steer the group in general forward and keep the majority engaged whilst the other can check individuals are OK and following the activity. It also means that you can work like a relay race, taking it in turn to lead the activities, maintaining momentum and enhancing exercises with something different.[33]

In the Storybox workshop that I observed, I saw some residents had dementia, some had sensory impairments and some had physical health needs, each of which affected their participation in the workshop in different ways. The workshop demonstrated that creating opportunities for group and one-to-one encounters is an important aspect of theatre practice in care homes, as it enables practitioners to address the diverse needs of participants, supporting different forms of participation. Crucially, the 'relay' approach to facilitation can also enable artists to take a break from the task of continuous improvisation.

The way that the workshop started was typical of the uncertainty that theatre artists can face when working in care homes; it took place on Remembrance Day and as such the care staff were not sure how many residents would participate. As we entered the room, the residents were seated in different places around the space. Some were watching television, one was reading a TV magazine and some were seated on the other side of the room away from the hub of the group. I wondered how Evans and Cocker would address the group as a whole as everyone was so spread out. There were no care staff to be seen and it would have been difficult to move residents as they were seated in heavy backed chairs. The workshop began hesitantly as Evans' suggestion to turn off the television was met with resistance. Another resident was visibly distressed, and told us that she had been taken away from her family. At this point Evans turned to me and said 'I think today is going to be difficult, I think we're going to have to go with it.' Rather than ploughing ahead with the warm-up activity they had prepared, they decided to sit down with the residents and watch television. After a few minutes, the TV prompted everyone into a two minutes silence for Remembrance Day and we watched in silence with the residents. After this had finished, Evans took the opportunity to turn the volume down on the TV and asked if anyone would like some music. One man looked at Evans' boots and said 'these boots are made for walking'. The artists accepted his suggestion by playing the song and as Nancy Sinatra's voice drifted into the space, Evans led the group into a physical warm-up. The uncertainty around getting started in the workshop highlighted the importance of improvisation when working in care spaces. As arts workshops typically take place in communal spaces, artists are often required to work alongside other activities that are taking place at the same time. Rather than attempting to compete with these activities, Evans and Cocker engaged respectfully with them by joining in.

There was no official start to proceedings, no 'ritual' which marked the beginning of the workshop. Instead, the fact that it was Remembrance Day meant that the workshop began by watching television with the residents. Evans' remark that they would have to 'go with it' drew attention to the wider significance of improvisation when doing theatre practice in care homes. It suggested that working creatively with residents also requires artists to respond to what is happening in the space outside of the workshop. Furthermore, the notion of 'going with it' is pertinent to participants with dementia, who may not necessarily fully understand what is happening in a workshop and may be required to improvise in order to participate in the session. Over the course of the workshop, the artists and residents evoked a fairground through props, songs, storytelling and role-play exercises. One exercise that stood out involved residents in role as fortune tellers. Each participant was offered their own balloon and invited to use it as a crystal ball that let them see into the future. As mystical music played, Evans asked if anyone wanted to tell her fortune. One of the residents said she was going to meet a tall handsome man. Another said that she would have seven beautiful children. Someone else piped up that she was going to live 'til she was 100'. One of the most memorable moments was when a resident really got into role, putting on an accent and eliciting giggles from the woman who was seated next to her. Her performance was received appreciatively by the other residents who made comments like 'She should be on stage' and 'Can you take her back with you?' The exercise validated the status of people with dementia as skilled improvisers who could lead the facilitators in creative scenarios. Additionally, the opportunity that the exercise provided for them to predict happy future lives for each other emphasized the creative potential of improvisation in supporting people with dementia to imagine the future rather than remembering the past. This was apparent when the residents went on to tell each other's fortunes and predicted 'good health' and 'long and happy lives' for each other.

Storybox highlights the need for artists to be constantly improvising: in their approach to facilitation and in negotiating the challenges of working in care homes. In the workshop that I saw, improvisation was both the mode of performance and a strategy that enabled the facilitators to work alongside the other activities in the space. One of the limitations of improvisation, however, is that it can be difficult to accommodate the diverse contributions of participants, as it is not possible to take up every contribution that is given in one workshop. This is to an extent true for working in any participatory theatre setting, but here it is complicated by the fact that people with dementia may not be able to contribute verbally. This difficulty was alleviated somewhat in Storybox by the fact the Evans and Cocker skilfully incorporated one-to-one work within the session. However, there is greater scope to explore the possibilities of improvisation in relation to one-on-one encounters between theatre artists and residents with dementia. This improvisation may include, for example, movements instead of words, or improvisatory engagements with objects.

I would like to conclude by suggesting that theatre practice with people who have dementia can encourage researchers of performance and health to think more broadly about the value the arts in health settings. In a climate where much of the creative work with dementia patients is funded by health and wellbeing agendas, arts practitioners are often required to communicate the value of their work in measurable terms.[34] While this information can be extremely valuable in understanding the health benefits that come with participation, by focusing on medical outcomes it inevitably offers a partial understanding of the value of the work. Although this is a general problem with health-related arts practices, the attempt to measure the impact that a theatre project has on the wellbeing of participants by scoring mechanisms poses particular problems because it does not necessarily 'fit' with a performance process. This issue is taken up by Andrea Gilroy in her investigation into evidence-based practice in arts therapy. Gilroy suggests that 'outcomes are particularly problematic when the "treatment" being evaluated cannot be broken down into measurable component parts'.[35] In dementia care settings this task of measuring wellbeing can be hampered further by the fact that participants may not remember having taken part.

In 'The Usefulness of Mess', Jenny Hughes and colleagues refer to the process of improvisation that is necessary for conducting practice-based research in Applied Theatre settings. Improvisation, they suggest, refers to 'actions that take place during a research process that are spontaneous responses to the unpredictable events and ventures beyond the confines of predetermined design'.[36] Rather than seeing these moments as an obstacle to conducting research, they argue that they are 'a troubling and potentially enriching part of the research process'.[37] The Storybox project disrupts predetermined notions of value and impact in arts and health research by drawing attention to the creative discoveries that can emerge from difficult moments and unpredictable events. By focusing on these creative encounters in the moment that they occur, arts practitioners may find ways of articulating the value of their work in dementia care settings in relation to its aesthetic potential. Furthermore, by celebrating the words, fragments, repetitions and sounds of participants in the way that they are expressed, theatre practitioners may, as McAvinchey suggests, be inspired to explore new and innovative approaches to theatre practice both inside and outside of care settings.

3.3 Interview – A discussion about death? 'I feel more alive now'[38]

Sue Mayo in conversation with Liz Rothschild (LR), Director of Kicking the Bucket: A Festival of Living and Dying, *Oxford, 16 September 2014*[39]

The first *Kicking the Bucket* Festival took place in 2012, and the second one in 2014. Events took place over two weeks right across the city of Oxford, with a variety of small, intimate gatherings, open lectures and performances, drop-in events and information sharing, and focused events, looking at, for example, dementia care and planning a funeral. The Festival offers opportunities to get involved in music, dance, poetry and song, to hear debate, or to drop in to the 'Death Café'.

Liz, how did you come to initiate the Kicking the Bucket *Festival?*

LR: Alongside my work as a theatre practitioner I'm also a celebrant, someone who works with people to mark significant events in their lives. This might be a wedding, funeral, naming ceremony, the end of a relationship, retirement, or menopause. I'm the Manager of a Green Woodland Burial ground,[40] and with those hats on I obviously come across people frequently who have experienced a bereavement, or are living with someone, or living themselves, with a life-limiting illness. I have been passionate for some time about improving the way we mark a death, through the way we use the rituals of funerals, and the processes that follow after a death, and about changing our experience of burial grounds, and I began to realize that this was all coming a bit too late – that the way in which people experience death and bereavement is affected by the amount of thinking about death that has happened beforehand. I suppose the third strand in my interest in this area became what I might call death education, to try to encourage people who are not being forced to confront death to see it as part of their everyday life. That's what led me to create the Festival and to emphasize the connection between the words life and death – to try to re-couple them. I think that here in the UK our culture has disconnected them in a way that is unhelpful, not only for us when we come to deal with our deaths, but actually in a way that affects the way in which we live our lives.

In 2012 I attended a vivid and moving rehearsed reading of Nell Dunn's play *Home Death*,[41] directed by Liz, at the Pegasus Theatre. The play tells the stories of three couples, all dealing with the realities of one partner dying at home. I noted that the discussion after the show was marked by a sense of relief that it was possible to talk about death and dying in a public space.

Liz, was this reaction typical of the feedback you gathered from the first Festival?

LR: Individually, people repeatedly reported a sense of 'relief'; a sense of 'reduced anxiety' and a sense of 'lightness'. So this was the opposite from what might culturally be expected about discussing death, when words like 'morbid' and 'depressing' tend to be the currency. Again and again, people were saying absolutely the opposite to this. People who came with others talked about a sort of openness, a dialogue that had been initiated that they could then maintain. This might be with friends or with family members. They were finding a public forum in which to begin a very private conversation. For the people that were coming on their own, one of the things that was expressed frequently was the anxiety felt by people who were not in conventionally recognized relationship structures, about coming towards their death. That, I think, exposes something about how we are supporting people in our society. The experience of the Festival for them was one of reduced isolation. I was aware that all of us who were there had already taken a step; it was as though we had removed one mask, we had said 'We know we're mortal, that's why we're here.'

After Home Death *one audience member spoke about rediscovering Oxford as a community during the Festival. There is a sense of celebration inferred in the word Festival. How important was this to you?*

LR: To a lot of people I had to repeat the fact that it wasn't a conference, because the understanding initially was that this must be a conference. I kept having to say 'No, it's a *festival*, and it's a festival of living *and* dying.' The only resistance I encountered in a few places was actually from professionals, about the name of the Festival. There was a discomfort about that, because I think it was felt to be a bit 'in your face' and a bit crass by those who didn't like it. Yet that was almost exactly why I did like it, because I felt it was sending a signal that was like a big blast of fresh air and that it had energy and vitality and humour in it, so I stuck by it. And I have to say I've had far more positive feedback than negative about it overall. I suppose the other bit of that is that it's a euphemism,[42] and, quite rightly, within the world of people thinking about death and bereavement, there's a great desire to get away from all the damaging euphemisms that cause all kinds of problems – like 'going to sleep' or 'gone away' – which, particularly for children, have created any number of unnecessary traumas on top of the actual reality of the death.

This sense of celebration also seems to have provoked all sorts of formal and informal conversations. In British culture it is unusual to talk much about death and dying.⁴³ *Did the Festival somehow give permission for this dialogue?*

LR: An important element of the festival nature of the event is to be really visible in the city. In 2014 we built on the idea of having a hub of activities in one place, which was easy for us to manage, and worked well at building up that atmosphere we were talking about, but we've also continued being out in a variety of venues, because we wanted people to stumble over us. It is my impression that some people attended one thing and then decided on the spot to attend another event and very much enjoyed the fact that they were combining and recombining with familiar faces. So you could argue a temporary community was created – not just a community of one event, but a festival community. As one audience member commented:

> It felt like being in a club or on holiday. At every event you would meet up with some of the same people you had met at an earlier event and because we had shared something truthful and real and heartfelt you felt a connection with these people and each event started with a joyful reunion. It was a lovely, rare thing and rather sad when it ended.⁴⁴

Indeed, some audience members felt that these conversations would not have happened had the festival not taken place, that there was a sense of it being opened up, beyond the events themselves. Even though every element in it focused on death, it is back to this point that when you focus on death, you're actually focusing on life.

Like Liz, I have worked a lot on theatre projects that include older people, including those experiencing dementia. This work has increased my awareness of a hidden and unquestioned assumption that life equals success, and death equals failure. Medical professional Atul Gawande writes about this binary: 'The shock to me, therefore, was seeing medicine not pull people through. I knew theoretically that my patients would die, of course, but every actual instance felt like a violation, as if the rules I thought we were playing by were broken.'⁴⁵ He observes that this sense that dying is a failure permeates attitudes to the later stages of life: '[W]e regard living in the downhill stretches with a kind of embarrassment. We need help and regard that as a weakness.'[46]

I wondered if Liz believed that this level of anxiety about accepting the inevitability, the natural order of the life cycle, comes from the sense of failure associated with death.

LR: One of the reasons we in the UK have such difficulty with death is that we don't witness it or experience it in any way, so we're totally removed. People experience the death of a pet, but in most people's lives the only death that they're close to is an extremely upsetting and distressing death that comes very close into their life. When a neighbour dies we don't go and view them, as one would have done in traditional societies. It still to some extent prevails in Ireland, but here it's just not what you do. Therefore death is a strange territory to us. Plus, we live in a capitalist culture that has the sense we can infinitely consume and infinitely grow, and everything is always just going to get bigger and better. Medicine has been absolutely focused on healing and recovery, and hasn't really acknowledged the idea that there's going to be a stopping point. The whole emphasis has been on maintaining life and not allowing death. There is a superstition that if we go near death, death will come towards us.

Stephen Jenkinson, one of the speakers at the 2014 Festival, speaks about 'death phobia'. Like Liz, he has moved from only working with people as they faced death, to understanding

> that all of the people I was working with were on the receiving end of this dominant cultural understanding about what dying is ... Life has to continue, but you don't ... It's the end of life that gives life a chance.[47]

This theme is echoed in the puppet play by Karin Andrews Jashapara,[48] based on a traditional folk tale 'Death in a Nut', which was part of the 2014 Festival. Why this story? Are there difficult things that we can talk about more safely through art and creative encounters?

LR: ['Death in a Nut'] is a very lovely story in which a child defeats death and puts him into a nut. Then of course nothing will die, with the result that there's nothing to eat. The story is just trying to show that, however painful, death is a necessary part of the cycle of life. I passionately believe, and have done all my life, that the arts are a way of helping us live our lives better – that through artistic experiences as participants or as audience (which is also a participation of a different kind) we can gain new perspectives, new understandings, fresh ideas, renew or gain new empathies and understandings about the way the world works, about what we feel or think and about other people. So, to me, trying to deal with difficult subjects only throughout the head is not a helpful place to go, especially when it's very complex and emotional stuff. I would never have considered not using the arts.

Is it hard for people who are in the later stages of life to reflect on their own and other's deaths?

LR: I think the answer is that sometimes it is riskier and scarier but, also, so is the silence. Because it's so omnipresent in some ways for those people, the silence can be creating as much fear as the reality. 'Not talking' prevails; both with the dying and with the bereaved. There is this double isolation – the isolation of losing somebody that's very significant for you, and the isolation of the fact that people feel unable to offer support and, in our culture anyway, are self-conscious about that. So for fear of doing more damage they do nothing, and actually they do worse damage. The prevailing wisdom is to just ask the person what they want. They are not expecting you to be the Buddha, but they wouldn't mind a bit of contact!

This focus on 'contact', on noticing rather than ignoring, reminds me of Nicola Shaughnessy's unpacking of the word 'Applied' in Applied Theatre, where she explains that 'Applying is derived from the Latin applicare, *its etymological sense being "to bring things into contact with one another", to "join" to "connect."*[49]

The Festival provides many opportunities for contact, for noticing and for awareness. The relief expressed by so many participants and audience members is the relief felt when notice is taken and care is given, something that we all hope for in our dying and in our death.

Further reading

Earle, S., Komaromy, C. and Bartholomew, C. (eds), *Death and Dying: A Reader*. London: SAGE, 2009.

Gill, S. and Fox, J., *The Dead Good Funerals Book* (Dead Good Guides). Ulverston: Engineers of The Imagination, Welfare State International, 1997.

Levine, S., *Healing into Life and Death*. New York: Knopf Doubleday Publishing Group, 2010.

Luper, S. (ed.), *The Cambridge Companion to Life and Death*. Cambridge: Cambridge University Press, 2014.

4

Communicable Diseases: Tuberculosis (South Africa), Malaria (Malawi) and Dengue Fever (Brazil)

4.1 Introduction

Katharine Low

Communicable diseases, which are sometimes called contagious diseases (referencing the mode of infection), are parasitic and infectious diseases transmitted between humans or from animals to humans. Outbreaks of communicable diseases can occur in particular circumstances in high-risk situations or groups, and as a result of humanitarian emergencies or ecological disasters; for example, elders and young people are at increased risk of influenza in the winter months, and an outbreak of cholera in Haiti followed the destructive earthquake in January 2010.[1] *The Global Burden of Disease Study* concluded that in 2013 over a million deaths were due to parasitic diseases, of which 854,600 were related to malaria, 1.3 million deaths were caused by HIV/AIDS, 1.3 million by diarrhoeal diseases, and 1.3 million by tuberculosis (TB).[2]

However, diseases are not experienced equally across the globe. Severe health inequalities mean that poorer and vulnerable communities are more likely to be affected by deaths related to communicable diseases. For example, of 9.6 million new TB infections diagnosed globally and the 1.5 million deaths in 2014, 95 per cent of those TB deaths were located in developing countries and it is estimated that in 2015 1 in 3 HIV-related deaths were linked to TB.[3] Yet, as Veronica

Baxter and Michele Tameris examine in their essay, it is the African continent that is most affected by TB, with an estimated 281 cases per 100,000 people in 2014, a significant increase from the global average of 133.[4] Furthermore, the presentation of increasing numbers of multi-drug resistant tuberculosis (MDR-TB) highlights the need for diverse and multiple discussions about approaches to prevention and control. In their analysis, Baxter and Tameris discuss how a comic book, created to raise awareness around TB in the Western Cape, South Africa, has been developed into a performance by a local school and has since been performed to over 8,000 school pupils in a remote area of South Africa.

Similarly, parasitic infections like malaria and dengue fever are mainly concentrated in developing countries. Infected mosquitoes are responsible for transmitting several communicable diseases, from the female *Anopheles* genus which transmits malaria, to the *Aedes* genus which carries dengue, chi and yellow fever and which has recently extended to the Zika virus.[5,6] Although prevention relies on relatively simple and low-cost strategies to reduce contact between mosquitoes and humans, death and infection rates remain high and at times preventative knowledge is limited; for example, with malaria it is often reported that people distrust those who distribute the protective measures and are sceptical about the protective barriers' potential toxicity.[7,8] Zindaba Chisiza addresses malaria in his snapshot of Theatre for Development approaches to Malaria prevention in Malawi where he argues for the importance of sharing accurate information and avoiding simplistic performances which can alienate and confuse audience members. In contrast, Jan Onoszko's interview with the Artistic Director of the Brazilian AfroReggae company, Johayne Hildefonso, epitomizes the development of a street performance which was engaging and relevant to its intended audience. In their interview, they discuss the development and the successes of the 2009 performances of *Public Enemy No. 1 – Dengue* in reaching and engaging with their audiences.

4.2 Essay – Tuberculosis: The forgotten plague
Veronica Baxter and Michele Tameris

Tuberculosis (TB) has long been a scourge in history, from at least the time of Hippocrates around 460 BCE[9], and was observed in mummies in Egypt dating back even further, to approximately 2400 BCE.[10] Closer to the twenty-first century, tuberculosis (called consumption in earlier times) has been a feature of, and even romanticized in, literature and the arts. Probably most famous among these are Edvard Munch's paintings *The Sick Child*[11] and *The Dead Mother*,[12] and Claude Monet's portrait of his wife, *Camille on her deathbed*.[13] However, it is the history of tuberculosis in literature and performance that present extraordinary narratives of the 'wasting disease' as one associated with lovesickness and an artistic inclination from as far back, at least, as the Renaissance.[14] In this essay the historical and contemporary associations with tuberculosis will be discussed with reference to classical opera and contemporary adaptations, as well as South African examples of performance about TB.

Lawlor argues that 'by the end of the eighteenth century, consumption is not only the symbolic disease of the lover or a desired condition for the dying Christian, but also the glamorous sign of female beauty'.[15] In European opera the story of the heroine who dies from consumption has been interpreted by several composers, including Verdi's *La Traviata*[16] and Puccini's *La Bohème*.[17] Although the music is striking in these operas, the romanticized tale of a consumptive death is perhaps misleading, as is the contemporary adaptation in the film *Moulin Rouge*.[18] In fact tuberculosis then, as now, was painful and scary. But consumption was aestheticized in the eighteenth and nineteenth centuries, with literature and performing arts showing 'glamorous representations' of death, usually tied in with 'love melancholy' and the idea of a religious 'good death'.[19] Clark Lawlor suggests that despite the majority of horrendous deaths from consumption (specifically when referring to pulmonary tuberculosis), occasionally, 'people *did* die beautiful and easy deaths'.[20] A 'beautiful' or 'easy' death seems to have happened in sufficient numbers to make the romanticizing of a consumptive death possible, and for Romantic poets (Keats died in 1821 of consumption) to be seen as sensitive, refined, intelligent creatures by virtue of their maladies. In short, 'consumption has been described as the most intellectual and the most mysteriously psychic of all diseases'.[21] The romantic mythologizing of consumption continued, at least, until Robert Koch identified the tuberculosis bacillus in 1882.[22] However, thereafter, social attitudes shifted slowly to identify tuberculosis with the poor, the foreign and the unclean. Tuberculosis has become stigmatized in the Global South, where it remains an epidemic resulting in 9 million new infections and 1.5 million deaths as reported in 2014.[23]

One of the performances that aestheticizes tuberculosis is the late nineteenth-century tragic opera *La Bohème* and its contemporary adaptations *Rent*, *Moulin Rouge* and *Breathe Imphefumlo*. In *La Bohème* and its adaptations, the associations with tuberculosis are expanded to include the characters' poverty, their student bohemian lifestyles and their belief in romantic love. Rodolfo, a student, falls in love with Mimi, who has tuberculosis. Because he is poor, he feels that he cannot take care of her properly. Mimi leaves him, only to return later and die in his arms. The stage musical and film, *Rent*, has the same storyline except that several of the characters are infected not with tuberculosis, but HIV.[24,25] The characters in *Rent* are also protesting a neoliberal takeover of their shabby bohemian apartments, in order to gentrify inner-city New York. The characters also fall in love and suffer loss, linking HIV to older notions of 'consumption' (TB) as the lovers' disease.

In South Africa a new film adaptation of *La Bohème*, distributed under the name *Breathe Umphefumlo*, is set in a sprawling, poor township called Khayelitsha, near Cape Town. Isango Ensemble's film adaptation of the opera, *Breathe Imphefumlo* has been released at international film festivals. Reviews of the film acknowledge the timeous adaptation that illustrates the tuberculosis epidemic in South Africa, as well as the poverty surrounding its spread.[26,27] The film has translated the libretto into the Xhosa language and the musical instrumentation is resoundingly African, but much of the opera remains Puccini. Similarly to *Rent*, *Breathe Imphefumlo* situates itself in a contemporary urban setting. The original characters of Rodolfo and Mimi are now presented as politicized students existing in a derelict residence, a jazz singer (the Musetta character) and the South African reality of constant electrical power outages and corrupt politicians. Much of the action takes place inside cramped and poorly ventilated rooms,[28] although occasionally the shack land in which the characters live is shown, emphasizing the close quarters and lack of sanitation. The political implications of *Breathe Imphefumlo* are clear – poverty, poor sanitation, poor ventilation and cramped living conditions, lack of service delivery in the form of electricity and health services are major causes of Mimi's illness. In this case the characters do not embrace the bohemian lifestyle, but their lives and love are betrayed by corrupt politicians.

There is a great deal of irony in the appropriation of a Western opera classic to comment on South African 'consumption' in current times, because, to a greater degree tuberculosis has been eradicated in the 'developed' world. Like opera, tuberculosis was brought to Africa (and other colonized parts of the world) from Europe, ironically from those who came for the sun and fresh air to counter the disease. Tuberculosis swept through the indigenous population of southern Africa.[29] Local indigenous people did not have the immune systems to resist tuberculosis, and by the end of the nineteenth century the rates of infection were very high, exacerbated by the poor migrant workforce on diamond and gold mines. Poor nutrition, cramped living conditions, few medical facilities, alcohol misuse and silica dust made the spread of tuberculosis bacteria worse. Fast forward to after the end of legislated apartheid in 1994, and the statistics revealed that tuberculosis infection rates remained at approximately 750 people per 100,000. This increased rapidly thereafter due to co-infection with HIV.[30] It was evident that the impoverished and unequal medical systems in South Africa could not cope with either epidemic, and treatment failures were high. Edginton[31] argues that it is well established that a no-treatment situation is better than a poor-treatment regime, owing to the resistance to medication that develops in the context of patient non-compliance, or the unavailability of the medications in clinics and hospitals.[32] The treatment success rate in Africa is 70%, well below the World Health Organization's target of 85%. Unsuccessful treatment results in relapse, as well as a growth of drug-resistant tuberculosis.[33] Co-infection rates were worsened by the delay in effective treatment for HIV. HIV/AIDS treatment in the form of antiretroviral medicines was only rolled out in 2004, after disastrous years of the previous Health Minister's suggestions of beetroot, garlic, the African potato,[34] olive oil and lemons as an antidote.[35]

For now, tuberculosis presents a great challenge to many of the world's health systems, with South Africa claiming 306,166 new notified[36] infections in 2014. Of these, 10 per cent were under the age of fifteen years, and three times as many women were infected as men. National prevalence is measured at 834 cases per 100,000 of the population, but in the region of the Western Cape, where the *Carina's Choice* study took place, prevalence is almost twice this rate: 1,400 per 100,000 in general, and for adolescents, 500 per 100,000.[37] The rural town of Worcester (South Africa) is well placed as a test site for tuberculosis interventions, as borne out by the presence of the South African Tuberculosis Vaccine Initiative (SATVI), part of the University of Cape Town.[38] This site has conducted 20 clinical trials to test nine novel TB vaccines against tuberculosis, and modelling has shown that an effective vaccine for adolescents would interrupt the tuberculosis epidemic.[39]

Carina's Choice (in Afrikaans, *Karina se Keuse*) was initially a comic book produced in the three languages of the region: Afrikaans (85 per cent), English and Xhosa.[40] This comic was designed to disseminate information about tuberculosis prevention and infection, and to raise awareness of the value in participating in vaccination trials with SATVI. The comic showed a family of mother, father and their children, late adolescent Carina and her baby, and Tupac, their younger son. The narrative shows Tupac with an ongoing cough requiring a visit to the doctor at the clinic. His mother and sister accompany him, and while waiting for him, Carina encounters a member of SATVI's team.

Upon hearing about the prevalence of tuberculosis in the community, Carina enquires about her baby's safety. She is reassured by the information that her baby received the existing vaccine for infants, Bacillus Calmette-Guerin (BCG). She signs up herself and her baby for SATVI as a volunteer for clinical trials. Tupac is diagnosed as having a chest infection, but Carina uses this opportunity to persuade her family and friends to consider signing up for clinical trials. Queries are raised about the benefits to them, and a member of the Community Advisory Board outlines the benefits to the community and the ethical safeguards in place to protect their interests.

In 2012 a local school's drama teacher, Natasha Africa, decided to dramatize the comic book with a select group of her pupils. This performance played at their school, which is a SATVI site for community health. Based on the success of this performance, SATVI clinician Dr Michele Tameris approached Amber Abrams from the South African Medical Research Council to conduct focus groups and to analyse the data generated from each performance. Tameris contacted the University of Cape Town's Drama department which joined the project, providing an Applied Theatre practitioner. In some ways this role was that of dramaturg to work with the comic book 'script', to develop the performance capacity of the actors from the local secondary school and to design a performance that could travel to various schools, and oversee that the information carried through the play was accurate. Since this was an ideal learning opportunity, the project involved several university students in the development of the performance.[41] Natasha Africa, from Worcester Senior Sekondêr, and her drama pupils made up the rest of the team.[42]

The result of this collaboration was the production of *Karina se Keuse* (*Carina's Choice*), which was performed in Afrikaans to 8,000 high school pupils in the area of Worcester, from July to September 2013. The themes for the performance's development had emerged from adolescent focus group discussions that generated transcripts, which were inductively coded by two researchers.[43] These themes also informed the pre- and post-performance questionnaires, which were administered by the individual schools. In summary, the researchers report that overall just under 8,000 pupils responded to questionnaires about *Carina's Choice*. The performance had a few key goals in terms of education:

- What are tuberculosis symptoms and how to access treatment?
- Reinforcing the message that tuberculosis can be treated effectively, once diagnosed.
- There is a need for a new, more effective tuberculosis vaccine for adolescents and older.[44]
- SATVI is a site that conducts clinical research to test new tuberculosis vaccines.
- SATVI emphasizes safety and ethical conduct in their clinical trials.
- Participants have rights in clinical research, and SATVI works with a Community Advisory Board which helps to protect those rights.

Part of the intention of the project was to encourage adolescents to volunteer as potential participants in clinical trials. The play was developed through workshopping[45] from the comic with a group of adolescents from the Worcester Senior Sekondêr, some of whom had performed in the performance of the comic in the previous year. The cast members were taken through a deep learning process of theatre training in a very short period of time, including voice and movement training, improvisation and characterization. Most of the pupils were studying drama in their syllabus, and therefore benefited from this learning experience. A range of rehearsal and improvisation techniques were used, such as improvising from analytical still images, using physical theatre in a 'comic book' style to dramatize the vaccination process for babies, and working from costume to create characters – that is, from the outside in. The 'comic book' style[46] was reinforced by bold Pop Art images on moveable flats providing a basic design, and engaged the audience with the core messages of prevention: keeping the windows open, not smoking, ensuring that babies are given the BCG vaccine, washing hands and coughing into the elbow or clothing.

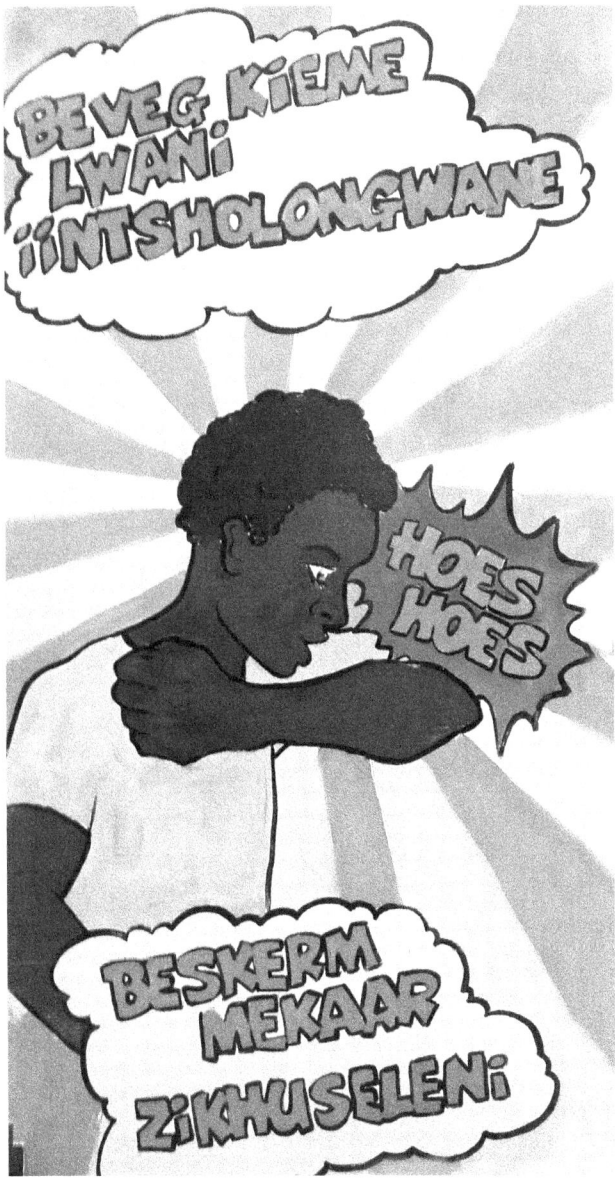

Figure 2: Pop Art image from *Carina's Choice* advises coughing into your elbow (not hands) to prevent the spread of tuberculosis. Photo © Veronica Baxter.

Heightened physical action was used in a sequence showing the administering of the infant vaccine, humorously demonstrated by actors making a slightly scary, machine-like conveyor belt, dressed in white coats, laboratory glasses, surgical masks and blue gloves. The actors embodied the protective benefits of the vaccine and fought off the tuberculosis bacteria, while the baby was passed along the conveyor belt. The baby (a doll) emerged unscathed but vaccinated, and was returned to her mother's arms.

Songs used familiar tunes with new words, and an original rap was collectively devised, performed in English and Afrikaans. The words of the rap described modes of transmission (coughing, sneezing), prevention (hand hygiene, coughing into elbow, clothes or handkerchief, immune boosting nutrition, and ventilation of spaces) and symptoms (night sweats, fever, coughing, weight loss, fatigue and weakness), as well as hinting at the problem of co-infection with HIV, and unwanted pregnancies. The rap ended by advocating participation in the clinical trials for an adolescent vaccine.

> Now with a **lack** of sanitation and **poor** ventilation
> With the *hubbly* going round and round
> **You** can get the **V.** –
> That's TB, not H-I-V.
> But **while** we're on the **subject**, always use a **rubber**
> Cos **un**protected sex could **make** you a **mothe**r (or father!)
> so **guard** yourself **against**, **HIV**
> take **part** in the trials with, **SATVI**
> and **help** us with the **fight** against – **TB**
> (Beat TB!) repeated 4 times

It is evident from the above descriptions that *Carina's Choice* was instrumentalist in its form, delivering set messages about tuberculosis and advocating participation in clinical trials through SATVI. Its non-participatory format ran the risk of implying that if you contracted tuberculosis, it was your fault because you were poorly informed, and that if you followed the preventive measures, you would not be infected.

The reality is that researchers are still unsure of what causes this region to be an infection hotspot, but what is clear is that poverty, poor nutrition, crowded living conditions and a grossly unequal, dysfunctional health system contributes greatly. A complicating factor is that about 80 per cent of South Africans have latent tuberculosis, although in only 10 per cent does the bacteria become active.[47] A longer participatory theatre process in each site may have yielded more engagement with the contradictions inherent in tuberculosis causes and cures, and participation in clinical trials. This was not possible because of the cast's schoolwork responsibilities, and the time given to the performance by individual secondary schools. Additionally there were hundreds of adolescents at each performance, and the time frame for development of the learners had not allowed for training in facilitation by Q and A or participatory theatre methods. However, the notion of participation is much contested in Applied Theatre, as outlined in Chapter 2. In most South African and African schools, the dominant mode of education remains 'teacher-talk' or teacher-centred.[48] However much this may depart from education theories, Irmhild Horn warns of the dangers of displacing content over form by assuming everything can or should be done in a learner-centred manner. The *Carina's Choice* project was designed with fact-giving in mind, but also was conscious of the difficulties in challenging the existing hierarchy and mode of education, essentially also undermining the difference in status between pupils and teacher. To invite participation in schools where interaction was unfamiliar was not possible in this project. Also in teacher centred learning contexts, participatory work has the potential for pupils to misread the facts of TB as open to interpretation. This meant that aside from the actual performance, interactive aspects of the project were confined to the cast of the production and in focus groups.

Despite the limitations of a fact-giving performance, questionnaires administered pre- and post-performance yielded a few statistically significant findings. For example, pupils were more accurately able to identify the causes of tuberculosis as a bacterial infection. After the play had been performed, more pupils were able to identify symptoms of tuberculosis, although this varied between different schools. The most significant positive finding was in awareness of the prevention of transmitting tuberculosis by 'covering the mouth'. There was also a statistically significant drop in post-performance questionnaires of the number of pupils who associated or equated tuberculosis with sexually transmitted diseases. Fieldworkers from SATVI reported that the performances had facilitated a smoother recruitment of adolescents for the clinical trial that started shortly after the tour. In short, 'theatre, presented and motivated by adolescent peers, can raise awareness of tuberculosis, and assist clinical trial preparedness and further engagement between trial staff and their trial community'.[49]

A key focus in the development of the performance had been my emphasis on the cast having an age-appropriate, developed understanding of the causes, symptoms and treatment of tuberculosis in their community; for example, they were asked to internalize the information about tuberculosis, and specifically to their area, the *Boland* (translated as 'land above'). The main task of the workshop process was to develop the performance piece, and initially some participants questioned why it was necessary for the school actors to have as much subject knowledge because this took away time from rehearsal. This was particularly true because the cast would be doing a 'closed' performance piece, with no workshop elements added.

The school cast was effective in absorbing the core facts about TB prevention, risks and symptoms – and this proved to be pivotal in the workshop process. The designer wanted to see the effects of main costume items in an earlier stage of the process, and the team was attempting to cast the parts in the play. Cast members were asked to choose one of six tables on which were several costume items like hats, wigs, nursing uniform items, peak caps and a 'gangsta' medallion. Each actor selected items and assumed the character that the costume items suggested. From this character's point of view, they then had to put across five aspects of information about attitudes to, and facts about, prevention, transmission and treatment of tuberculosis. They repeated this process at three different tables, playing other characters and presenting another five key points. This exercise not only worked well to cast the actors, but also demonstrated their ability to integrate the information with their understanding of the community context. They created broad comic characters, and several of these were kept for the final performance. This exercise also developed the pupils' ability to improvise. However, some of the characterization was lost, in particular at the end of the play. The presentational form of this became about 'telling' rather than 'showing' – undoubtedly owing to the inexperience of the actors to sustain role and the time constraints to create a more satisfying conclusion to the play than that of the comic book.

However, as a result of the process, the cast developed peer educator skills and a reputation in their community, expressed by two of the cast members as 'ek ń verskil kan maak in my gemeenskap om TB te geveg' ('I can make a difference in my community to fight TB') and 'ek weet nou baie meer van TB as voorheen' ('I know much more about TB than before').[50] This proved to be a valuable outcome for the project, and several of the actors reported that in their school and immediate community (Roodewal in Worcester) not only were they minor celebrities, but they were asked and were able to answer questions about tuberculosis.[51] There were no longitudinal studies conducted to measure the retention of the knowledge by audiences, nor evidence of the play's effectiveness in reducing stigma within the communities most affected.

Although there were clear benefits for the audiences in being given information about tuberculosis and SATVI, advocating participation in clinical trials is not without its contradictions. Poverty, unemployment and their concomitant cramped living conditions, poor nutrition and substance abuse are major causes of the epidemic. Clearly the Worcester area is an ideal site because of the prevalence of tuberculosis, which provides pharmaceutical companies with low-cost clinical trials. If new and effective drugs were found, could the South African government or people of Worcester afford them?[52] In 2013, for example, activists were 'crying foul' about the drug rifapentine, which had been tested in southern Africa, but was not available to the communities in which it was tested.[53] Sonafi-Aventis (or Sanofi), the pharmaceutical company, was then charging $1.60 per tablet, taken weekly. This was deemed too expensive for the southern African market, even if this were available outside of the USA. The same company stopped manufacturing the BCG vaccination for infants and children, causing a global shortage.[54] In 2015, the US-based Treatment Action Group released a report that research on tuberculosis was underfunded by US$1.3 billion.

Pharmaceutical companies engaging with research are not obliged to contribute to the community's socioeconomic development, which raises the question of who benefits from the clinical trials, and whether the site would become unfavourable for pharmaceutical companies if improved socioeconomic factors resulted in fewer infections. Participants in the clinical trials are recompensed for their travel and food for each visit, which does contribute a small amount of money into an impoverished community. However, SATVI, to its credit, organizes a social responsiveness programme funded though their own endeavours, recognizing that biomedical research on its own does not address the problem of TB.

Political questions arise from this discussion, such as who funds biomedical research and what is the ideal reciprocity, what is at stake for the community participating in the trials, who should invest in developing the community's social needs, and what role should the national Department of Health play in the region. These issues were not raised in the production of *Carina's Choice* other than in the form of mild criticism of socioeconomic disparities, such as a few lines of dialogue about food. For example, where the play advocated good nutrition, one of the characters pointed out that they were the fruit pickers who could not afford to eat that which they picked. Tupac's mother and father bickered about how little money there was for transport and clinic fees. While the Community Advisory Board (CAB) was shown to represent the trial participants' interests, this was not taken up in any significant way in the drama.

Carina's Choice was not the only educational performance work being done in the Western Cape in 2013 – a touring piece by Delft Youth

Theatre in Cape Town also sought to educate communities about the TB problem, performing at clinics and community centres in the area. This performance resulted from an improvisation workshop process and a scriptwriter collectively devising a theatre piece called *Bad News? Good News!* The project was led by Jill Black of the Sustainable Livelihoods Foundation,[55] and while *Bad News? Good News!* was completed in 2013, it has continued to be a calling card for the Delft Youth Theatre group in Cape Town who have sustained their work. Similarly to *Carina's Choice*, the project used local members of the community to create and perform the piece, creating a tier of leadership around activism through theatre as well as health knowledge.

Performance projects like *Carina's Choice* offer some entertaining relief from the grim reality of TB in the Western Cape, while developing understanding of and activism against new infections and for finding an effective vaccine. The conundrum of why the region has such a high burden of tuberculosis infection will not be easily solved. Until the socioeconomic conditions and education improve, tuberculosis will continue to spread. The overall dysfunctional state of both the health and education sectors plays a facilitative role in the spread of the disease and lack of access to treatment for the infected. The statistics and reality of the disease in South Africa and other Global South contexts belie the romanticized performances of the 'good death' prevalent in the nineteenth century. Ultimately TB remains a disease stigmatized by perceptions of dirt and shame, HIV co-infections and poverty.

4.3 Snapshot – Dialogical theatre: Reconsidering the role of Theatre for Development for malaria prevention in Malawi

Zindaba Dunduzu Chisiza

Malawian Theatre for Development (TfD) in recent years has become reduced to advancing the agenda of the funders of NGOs, rather than a process of community transformation. This snapshot argues that dialogical TfD is more effective at empowering ordinary people. In the 1980s the first iterations of the practice in Malawi were attempts at a dialogical practice, but Hasting Banda's dictatorship (1964–94) made it difficult for such a theatre to develop. In the early 1990s, NGOs began to use actors – who got paid large sums of money – to make TfD that promoted their agenda.[56] Jane Plastow says that the emergence of donor-funded TfD in Africa changed the practice's socialist ideology found in early TfD practices.[57] This ideology was informed by Paulo Freire's (and Boal's) problem-posing education – a method of learning where teacher and learner, as equals, engage in a collaborative process of problem exploration and solution finding.[58] In Malawi, contemporary practitioners do not know about Freirian principles, and this has resulted in them using the practice to promote donor and NGO messages.[59] Another problem affecting existing TfD practices is what Patrick Mangeni identifies as the simplification of TfD to messaging and providing solutions to communities.[60] This is happening because practitioners do not know the principles that underpin real development, but think that they go into communities as experts on local people's problems.[61] Plastow argues that there is a trend for self-appointed trainers of TfD to conduct five- to ten-day TfD workshops, where participants are hurriedly taught particular TfD methodologies, and thereafter these participants pose as experts.[62] The danger in this kind of theatre practice is that practitioners have a limited theatrical toolbox and no grounding in participatory approaches to practice.

I illustrate my argument with a look at one particular NGO's use of message-based TfD. Malaria is one of the major health burdens affecting Malawi.[63] In 2010, the National Malaria Control Programme reported an estimated 6.9 million cases of malaria out of a population of 14 million people.[64] From 2005 the Malawi government has sought to reduce malaria prevalence in part by the distribution of free Long Lasting Treated Nets (LLTNs), and through behaviour change communication methods like TfD.[65]

In 2011, I conducted research on a case study, the *Malungo Zii* (*Let's End Malaria*) malaria awareness campaign by Population Services International (PSI) Malawi.[66] The campaign used TfD as a tool to raise awareness and increase the uptake of prevention services.[67] On 6 August 2011, I observed a *Malungo Zii* performance by Kamphiritiya Theatre Arts at Namadzi Trading Centre, in the southern region of Malawi.[68] The story pitted the 'wise', urban Mr and Mrs Heneke against the 'stupid', rural Mr and Mrs Chipika. The latter couple refused to use LLTNs – even though Mrs Chipika was pregnant – and were not aware that health care facilities were offering free anti-malaria prophylactic drugs to pregnant women. The Chipika family believed LLTNs caused stillbirths in pregnant women.

The play used a comic style of performance with characterization that drew on Malawian stereotypes: the village drunk versus the wise and modern town dweller.[69] In the play, Mr Heneke knew everything about malaria prevention, while Mr Chipika's ignorance was exaggerated for comic effect. The comic depiction of Chipika was a theatrical device, but the actors exaggerated their performances to elicit laughter. Although my impression was that the audience enjoyed the performance, the mockery of rural characters as 'stupid' or 'backward', compared to urban characters, reinforced 'domestication' and 'blaming the victim' rather than being emancipatory.[70]

The performance also made use of posing questions to the audience at various points in the action.[71] For example, at one point in the play an actor asked the audience if people sold LLTNs to purchase beer, which was met with a 'yes' in chorus. Although this superficially enabled audience participation, it did not allow for any meaningful debate. For example, the actors would ask questions that would get one-word answers, perhaps so as not to disrupt the flow of the play – in my opinion demonstrating the absence of understanding and training in TfD and Freirian approaches to dialogical theatre.

After the performance, the actors waited for the audience to settle for a post-performance discussion, but the audience began to disperse. However, nothing to that point in the theatrical event had indicated that a participatory discussion was desirable, and the play itself had not demonstrated that the audience's opinions on the uptake of LLTNs and the myths around them were valued. The actors (and through them, the NGO) simply imposed 'solutions' on the audience. For example, the 'modern' characters told the 'backward' characters that they should not sell LLTNs because they prevented malaria. In my view, it would have been empowering if the performance had used techniques like Boal's Forum theatre to engage the audience on the causes of this problem. In devising the project, the initial research processes may have been seen as sufficiently consultative with the beneficiaries of the malaria campaign,[72] therefore the structure of the theatre piece did not create spaces for discussion that could have revealed why communities are not using preventive measures.

I argue that the *Malungo Zii* performances sought only to communicate donor messages and was not interested in initiating real transformation. The problem with this kind of theatre is that it 'domesticates', serving only to sustain a culture that views local communities as incapable of self-transformation, flies in the face of Freirian principles and does a disservice to the value of TfD. I argue that we need to return to an appreciation of TfD that seeks to create dialogical processes that aim to empower local communities into initiators of their own change, but there is little evidence of this happening in current NGO-funded arts work in Malawi.

4.4 Interview – *Public Enemy No. 1*: Dengue fever in the *favelas* of Brazil

Johayne Hildefonso (JH) is interviewed by Jan Onoszko, July 2015

Johayne, how did the Dengue Fever project come about?
JH: In 2009 AfroReggae was invited by the State Education Department and the State Health Department because, as you know, these days dengue [fever] is a really serious problem, it kills a lot of

people.[73] People, despite the strong campaigns, still don't believe that a mosquito can kill.[74] So there's a lot of rubbish around, water butts that aren't covered, a series of problems that result in this dengue problem. We created this project and spent four months doing 200 performances. The play was called *Public Enemy No. 1 – Dengue*.

What was the form of the performance?

JH: First you have to grab people's attention. We used a percussion group because the whole text is punctuated with music. And so we had this along with the information, which is important because we were talking about a serious topic, but we did it with humour. We created a text where we had a battalion to combat dengue which entered the body to show how dengue works inside people's bodies but always with a lot of humour.

Were there any influences from a particular tradition or cultural approach?

JH: No, no. We just began by playing around with it. I asked a friend of mine to write the text.[75] She already knows how I like to work. I told her roughly what I wanted to include and she produced the text which was great, and we began to improvise and found it was fun to do and that's how it worked. As well as talking we used a lot of signs, banners with things written on them – words, slogans – because that works very well on the street.

Was the type of performance that you did different to the usual style of AfroReggae's work?

JH: AfroReggae's theatre troupe began by doing this type of work. It was a troupe that only did prevention texts: how to prevent cancer, for example, we talked about breast-feeding, about sickle cell anaemia. We only dealt with diseases. And it was only after that [dengue tour] that we decided to change and become a theatre group working on theatrical texts, which doesn't stop us from still doing this type of work today. In the past its original name was Trupe da Saúde (Health Troupe). Today it's called the Trupe de Teatro AfroReggae.

Why did the project stop?

JH: It stopped because it was a commissioned project. There's nothing to stop us doing it again, because the text is very pertinent because dengue is back again [in 2015], except that now we're working on new texts. It's not a performance that we would put on of our own accord, but if a commission emerged, a sponsor, then yes. It was an expensive thing to produce: there's transport, costumes, food. We drove all around Rio de Janeiro state with this.

What do you feel about this direct way of working?

JH: You used a word that I was going to use. It really is a direct way of working. The best thing we saw which shows it worked, is that people stopped to pay attention. There were moments – I've even got goose bumps now – there were some really powerful moments. I remember at one performance in the Complexo do Alemão, a gentleman began crying during the show; at the end he came to speak to us and he said, 'I want to thank you for the work you're doing, because it's important work to bring this information. I lost my son because of a dengue mosquito.' People would shout at the end of the performances saying 'It's really important. You have to do it more.' We were dealing with a serious topic and doing it with humour to make it lighter, but the information was getting through and it worked.

Remember also, this is how we began working in the field. We played the scenes with the audience, which is different to a play when you create the fourth wall – you don't interact with the audience. The audience follows the story but you only play the scenes with the actors. In *Public Enemy No. 1* we broke down the fourth wall and spoke directly to the audience.

Is dengue a disease of poverty, do you think?

JH: I think that dengue isn't just a disease of poverty. Obviously in poverty it's easier [to become infected] because if a *favela* doesn't have an infrastructure, there's standing water, lots of uncovered water butts, areas with lots of rubbish. Obviously that's where you'll find mosquitoes. You also see them in districts that aren't so deprived.

How do you feel about this way of working where you have to give a direct message and perhaps include medical and sanitation data? How does this fit into your methodology?

JH: There's no secret to it – if you have a great text with a great idea, the rest falls into place and works. It's something we like doing. It's something we already do on a daily basis.

Who were the actors? How did you choose them? How were they paid?

JH: They were our theatre troupe. At the time the troupe was larger. There were almost thirty of us, including the percussion group. Each one of them was paid exactly the same fee, plus an allowance for food because this took up the whole day.

The selection was a process. We took the text, read it through and worked out who fitted with which character. So-and-so is a great sergeant, another one a mosquito. We decided to make the mosquitoes all fat, and women because it is the female mosquito that transmits dengue fever – which was fantastic because they did it beautifully and made it humorous.

Considering more broadly the work of AfroReggae, why aren't there any outside agencies working like you do?

JH: This is my opinion, but the work we do is among the most difficult work you can do. First because if you're working in a *favela* you have to know that community, and people you can depend on so you can carry on developing the work. If you go into a *favela* without really knowing it, you won't succeed in doing anything. You need to know if it's safe and calm. If it isn't, it's even more difficult because you need to mediate with the drug traffickers.

Does the state care about the favelas?

JH: I think they do care but they aren't capable of solving the

118   Applied Theatre: Performing Health and Wellbeing

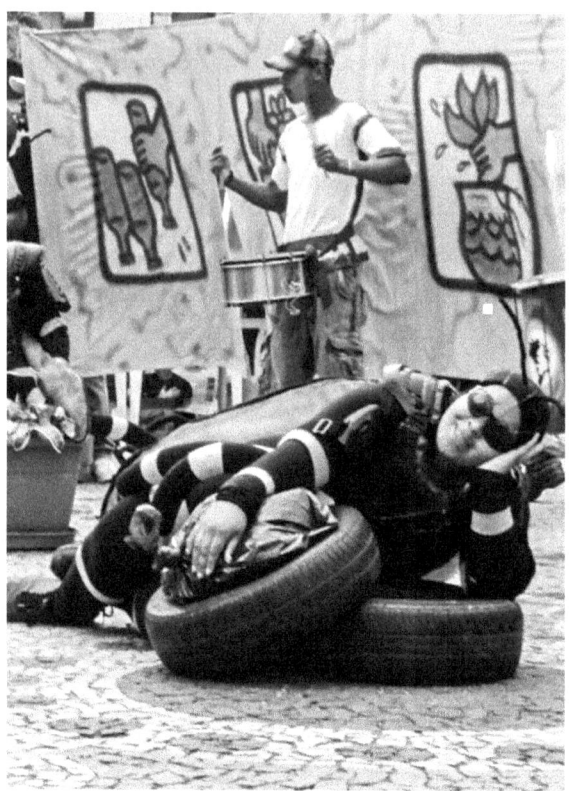

Figure 3: An *Aedes aegypti* mosquito looking satisfied at causing dengue fever, *Public Enemy No. 1*, 2009. Photo © AfroReggae.

problems of all the *favelas*. I think that they could if real work was done focused on the *favelas*. One thing we know only too well is that during election campaigns they go into the *favelas*, do lots of things, promise lots of other things, but on a day-to-day basis it is the institutions who've been in the *favelas* for years who end up doing the work.

How does AfroReggae's practice differ from the work an external agency might do in the same setting?

JH: AfroReggae offers workshops to children in theatre, dance, circus, percussion, violin, cello, drumming, electric guitar, singing,

Afro-dance, ballet, among other disciplines. We also work closely with the families – there aren't many institutions who are willing to endure the headaches we do, so that's our difference – we're genuinely worried about the children who are not in school and try to get them back in. We work with issues which other institutions don't want to deal with because it's a lot of work to mediate with the drug traffickers, but we do it because it's important.

What do you think are the health benefits for a child being part of AfroReggae?

JH: First, any of these activities raises self-esteem. Any of these activities makes you happy. I could be talking about any of the *favelas* where AfroReggae has activities, but here I'm talking about Vigário Geral because it's where I spend most of my time – it used to be a really sad *favela*. These days you see children singing, playing, dancing, people there have access – they go to the theatre, they go to shows, they welcome people from outside the community. These days there are young people who would never have thought about going to university but they're going. Alongside this, we work on other issues – showing that it's important to look after yourself, it's important to wear clean clothes, it's important to know how to wash yourself. We deal with various issues, sexual health issues, all these things are talked about. There are lots of taboos at home, parents won't talk about things, but we talk about them at the workshops and all this creates health.

5

Non-Communicable Diseases: Lifestyle and Post-Colonial Stress Disorder (Canada), Nutrition and Health Eating (Denmark), Diabetes (UK)

5.1 Introduction

Katharine Low

Non-communicable diseases (NCDs) account for nearly 38 million deaths globally per year and 40 per cent of those deaths are described as 'premature', that is, they occur before the age of 70.[1] NCDs include cardiovascular diseases, cancers, chronic respiratory diseases and diabetes. The treatment and potential burden of diseases resulting from NCDs is seen as 'a major public health challenge that undermines social and economic development throughout the world'.[2] NCDs are often described as lifestyle diseases in that they are perceived to result from particular choices such as unhealthy diets, exposure to tobacco or alcohol, and physical inaction, yet the underlying causes of these lifestyle 'choices' are not always addressed or challenged. In the examples of practice that follow, there exists a clear emphasis on the importance of not solely responding to 'symptoms' via a medically inspired prevention approach. Instead, the authors in this section make the argument for taking the space to better understand the causes and underlying cultural connections that have an impact on lifestyle diseases and consider how culturally based responses may provide a way into a particular community. Furthermore, the 'choices' facing the poor in the Global South[3] are often limited to the consumption of bulk carbohydrates, frequently the cheapest option, leading to a peculiar form of obesity, something that Julian Robbins and his colleagues address in their essay in the following section.

As a research partnership formed of Indigenous and Settler scholars, Julian Robbins, Warren Linds, Linda Goulet, Jo-Ann Episkenew and Karen Schmidt offer a unique perspective on the impacts of post-colonial stress[4] on Indigenous Canadian youths and the youths' understandings of their own wellbeing and health. Working with Indigenous communities in southern Saskatchewan, Robbins and his colleagues address questions of how colonization is felt and held in the body and the impact it has on day-to-day living, and begin to make links between culture and health through theatre practices.

Understandings of health and wellbeing are important connections to make, specifically when addressing some of the factors influencing diet and physical activity. The 2015 WHO report on European Health noted a need to better understand the cultural contexts and influences of culture on wellbeing, and the resulting impact on health. In particular, the authors note that in improving the reporting on health and wellbeing they 'could include cultural outputs such as historical records or anthropological observations, and may comprise quantitative and qualitative evidence, as well as narrative case studies.'[5] Here the WHO could consider the following two snapshots from Europe as examples of case studies that address some of the key causes of NCDs, namely diet, obesity and physical inactivity. Contextualized by a study from 2010 which found that globally 43 million children were overweight,[6] Dan Grabowski and Jens Aagaard-Hansen discuss the development of a theatre project in collaboration with a diabetes research centre in Denmark. Supported by the Danish Heart Foundation, the researchers worked alongside a long-standing theatre company, Milton-Sand & Søn, to develop a series of short health-related plays for young children in Copenhagen. Grabowski and Aagaard-Hansen deliberate the success of the theatre approach with the children in terms of the health promotion knowledge gained and argue for the importance of considering the identity and involvement of the audience in such performances.

Finally, the importance of linking culture and health is something that Geetha Upadhyaya considers in her snapshot on the work of Kala Sangam, a South Asian arts company based in Bradford, UK. Here, Upadhyaya offers an account of a drama-based project that began conversations about diabetes in a manner that was both culturally sensitive and inviting to its target audience.

5.2 Essay – 'Acting Out' our health: Assisting youth in making healthy lifestyle choices through linking Indigenous perspectives about wellbeing with Applied Theatre

Julian Robbins, Warren Linds, Linda Goulet, Jo-Ann Episkenew and Karen Schmidt

Introduction

We are a collaborative research partnership of Indigenous and Settler scholars from three universities and health professionals from the File Hills Qu'Appelle Tribal Council (FHQTC) Health Services. FHQTC Health provides services to eleven First Nations[7] representing five cultural and linguistic groups situated in southern Saskatchewan, Canada. Our research explores the impact of the arts on the wellbeing of Indigenous youth, and it is informed by Indigenous perspectives. Our shared goal is to adapt Forum Theatre[8] workshops for Indigenous youth and use theatre games and other arts activities to create spaces in which youth can explore and develop their own sense of wellbeing. Our workshop processes develop the youths' individual and collective self-determining actions, an important concept in Indigenous thought.[9] We have found that as youth begin to question habitual thinking, they become aware, acquire knowledge and are, therefore, better equipped to take appropriate independent action.[10] Our work is informed by theories of colonization–decolonization,[11] Indigenous research[12] and embodied knowing[13] in the contexts of arts, education and health.

Colonization is present in our bodies and in the bodies of those with whom we work since it restricts and shapes our thinking, our actions and interactions, especially how we interact with those who have power. Augusto Boal has written that our day-to-day living affects us bodily but we are not aware of it, as, '[i]n the body's battle with the world, the senses suffer. And we start to feel little of what we touch, to listen to very little of what we hear, and to see very little of what we look [at] ... In order for the body to send out and receive all possible messages, it has to be reharmonised.'[14] In our work, Applied Theatre is used to reharmonize and decolonize through actions and interactions. Our collaboration strives to deconstruct colonial relationships and develop more equitable, respectful, honouring relationships between and among the youth and facilitators.

Our collaborating participants include youth ages twelve to eighteen from various First Nations within the FHQTC area. We follow the cultural protocols of the different communities as elders from the communities are included in our workshops to support our process and share traditional Indigenous understandings as well as speak to, and model, First Nations values that inform workshop norms. The elders also serve to remind us to pay attention to the cultural and historical context of our work.[15]

Contextualizing health issues for Indigenous youth in Canada

Ashley Ning and Kathi Wilson[16] conducted a comparative review of health literature from 2000 to 2010 on Indigenous youth and their non-Indigenous counterparts in Canada. Their central conclusion was that current research does not appropriately reflect the unique concerns of Indigenous youth. Ning and Wilson's research indicates that the health profile of Indigenous youth in Canada is not only incomplete but also unacceptable. Compared to their counterparts, Indigenous youth are disproportionately burdened by health disparities, resulting in more suicides, addictions, diabetes and sexual transmitted diseases caused by social inequalities, such as racism, poor educational outcomes, low-employment and poverty.[17,18] Currently, Indigenous youth in Canada have a suicide rate five to seven times higher than their non-Indigenous counterparts.[19] In addition to documenting the many health disadvantages for Canadian Indigenous youth, Ning and Wilson identify significant gaps that exist with respect to the inclusion of cultural elements in contemporary research. Notably, none of the studies on the health care of Indigenous youth examined the role of traditional healing or the cultural appropriateness of care. Our work is beginning to make the link between culture and health through exploring wellbeing through the arts.

Health and wellbeing in Indigenous contexts

'Wellbeing' is a term being used more frequently in conceptualizations of health to portray the idea that an ideal state of health refers to a holistic understanding rather than mere physical absence of disease. Furthermore, Indigenous perspectives are unique, differing from definitions that flow primarily from modern Western medicine. For example, perspectives on health and wellbeing from within Indigenous communities often make reference to the interrelatedness of all things.[20] Arvol Looking Horse highlights that Indigenous health perspectives 'view the earth as a "source" of life rather than a "re-source".'[21] While recognizing the benefits of other approaches to health and healing in contemporary times, many Indigenous viewpoints recognize the benefits of healing practices that predate the spread of Western scientific bio-medicine.[22] Within Indigenous communities, links to ancestral knowledge and traditional systems of health and healing continue to provide foundational philosophies about living in a good way and maintaining health, while local contexts are also important.

With particular reference to the local context, the research team administered surveys to FHQTC Indigenous youth[23] to identify some of their top health priority areas. Top ranked areas of concern were lack of access to healthy role models and healthy foods as well as abuse and suicide. These priority areas are currently being integrated into the curriculum of FHQTC schools, so we continuously aim to harmonize the material of our arts-based programmes with the health objectives identified by the youth.

Elders from local Indigenous communities speak about health and wellbeing

The teachings of community elders – who hold community knowledge and are responsible for transmitting Indigenous knowledge through oral teachings to the next generation – have influenced our programmes. Elders shape their teachings through an intergenerational cultural dialectic that both looks to the past while also being engaged in dialogue with younger generations. As Joseph Couture has observed, '[The elders] are propelled by the past, and are drawn absolutely towards the future.'[24] The elders and their insights into the health of the youth in their communities shape our research. Thus, in addition to elders attending our workshops, we report to and take direction from them on an annual basis. To further our understanding of the traditional view of health in the communities in which we work, three elders from different First Nations in the FHQTC area who had previously participated in our work were asked to share their perspectives on health and wellbeing. Joe O'Watch is Nakota from the Carry the Kettle First Nation; Lorraine Yuzicappi is Dakota from the Standing Buffalo First Nation; and the late Ron Keewatin is Nêhiyawin (Cree) from the Peepeekisis First Nation.[25] All spoke about the importance of their respective Indigenous languages as a 'doorway' into being able to understand more robustly how their cultures viewed health and wellbeing and that Indigenous conceptualizations about health and wellbeing are not always directly translatable into English.

All three elders had different ways of talking about health, but all three viewed it from a holistic perspective. For example, one elder talked about health as the 'spirituality' of an individual, but defined it in the following way: 'when we say spirituality, we're talking about the health, body, mind, spirit ... In order to have a good spirit, a spiritual mind, is that you have to have all these things, a good mind and good lifestyle ... [I]f you believe in your ways, spirituality, it talks about how you should live.'[26] Health is holistic. As another elder explained, '[Health is] like when you have ... your life in balance: your physical, emotional and all that ... And if one of those goes out of whack, you're sick.'[27] With respect to the FHQTC youths' identified concern about healthy foods, elders spoke about how a traditional way of life played a role in the treatment and prevention of illnesses to attain a long, healthy life.

Elders talked about using traditional medicines and understandings of wellbeing to manage and even overcome various illnesses. However, as one elder explained, an Indigenous perspective of managing a disease like diabetes does not necessarily entail the exclusion of mainstream medicine. A holistic understanding of health and wellbeing allows for the use of understandings that come from other systems of medicine. In reference to some of the potential causes and management of diabetes, this elder noted that by living an

> ... imbalanced life ... you have to do things right which your doctor tells you or your parents or the nurse or something like that, you know. They're not eating right, they're not living right, you know. They're just living with drinking and doing drugs and stuff and [things like diabetes], that's what they end up with.[28]

Health and wellbeing as 'right relationships'

Youth prioritized positive role models, abuse and suicide, which are impacted by the nature and quality of interpersonal relationships, and these relationships are affected by the impact of colonization.

When specifically asked about how theatre games activities could have a positive impact on FHQTC youth-prioritized health issues, such as suicide and abuse, one youth responded 'I keep going back to that relationship thing ... [because the workshop] broke those barriers we had as students.'[29] Indigenous traditional healing does not occur in isolation. Willie Ermine, a Nêhiýaw (Cree) scholar and ethicist, views Indigenous Knowledge and traditional healing through a lens of 'community mind and thought'.[30] Ermine suggests that traditional approaches to health and wellbeing arise from this 'community mind', and that the reward for maintaining this approach 'is not for us, but for our children because they are the future'.[31] One elder pointed out:

> I'm raising two grandchildren ... I'm telling them how my father and mother raised me and my grandparents and that was to love one another, to respect one another, to respect Mother Earth, respect our ways and to live a good life, and to leave those drug[s] and alcohol alone. There are better things in life.[32]

Healthy living in the community mind is based on the traditional value of respect that is as applicable to health today as it was in the past. Conceptualizing health and wellbeing as community mind is also an important element to consider in helping to guide relationships that youth form amongst each other. One elder spoke about this:

> ... there will always be a sort of a leader ... If they start drinking, well, they will all drink. If they start smoking marijuana, they all smoke. But if that leader or popular person, you know, would stay away and set examples for the rest of the group [it can also have positive effects on the whole group].[33]

Links between wellbeing, traditional knowledge, and Applied Theatre and Arts Processes (ATAP)

A familiarization with, and respect for, local understandings about health and wellbeing are essential for programme success. As in the case with our relationship with FHQTC, this result is achieved by building and maintaining relationships with communities over an extended period of time.

The elders we spoke with voiced a desire to continue these sorts of programmes as part of their community-based health and wellbeing initiative for youth. One elder noted that introducing youth to their traditional ceremonies in concert with ATAP programming could help combat some of the more non-productive influences that exist today.

Reflecting on her experience, a youth who attended one of our workshops explained how she saw the connection between traditional ceremonies and theatre games:

> I grew up pretty traditionally too. I was quite blessed to have elders take me in ... and the way you do things, is you don't question what they do, you just do it. And that's a model. And that's kind of what the theatre games are doing. We kind of had them [the workshop leaders] model this is how we do it, then we would do it and add your own flair to it. To me that's what tradition is, it is ... a lot of physicality and a lot of just doing without having to feel ashamed or scared. Because that's what theatre forces you to do, right ... to work together, just do it ... But there was no judgement though if you got something wrong. And in that way, it is theatrical, right, because you're just expected to come out of your shell.[34]

Ron Keewatin told us that Indigenous youth, like most of us, are well aware of what they 'should' do to be healthy but find it challenging to put into practice. In one of our early workshops, we asked for the youths' view of health. They gave us the 'pat' answers, responses that we think they thought we wanted to hear – don't drink, don't do drugs – yet when asked to create stories of their lives, their portrayals all illustrated incidents of peer pressure where alcohol and drugs were an integral part of their reality.

Applied Theatre as a decolonizing practice

While developing an approach that aims to use Applied Theatre as a decolonizing practice, it has become essential that we understand the history of Indigenous people and the creation of the colonial state of Canada. To Cherokee Theatre of the Oppressed facilitator Quo-Li Driskill, colonization is an act 'done to bodies and felt by other bodies'[35] ... [that is] damage done to our skin, flesh, muscles, bones and spirits'.[36] Colonization imposed a set of beliefs and moulded the body 'through direct behavioural influences and physical environments'[37] such as confinement to reserves and in residential schools.

It follows then that decolonization requires healing through a kinaesthetic process that is central to Applied Theatre practice. Decolonization is about self-determined action, but agency is dependent on having a well-developed imagination.[38] Before taking action one must first imagine what change might look like and envision the steps required to achieve it. One also needs to have the volition and agency to enact the imagined changes. But the history of residential schools in Canada shows that Indigenous children's imaginations and actions were suppressed as a component of socialization into a colonial world. Gwich'in writer Robert Arthur Alexie described children's experiences in residential schools in these terms: 'something is happening to them, but they don't know it. They are developing a routine and someone else is making decisions for them. Somewhere in the far distant future, they will be unable to make decisions for themselves and will rely on others to do it for them.'[39]

The theatre games structure behaviours that challenge youth to make decisions and take positive risky actions in order to participate in the games. This participatory decision-making and action develops a 'safe enough'[40] space where the youth can exercise their imaginations, practices making decisions and then enact those decisions. The creative space also facilitates new possibilities to be negotiated and enacted in relationships among the youth and with adults, where different kinds of relations can be negotiated. The 'safe enough' creative space allows the youth to tell their stories through collective images that involves an embodied process of interaction where the future is modelled and transformed through an aesthetic and playful process. For example, one youth shared the following:

> You gotta take risks in order to get ahead, I guess. But you also gotta take precautions. Gotta be safe about what you're doing. Yeah. Sometimes you do have to take risks to go to where you wanna get. That's what you guys taught me.[41]

At the same time, as facilitators, we continually reflect on the reality of colonial relationships, questioning when we might be perpetuating oppressive ideologies and behaviours rather than being engaged in a collaborative process with community partners and youth participants.

Embodied Applied Theatre and wellbeing

Theatre games, such as blind games, energizers and community-building activities, develop trust within the group and with us as facilitators.[42] An embodied and performative aesthetic emerges, since '[however] small, any physical/mental engagement in a theatre process will have developed phrases and traces that will be interventions in the embodied lives of participants.'[43]

In theatre games, 'control achieved through release in play frequently creates a confidence that can be carried over into real situations in the world outside. Games are a means of education and personality growth.'[44] Cooperation, communication games and image creation provide a context for relationship building, participation, collective action and social learning, and the emergence of community.[45] The youth have shared that the theatre workshops helped them express themselves, to get out of their 'box of oppression'.[46] One student had a particular insight on how that was achieved:

> People are kind of sheltered in, and it's hard to let that emotion out without being afraid that people are going to judge you ... But through your games, you guys were letting us out that way. Like we were actually coming out, but [the youth] didn't know it ... cause we're just trying to have fun, but yet we're letting it out.[47]

Theatre games are active – the rules require action on the part of participants. The games are often playful and fun, but you are not 'centred' out because everyone is moving together. As a young woman in another workshop stated, 'I learned that ... I'm a very shy person. More when I have to like, talk in front of people and everything like that. That I don't like. And ... what I learned from people is ... or from the group was that everybody came out of their shells more and more each day.'[48]

The exercises we use are traditionally seen as a prelude to theatrical exploration. However, in the context of an exploration into wellbeing, such kinaesthetic-based approaches are part of the development of wellbeing that emerges in theatrical work and can inform every level of the creative process. As one youth explained:

> You guys are finding ways to help us open up in these like fun ways. … I saw lots of people who usually don't step up in class and stuff, and when they have these little circles in class, they won't say anything. [But here] we were stepping up in these games and wanting to play, and we didn't care who we were playing with. Here we didn't just choose our friends. We could just be who we are. We could take off our masks.[49]

In several workshops we introduce the 'circle of knots',[50] which is an activity where group members, with closed eyes, join hands randomly in the middle of the circle. Participants open their eyes, and without talking, look at their randomly linked hands with bodies attached, and cooperate to untangle the 'knot'. Multiple times in our workshops, they untangled their knotted hands and bodies and then, without prompting by facilitators, reform a more complicated knot and try again to untangle themselves. We now call this 'collaborative competition', where leadership is dispersed among the group as each person contributes to solving the problem faster and different participants take leadership at different times.

We have used several games to explore collaborative leadership as elements of wellbeing, and some have challenged us as facilitators and the youth as participants. For example, in a game called 'Follow the Leader', there was no problem for participants to follow each other around the room as they took turns leading others with a gesture and rhythmic sound; however, when the direction was to find a common rhythm and sound and then go around the room attracting other groups to this, things came to a standstill as youth leaders chose to be followers of the adult leaders. Engaging in the play[51] of the game was acceptable, but when asked to declare themselves the leader, there was resistance. One youth put her reaction this way: 'I don't know, through these games I kinda learned that, you know, you can make a decision to do something or you can't, and I learned through these games, like how it feels, like the pressure of it, even though these were just little games.'[52] In contrast to this resistance, in another workshop there was an unexpected leadership in the group when we were engaged in simple image theatre activities as part of the preparation for the youth to imagine an 'ideal' community and what they would bring to it. We asked them to identify and portray through tableaux important parts of the participants' community. The facilitators asked for a list of cultural objects. The youth identified tipis, buffalo and pow-wow grounds, and created tableaux of these elements. Then, spontaneously, some of the girls in the group suggested that they portray a pow-wow. They organized themselves and created a full performance of a pow-wow grand entry where all the dancers enter to the sounds of drums and song, followed by individual competitions like the grass dances and jingle dances. Normally in a pow-wow in this community the 'caller' is a man, but in this case, the girls in the group chose to be the callers, and the boys played the drums and participated as dancers. The workshop created a space where the youth initiated a theatrical exploration to express their strong connection to their culture and enacted what was important to them through the selection of the 'scenes' of the pow-wow. The participation in theatrical expression allowed the youth to explore and bring their own meaning to ideas of leadership. One youth described how the games transformed his understanding of what it meant to be a leader:

> It changed my whole perspective on what leadership was ... in these theatre games it was about all of us working together ... and that is what it was for me. And another thing about leadership was, I always credited the person who got up right away to do it or that person to be the one to break the silence or to be the one to start [and that was the

leader]. And I realized that I was being *that* person but it didn't mean that I was the leader.[53]

The spontaneity of theatrical expression prompted us to investigate further what activities engage the youth and what didn't and to make links between these aspects and the search for culturally meaningful wellbeing with Indigenous youth.

Conclusion: Indigenous perspectives in Applied Theatre

Ermine has proposed that the intersection of Western and Indigenous ways of knowing creates an 'ethical space' which 'is formed when two societies, with disparate worldviews, are poised to engage each other'.[54] When those two sets of worldviews are brought to the encounter, a space of uncertainty exists where nothing is yet formed or understood. Turnbull[55] notes that this space of flux cannot be defined or predicted; it can only be performed. In other words, the practice of Applied Theatre and wellbeing emerges in the work we do with the communities and youth.

In the ten years we have been working with Indigenous youth using Applied Theatre and other arts approaches, this space of flux has been a space of learning for the youth and for us as researchers as we come to recognize its power and understand its potential. When youth are given the opportunity to reflect on their lived experiences and practise making decisions in a safe space, they develop an awareness of their decision-making processes as well as the confidence and potential to do so in other aspects of their lives outside of the workshop.

Arts-based learning is decolonizing, restorative and empowering.[56] While Western health tends to focus on an individual approach that emphasizes a biomedical model, this essay points to a holistic, more culturally meaningful approach to wellbeing for Indigenous youth. Although our arts practices are based on Western approaches to the arts, we believe the arts have potential in health programming when cultural knowledge is embedded in the programme design. As such, Applied Theatre contributes to the developing knowledge of the connection between arts-based pedagogies and effective practices in the development of health and wellbeing with Indigenous youth.

(This research was funded by the Canadian Institutes for Health Research and the Saskatchewan Health Research Foundation. We thank the Indigenous youth participants, the elders for their support and FHQTC for their willingness to collaborate with us and integrate our research project into their youth health initiatives.)

5.3 Snapshot – Health theatre for children
Dan Grabowski and Jens Aagaard-Hansen

Introduction

In recent years, non-communicable diseases (NCDs) such as type 2 diabetes have increasingly gained attention in the international public health community as a result of evidence that they have surpassed infectious diseases as the leading cause of death in the world.[57] The reason for this increase in NCDs of epidemic proportions is tremendously complex, with essential risk factors involving unhealthy eating practices and physical inactivity leading to overweight and obesity. In the Capital Region of Denmark, 30 per cent of the population sixteen years and older are moderately overweight and 11 per cent are severely overweight.[58] Urgently in need of being dealt with, this alarming health statistic has led to a surge in campaigns and interventions that have had varying degrees of success.[59]

In this snapshot, we consider the study of two health theatre plays for children in Denmark, one targeting pre-school children from three to six years of age and one targeting school-aged children from six to nine years of age.[60] Launched by the Danish Heart Foundation as a nationwide health promotion initiative and written and performed by the professional two-person theatre group Milton-Sand & Søn,[61] the two plays are based on the principle of communicating information about health through fun, dance and song. Both plays tell stories of the Rumlerikkerne, the heroes' quest for health in a classic tale of good (healthy) versus evil (unhealthy). Using a variety of creative and funny characters, the storylines communicate messages focusing on food and exercise. One of the primary catchphrases is 'Fruit is the best, sweets are only for parties' (which rhymes in Danish); it encapsulates the general message that occasional unhealthy behaviours are fine in the context of healthy choices most of the time. Children are encouraged to participate in the singing and dancing, and both plays contain dialogue between children and actors. The characters and storyline quickly motivate most children to take part in the dialogue with the actors and apart from the planned participatory dancing and singing, there is also a lot of shouting and wild gesticulations during the more dramatic parts of the plays.

Theatre can form the basis of engaging learning strategies for health professionals.[62,63,64] It has been used in health promotion with children,[65] but a need exists for theory-based studies addressing theatre in health promotion for children.[66] The various approaches to the prevention of lifestyle-related diseases and the promotion of healthy lifestyles often face difficulties in presenting health and health communication in ways that appeal and make sense to the target audience.[67,68,69] This often results in misconceived campaigns and approaches with little or no effect in terms of changes in health behaviour and/or acquisition of health knowledge. Research suggests that many of these campaigns and approaches only manage to appeal to people who are already healthy.[70,71,72]

The health theatre approach is studied with a particular analytical focus on identity, participation and knowledge[73,74] When employed like this, we believe that a focus on either of these concepts entails a focus on the two other concepts, and thus a more in-depth understanding of the mechanisms is possible.

The data material consists of twenty focus group interviews with a total of 98 children between three and nine years of age, twenty-two semi-structured individual interviews with parents and teachers, and observations of children at five performances. The interviews with children were intended to prompt children to discuss and reflect upon issues related to Rumlerikkerne, as well as their daily lives and health. Teachers were interviewed to give their initial opinion of the theatre as a health-promoting tool and their experiences, if any, of incorporating the play into the curriculum and daily health routines. The interviews with parents were made in order to find out whether the children had talked about the theatre or the health information and whether it had resulted in concrete changes in health behaviour in the home.

Findings

The performances rarely generate genuine participation. For the most part, participation is limited to singing, dancing and the collective answering of a few questions. The children have no influence on the storyline and there is no real improvisation from the actors. However, when dealing with very young children, a little may go a long way towards helping children develop a feeling of participation and the observations show that during the plays most of the children felt some sense of engagement. For example, one child noted the following: 'And then I got a high five from one of them when we danced at the end. It was fun' (girl, 5 years). Another child shared this example of participation: 'And then the big guy could not find her, and then he had to ask me and so I said to them that the Candyburb [the villain in the play] had taken her away' (girl, 4 years).

While these children may not have acquired concrete health knowledge from these two examples of participation, the interviews reveal that their attention has been focused in a way that presents teachers with an opportunity to incorporate Rumlerikkerne into the health education by referring to these adventures. With this participation-generated curiosity comes the possibility of linking the health information to the children's everyday life, providing them with an opportunity to see themselves as participants with valid and relevant identities.

To a young child a high-five from one of the actors may qualify as a participative action, while a child in third grade will have the capacity for quite another level of participation. This places great demands on the actors' ability to adapt the play to a given group of children observing the play and the health information in significantly different ways, particularly when children from the entire age span (3 to 6 and 6 to 9) are present at a single show:

> And then there was this guy, who was sorting out all the food. He showed us what a burger looks like, when it has been eaten. That makes you think about what things look like in your stomach when you eat food and stuff. I don't think it looked bad at all. Maybe it tastes good. He asked us, if we wanted to taste it and I said "yes". But then he wouldn't let me. It probably wasn't real food. (boy, 8 years, 2nd grade)

This boy remembers the incident because dialogue occurred between actors and children; this kind of participation has a positive effect. But he also sees through the gimmick, realizing that it was not real dialogue and that the offer to taste the food was not real. The data suggest that this kind of token participation[75] can create a fun environment and heightened entertainment but it does not make the boy reflect upon the health issues in a way that relates them to his own life and his own health.

In the pre-schools, the teachers did not have the resources or interest to try to incorporate the theatre into the daily routines or to use the curiosity generated by Rumlerikkerne to engage children in discussions about health and everyday life: 'We haven't had the time or the resources to prepare the children for the play or to talk to them about it afterwards. Actually, we didn't know that it was about health at all. We were just told to show up with the children' (pre-school teacher).

None of the pre-school children touched upon any health issues in their initial description of the play during interviews. This does not necessarily indicate a lack of knowledge about what is healthy and unhealthy; rather, it suggests that they were not prepared to reflect upon the health issues in the play. Without preparation and introduction the children acquired very little in terms of new health knowledge, new ways of connecting existing knowledge or of relating the health information to their identity.

In the schools, preparation and follow-up on health issues related to the theatre seemed to be a more natural extension of the teachers' core services. However, significant differences occurred in terms of creating meaningful and coherent contexts in which the children could understand the health theatre and themselves. Generally, the schoolteachers expressed an awareness of the complexity of this kind of health promotion: 'I've actually also used it, when we talk about lunch. Then I've asked them if they remember Rumlerikkerne and there are actually a couple of the boys, who normally don't want to eat the healthy stuff first, who have gotten better at it' (first-grade teacher). The response of this teacher is a good example of relating the information from Rumlerikkerne to the daily routines in school. The younger children seem to need this kind of help to make the connections between the theatre, health, their everyday life and their identities as active participants in their own health. The children, especially the oldest, seemed to have clearly defined identities when it came to their perception of themselves as healthy or unhealthy. The roles and expectations associated with these identities seem to determine how they understood and acquired health information. Many children identified with unhealthy lifestyles and unhealthy choices concerning food and exercise, describing themselves as unhealthy and therefore uninterested in information about health.

Observations of the children during performances revealed some situations where obese children, despite repeated requests, did not want to jump or dance along with their classmates. This happened in all age groups but was most evident with the children in second and third grade. This suggests that children at this age are very aware of being overweight and their unhealthiness, and, perhaps even more importantly, they are aware of how the other children perceive them. They appear to adapt to these roles and expectations to reinforce their health identities. Some obese children participated in the focus group interviews, and they all (albeit in different ways) confirmed how obese children were expected to fit into rigid predefined roles of being unhealthy. As one boy put it:

> I'm probably more like an indoor kind of guy. But sometimes I go a little bit outside and play with friends from my class, but that's not really my favourite thing. I really like to be indoors. I don't do healthy stuff. Me and Magnus we are kind of unhealthy, I think. We do not play as much football as the rest of the guys. But that's just who we are. (boy, 8 years, 2nd grade)

Throughout the interview this boy made it very clear that everything remotely concerning health was unimportant and irrelevant to him. A very large part of his identity seems to revolve around the fact that he is not healthy and does not need to be. It is equally striking that his classmates agree with this, thereby confirming his identity as one of the class's fat boys who is uninterested in health-related topics. He is, in other words, understanding his own identity in a certain way and at the same time he is observing the other children, confirming this understanding. This interpretation of his identity seems to affect all communication about health as well as the expectations associated with it, which appear to prevent him from relating the health information to his own life and may even be encouraging him to keep relating his identity and his personal expectations to an unhealthy lifestyle.

Conclusions

When teachers succeed in preparing the children for Rumlerikkerne and follow up on the curiosity they generate, children acquire more health knowledge than in the cases where the initiative stands alone without preparation or follow-up. It is significant that children acquire more knowledge and have greater ability to relate the information to their sense of identity when teachers incorporate the health messages into the health education and into the children's perception of everyday life. Children recognize and understand the health information that is meaningful in their everyday context and dismiss most of the information that does not immediately make sense.

Our findings suggest that the pedagogical context is important when trying to create a sense of consistency in the health information in order to give children a sense of cohesion and confidence that the health information is relevant and can be used across different contexts. This is most apparent in the teacher's statements about how information from Rumlerikkerne can be used in the everyday scenarios of, for example, lunch. This coherence seems closely linked with developing an identity that is connected to the immediate environment and the multitude of identities (e.g. other children, teachers) within it. If children become confused by conflicting health information within different contexts, it will be harder for them to feel connected to the communication within these contexts, which will inhibit both knowledge acquisition and the development of identities.

In our study, the health theatre served as an example of an alternative health-pedagogical context. Although the success in terms of acquisition of health knowledge and possibilities for relating the health information to self-interpretations and everyday life depended on the teachers' involvement and ownership, it is clear that the medium of theatre has potential in the field of school-based health education. The theatre presents an alternative context in which it is possible to twist health information and even existing health knowledge in ways that makes it possible to relate to – even for the children who normally interpret themselves as unhealthy. The key words in order to succeed with a health theatre approach seem to be participation, involvement and ownership – both from teachers and from children. The theatre group has recently used the recommendations from our study to expand and modify their approach and it now includes a homepage and a series of television shows filmed with children who attend the theatre. All changes have been made in order to create the best possible conditions for heightening participation, involvement and ownership.

5.4 Snapshot – Creativity and change in the lifestyles of South Asian communities in Yorkshire

Geetha Upadhyaya

Based in Bradford, Yorkshire, Kala Sangam[76] was, until recently, known for its challenging work in the field of arts, health and disabilities, particularly for the South Asian population. This snapshot will discuss one of its projects[77] to demonstrate the creative arts in health.

Over the past sixty years there has been a growth of migrant communities in the UK, and now more than ever, the NHS's health education and awareness of so-called ethnic minorities calls for cultural sensitivity. According to Anthony Barnett and colleagues, 'It is crucial to address specific communities individually according to cultural features such as customs, religion, lifestyle, food and languages.'[78] The arts in health work the company has delivered to date presents evidence that creativity is a non-invasive yet powerful medium (when used alongside biomedical approaches), especially in South Asian communities in tackling cultural taboos around discussing health. Our practice is informed by the following two principles: the World Health Organization's definition of health as 'a state of complete physical, mental and social wellbeing and not merely the absence of disease or infirmity';[79] and the idea that creative arts activities play a crucial role in restoring the equilibrium of psychosocial, biological and physiological parameters of holistic health.[80] This is borne out by Kala Sangam's work since 1993, responding to non-communicable or lifestyle health issues.[81]

In 2010, we worked with communities to address diabetes and the related health issues such as obesity, nutrition and a sedentary lifestyle. In certain South Asian communities, diabetes and related disabilities are not discussed openly. Barnett et al. argue that 'improvements in blood pressure and total cholesterol can be achieved with a structured, culturally sensitive, community-based care programme approach to cardiovascular risk management in a population of South Asians with type 2 diabetes'.[82] Our research and planning phase included identifying male and female participants with diabetes – with and without complications. We chose drama as the appropriate art form (including movement and song), employing an artistic director who would use interpreters to understand the core problems of the groups. Although contested in scholarship,[83] for some Muslim communities, a representation of living beings (acting) is still considered taboo; therefore from the outset we used great sensitivity. We also ensured that adequate continuous support and daily monitoring of the arts sessions was provided. Although this phase took longer than the usual approach, we observed a number of benefits in that the whole group bonded, developed trust and expressed a desire to work together to change their lifestyles.

Over a period of six months the group devised a short interactive piece, creating dialogues, music and movement. As it was the first time the whole group had ever acted or sung, the play was kept short and was a comedy. The message of wellbeing and health, especially in diabetes, had a tremendous impact on the audience and participants. The feedback from the participants revealed that the whole process was not just enjoyable, but through the play they could address negative emotions and turn it to a positive outcome. They also felt that their understanding of diabetes and the problems of non-compliance was improved through making the play, and was simplified for the audience. The short comic play was said to be easily understood and more accessible compared to the usual fliers, films or other information packs provided by community health centres. Some participants remarked that 'We did not know that diabetes will affect our children' and that 'Stigma is something that we can address through acceptance and handling our physical and mental status.' Another said 'I only had to give up sweets, not my life!' and another 'Thank God there are sweeteners and other alternatives – which I learnt through the group work.'

Overall, the play had a multi-pronged effect on the participants. It led to a change in their daily routines, including their dietary habits, exercises and medications. Participants formed an informal, mutual support group that built confidence, enabled acceptance of their challenges, strengthened social and family ties, and motivated participants (and audiences) to lead better lifestyles. While there is no further research evidence of the success of the project, the participants and their families engaged in collaborative documentation of their process in the project. For example, the overall project was evaluated through the administering of a daily thoughts diary written by the participants. To encourage family participation, we requested them to be involved in helping participants use the internet to maintain their progress. The daily routines were plotted as a simple graph to show the participants their progress, and all their meetings and discussions were documented by each one in turn. We believe that this approach ensured that they had collective ownership of the project.

This project has not been sustained owing to funding cuts, despite evidence that increasingly a 'dose' of the arts is being prescribed.[84] Kala Sangam has been unable to access any ongoing support from the Clinical Commissioning Groups (CCG) for such work to date. The benefits of using creative arts are sometimes hard to document, but they are sure to ensure changes in lifestyles and build healthier and stronger communities.

6

Sexual Health: Practice from South Africa and the Asia–Pacific Region

6.1 Introduction

Veronica Baxter

The Human Immunodeficiency Virus (HIV) was shown to be a predominantly heterosexual disease by the late 1980s, yet was still largely ignored by governments. In the words of one medical officer in Uganda, 'we just could not connect a disease in white, homosexual males in San Francisco to the thing that we were staring at'.[1] In the Asia–Pacific region by 2013, the prevalence of HIV had increased to 1.7 million infected, with the highest rates of infection in India, China, Indonesia and Thailand.[2] In sub-Saharan Africa, the prevalence is 24.7 million, with South Africa alone estimated by UNAIDS to have 6.8 million infections.[3]

With these statistics in mind, it is no wonder that HIV/AIDS became a subject of great importance, consuming funding and health resources in the Global South. As Katharine Low points out below, the first theatrical applications devoted to HIV and AIDS were sombre affairs; Lynn Dalrymple suggests that the earlier modes of Applied Theatre assumed that 'a change of knowledge and attitudes will result in behaviour change … Unfortunately it does not follow that information and attitude change will change behaviour.'[4] The earliest approaches to HIV in theatre were in line with what Jacques Rancière refers to as stultifying pedagogy, where 'what the spectator *must see* is what the director *makes her see*.⁵ Rancière contrasts this with what he calls the 'emancipated spectator', each individual with the power of exercising 'an unpredictable interplay of associations and dissociations' with the theatre performance.⁶ This suggests that what is gained from a performance is subjective and unpredictable. To some extent Rancière's words seem to contradict the point of theatre *applied* to a health issue, but they nevertheless call for a move away from overly didactic and stifling instrumentalism.

Katharine Low argues that the individual needs 'breathing space' when encountering theatre about sex and HIV, in order to allow for their 'associations and dissociations', according to Rancière,⁷ to unfold. She argues that in the context of HIV, the subject of sex is often asphyxiating because of the strong message that individuals are to blame if they contract HIV; that the sexual act is not only dangerous, but shameful and joyless. Helen Cahill follows up on this idea with examples from the Asia–Pacific region, arguing that fear-inducing stories may undermine the intentions of health promotion. Instead she argues that the good–bad binary must be resisted in theatre, instead focusing on using humorous, surreal characters to create opportunities for dialogue about solutions rather than dwelling on cause and effect.

While there are multiple other sexual health concerns highlighted by the World Health Organization, because of the alarming rates of new infections and the pull on financial and health resources, a focus on HIV and AIDS is still relevant.

6.2 Essay – 'It's difficult to talk about sex in a positive way': Creating a space to breathe

Katharine Low

Writing in 2012, Alain de Botton argues that '[d]espite being one of the most private of activities, sex is nonetheless surrounded by a range of powerfully socially sanctioned ideas that codify how normal people are meant to feel about and deal with the matter'.[8] It remains the case that irrespective of where we live, the general discourse of sex is often constrained, be it in everyday conversations, in popular films, in pornography or in public health campaigns. When a decision to address a particular sexual health concern is taken, it becomes even more apparent that we also struggle to speak about sex and relationships in a positive manner: themes regularly emerge about protection against inadvertent pregnancy or contracting sexually transmitted infections (STIs). Often, the discussion about sex is both frightening and stigmatizing. We see this in the historic AIDS campaigns, from the threat of a dangerous and deadly disease in the 1987 British 'Don't Die of Ignorance' monolith campaign, to the early STI awareness approaches used by doctors in Zimbabwe that used photographs of genitals with extreme cases of gonorrhoea and syphilis.[9]

Similar negativity around discussions of sex remains true today. Public health researcher Ford Hickson draws attention to HIV prevention within a context of homophobia in the UK, arguing that at times it appears that 'the point of HIV prevention is to find and fix the dysfunctional, to make them like us or to disable them as a threat'.[10] The term 'safe sexual health' is problematic as it presupposes a level of carelessness, that the person has 'failed' by not being healthy, deviating from a normative view of health, a position from which moral judgements are possible. Further, such a focus on protection, staying safe and keeping free of disease is heightened in a country like South Africa, where rates of HIV and STI infection, sexual violence and gender discrimination are high.

The historian Catherine Burns suggests that in South Africa most understandings of sexuality are 'deeply shadowed by the crisis that we face of the pandemic of HIV. We speak about sex pathologically, about its danger. It is very hard for us to speak about desire and pleasure. There is a lot of pain in the world of sex. And yet young people are coming into life all the time, and needing to touch, explore and be their sexual selves.'[11] Indeed, for many young South Africans, the journey of exploring and negotiating becoming a sexual being takes place within a landscape of danger of HIV infection, sexual violence and pervasive moral codes around appropriate behaviour, interaction and touch. All of this allows little space for playful experimentation, burgeoning desire or an acknowledgement of the emotional aspects of sexuality. An understanding of one's physical and emotional desires involves both a consideration of what it is that one enjoys and wants and how one might achieve those desires in a context where HIV and STIs prevail. Reaching this understanding is only possible through discussing sexual health matters openly, without shame or secrecy. Sara Ahmed's thinking around queer futurity and her unpacking of the term 'aspiration' feels poignantly appropriate here:

> We need to think more about the relationship between the queer struggle for a bearable life and aspirational hopes for a good life ... We could remember that the Latin root of the word *aspiration* means 'to breathe.' I think that the struggle for a bearable life is the struggle for queers to have space to breathe. Having space to breathe, or being able to breathe freely ... is an aspiration. With breath comes imagination. With breath comes possibility.[12]

Although Ahmed is discussing queer futurity, there are clear parallels with the South African situation around sex. In short, for South African youth, discussions around sex are suffocating – which causes an asphyxiation in that there is no 'freedom to breathe' and few spaces in which to breathe. Yet theatre-making can create such spaces and it is here that the exhilarating link between theatre and sex – intimacy, possibility and playfulness – is sometimes missed.

Alan Read suggests that it is 'self-evident' that intimacy and engagement form part of theatre, arguing that theatre 'requires an understanding of the dynamics of intimacy (the proximity of relations) and engagement (the conduct of association)'.[13] Read locates the moment of theatre within the negotiation between intimacy and engagement. Here lies the crux for theatre-making about sexual health: it needs to play more on the potential of intimacy and engagement within the theatre-making. It is important to recognize that understanding is not simply the transmission of knowledge. When the focus of learning is only on cognition, we miss out on the different subtle emotional and embodied understandings. If learning is explicitly the main driver for theatre work on sexual health, then the premise on which the work is founded will not work. The participants/spectators have to be able to emote, to feel it – sex is about feelings, bodies, juices and intimacy. Intimacy can mean a sense of belonging and being in a secluded particular kind of space that is created for you; it is a sense of collaboration or complicity; it brings about covert conversations. There is a frisson of excitement that comes through intimacy. Both sex and theatre can be exhilarating, dangerous and risky.

In this chapter I am making a case for work that plays with, and is about, bodies, juices and affect rather than dry didacticism and effect. Such work, I argue, is more comprehensible, inviting and recognizable for its audience. I explore ways of creating and inviting young people into spaces to breathe and be playful. I am interested in how these invitations may generate opportunities for audiences to make sense of the fluidity and flexibility of sex and sexuality for themselves. I am informed here by Josephine Machon, who proposes that active, intimate participation on the audience's behalf helps lead to opportunities where meaning-making, or 'sense-making', can occur. Specifically I am looking at how moments of intimate theatrical invitations or affect may lead to critical understanding and an engagement of the 'thinking body'.[14] I examine ways in which a theatre production creates moments of intimacy and space to breathe which I think can lead to sense-making for the individual, within the field of sexual health communication. In doing so I draw from two performances around sex, relationships and gender which formed part of the annual Drama for Life Sex Actually Festival, based at the University of Witwatersrand in Johannesburg in 2014. Devised and directed by Clara Vaughan with the Market Theatre Lab students, *Four Husbands for Ma Lindi*[15] interrogates sex, sexuality and gender. The play reflects how young people explore multiple perspectives in developing fulfilling, loving sexual relationships. *In Your Circle* is an adaptation of *HUSH*, written by Janet Buckland and the UBOM Theatre Company, which was based on Alex Sutherland's *Risky Business* (2008). In her adaptation and direction, Namatshego Khutsoane focuses on an all-female South African perspective, with an emphasis on lesbian sexuality. The play is a performed discussion between young South African women exploring questions around sex, sexuality and behaviour that occur in overlapping and intersecting social circles. Before engaging in the analysis, I begin by contextualizing theatre-making around sexual health in South Africa and will further unpack my thinking around the potential for sense-making in these kinds of performances.

South Africa: sexual health and theatre

In recent history, South Africa has been a sexually conservative country, undoubtedly reinforced by the apartheid regime's 'censorship and repressive policing' of sex and sexuality, the criminalization of homosexuality and the prohibition of sex across racial boundaries,[16] and the dominance of Christian thought and practices.[17] After the 1994 democratic elections, sexuality in South Africa has become increasingly politicized, with numerous constitutional rights around choice and desire put into place. Yet, as Jane Bennett notes, this is alongside escalating gender-based and homophobic-related violence as well as divisive debates around gendered and sexual norms,[18] which spill out into everyday life. It is estimated that half a million rapes occur per year,[19] while only one in nine are reported; so-called 'corrective rape' for lesbian women is widespread and a very real fear for many women,[20] and HIV prevalence is at 17.9 per cent, though this figure rises to 40% in the province of KwaZulu-Natal.[21]

As described in the Introduction to this book, there has been a long history of theatre-making around health concerns and, specifically in sub-Saharan Africa, sexual health concerns. Esiaba Irobi has argued that the emergence of HIV/AIDS created a new type of theatre-making in Africa, a 'theatre of necessity'.[22] In any case, the growing health concerns of certain African countries and the potentially lucrative opportunities for work has meant that Applied Theatre as a practice has been widely employed to address key sexual health concerns, although historically perhaps not always with the best intentions in mind.[23]

In South Africa there is a significant range of theatre-based activity from the long-standing Arepp:Theatre for Life (established in 1987 in Johannesburg and which now tours and works nationally) and DramAidE (formed in 1992 at the University of Zululand by Professor Lynn Dalrymple) to the more recent Themba Interactive and the Mothertongue Project. These organizations, often originating from university theatre departments, use a variety of different performance forms ranging from participatory-based theatre to interactive musical engagements.[24] When HIV/AIDS first emerged, in response to the statistics and, at times, lack of knowledge, productions would sometimes take a semi-didactic or 'gloomy' tone in their approach to the subject of HIV. There remained in these early works a strong focus on the mechanics around protection from HIV and an emphasis on behaviour change communication. Over time, however, there has been a growing focus on challenging and addressing stigma and, more recently, on exploring and celebrating diverse genders and sexualities.[25] Yet, not all approaches have managed to strike the balance of openness and dialogue and there are still productions and workshops where in the content, sex is not discussed in a positive way and is sometimes placed within a framework of disease, contagion and morals.[26] Such work is limiting and alienating as it does not engender a space for audiences to make sense, in one's own terms, and ignores the aforementioned similarities between theatre and sex. Thus it is important to examine those productions that tap into emotions and feelings around sex and invite the audience into a discussion and to consider how this happens.

What is interesting is what kinds of invitations are offered to audiences and how they make their own meaning from there. Here Gareth White's analysis of meaning-making as an aesthetic in *Audience Participation in Theatre* is a useful frame. Building on Bruce McConachie's discussion of the cognitive science of emotion, White argues that 'emotions and feelings tell us what to prioritise in our thinking, drive us towards certain kinds of thinking in response to stimuli, and organise our thinking about stimuli in the present moment and on reflection'.[27] I read this idea in the following manner: having a response to something may stimulate a conversation for both the body and the brain. So when we encounter something that resonates with us, it may trigger a series of responses. The questions this prompts are: how might this occur and what kinds of invitations are needed? Beginning with the first query, there are a number of ways of considering this.

Making sense on your own terms

Gordon Bilbrough, the artistic director of Arepp: Theatre for Life (Arepp),[28] argues that the company's intention within their productions is to leave the audience with a sense of incompleteness. Bilbrough proposes that it is that lack of resolution of the narrative that 'hooks' and 'snags' the audience's interest, which in turn creates a space for experiential learning[29] which he argues is 'how people can best learn from their experiences'.[30] As part of his argument, Bilbrough introduces Jack Mezirow's ideas of critical reflection on experience and learning, emphasizing how experiential learning, by being skill- and practice-based, can be 'transformative and emancipatory'.[31] For Bilbrough, in that 'hooking' and 'snagging' of the audience member's interest there is the possibility for engagement with one's own questions and experiences about the topic. In short, because its interest has been piqued, an audience member is reflecting and in doing so learning, as reflection is 'the act of cognitive engagement with the experience'. Bilbrough further argues that 'Fundamental to achieving experiential learning, however, is the fact that cognition occurred through some form of reflecting upon and engaging in discourse with the experience, its social context and the other participants.'[32]

While I appreciate how that moment of connection and interest can lead to further reflection, I think it is too simple to jump to naming this particular moment as learning. There is no narrative end-point, no incompleteness to encourage the spectators to make sense of for themselves, and there is not sufficient focus on the emotions and feelings that may emerge. Furthermore, how do we know that this moment of cognition has taken place? There is a more subtle and individual process that occurs in that moment when the spectator's attention is piqued: it is an individual making sense of the situation for themselves. It is also how we invite the audience and the participant into the event. It is finding a moment of recognition or intimacy within the theatre space, which resonates for a spectator and allows for a breath and a moment of sense-making.

I have borrowed the term 'sense-making' from Machon, who suggests in her theorization of the notion of (syn)aesthetics that the body is the conduit for the appreciation of the artistic experience. Machon argues that '[t]o experience (syn)aesthetically means to perceive the details corporeally' and 'that rich and *felt* quality of experience'[33] may provide a space for the senses to coalesce. It is having that space in which people can individually make sense of the experience that is most resonant from my perspective. The experience is more than just witnessing or recognizing one's own story on stage; it is about having an intellectual, emotional and corporeal understanding and engagement with the event. Machon further explains this moment:

> It is this fusion of the *felt* and the 'understood' in making sense/*sense* of intangible, inarticulable ideas that is crucial to (syn)aesthetics appreciation. Put simply, we *feel* the performance in the moment and recall these feelings in subsequent interpretation.[34]

This is not dissimilar to Bilbrough's description of why it 'works'; however, there is a greater emphasis on the emotion at play for the individual. Bilbrough focuses on the act of cognition and the intellectual reflection that can emerge from that act, while Machon focuses on emotion, felt and embodied experience. In essence, Bilbrough places the emphasis on making sense of the experience (making and drawing logical conclusions), while Machon is making a case for the embodied process of sense-making. Crucially, she argues that it is sense-making and not directly cognitive learning that occurs. Machon's idea of this experience is more held within the body: she describes the moment when the aesthetic practice 'activates the "thinking body" ... a sensory intellect which exists within the body and follows its own rules of logic that are both separate from *and often intrinsic to* cerebral intellect'.[35] It is this appreciation of a 'thinking body' that is fundamental when we examine theatre practices that engage with the issues of sex and sexuality. Creating ludic spaces that are intimate and playful are inviting (and not asphyxiating) for an audience: the topic feels 'possible', playful and breathable.

In order to start conversations around sex and relationships, we need to provide avenues for intimate moments of recognition with the audience, the participants and facilitators. We need to provide a space when exploring sexual health concerns through theatre, where the individual can appreciate the subject within their body and mind in a way that speaks to their experiences. Thus, a combination of Machon's discussion of 'sense-making' with White's discussion of that moment when Applied Theatre artistry results in an intense, intimate, consummatory experience, a space where an individual can experience themselves or an event quite differently; a (syn)aesthetic moment when bodily-thinking and sense-making can occur. In that intimacy and its inherent playful possibilities, an opportunity emerges: where an individual may want to be part of it, be in it, consider it and discuss it. This leads to my second query: what are the frames needed for these judicious moments of sense-making to occur? I argue that this can happen through different kinds of invitations, and in the second part of this essay I examine three of them: honesty, form and humour, using moments from *Four Husbands* and *In Your Circle* to illustrate how these invitations occur.

Honesty and recognition

As mentioned above, work that tackles sexuality and sexual health is often framed as urgent, in a sense that there is a crisis that 'needs resolving'. The subject under exploration is often negatively problematized. Clara Vaughan, the director of *Four Husbands*, describes this as sex being rendered pathological: '[T]he idea is that it [sex] has to be sick, it has to be a pathology; and if you talk about it you can only talk about it in terms of what's wrong with it.'[36] While the approach of graphically demonstrating some of the dangers found in sex is understandable because of the potential risks, the repeated negativity can be alienating for an audience. Whereas content that honestly depicts the complexity of negotiating one's own sexuality and the fluidity of sex as a young person is more exciting and inviting.

Such content was evident when I observed *Four Husbands*, where the audience's vocal reactions to the piece indicated that they recognized, emphasized with, and cringed alongside the actors. For example, in the scene entitled 'Breadwinner', Nosiphiwo[37] shares a story about meeting an older man who is hot, sexy and kind, who brings groceries and pays her school fees: she loves him. As Nosiphiwo describes the girl's realization that this is not a romance but rather, in the eyes of the older man, a transactional relationship, the vocal responses from young women in the audience demonstrated that they shared and understood Nosiphiwo's feelings of confusion, disappointment and sadness. This scene encapsulates a young woman's realization of her own naivety and offers it to the audience as fact. It is not turned into a model of how not to behave, but rather it shows the reality that these relationships happen without intent for young women. In doing so, a breathable space was created to talk about the indignity of such experiences without it becoming 'the worst thing' or resorting to victim blaming.

In his book *The Trouble with Normal*, Michael Warner notes that 'in those circles where queerness has been most cultivated, the ground rule is that one doesn't pretend to be *above* the indignity of sex … Only when this indignity of sex is spread around the room, leaving no one out, and in fact binding people in the room together, [does] it begin to resemble the dignity of the human.'[38] Here Warner is talking about queer communities, yet his framing could be applied to this context in that both *Four Husbands* and *In Your Circle* acknowledge that their audience members may choose to have sex. This is why both productions are successful with their audiences in forming connections. There is an understanding inherent in both productions that sex and sexuality exist, that people may choose to have sex or choose not to have sex, and that people have desires. The indignity of sex and the many different kinds of sex are named. That it is a process that everyone may or may not choose to take part in, but forms part of who they are, is acknowledged.

The HIV testing scene in Khutsoane's *In Your Circle* further epitomizes this idea. In a highly stylized manner, using both chorus and identifiable characters (young people being tested and different kinds of nurses), the scene illustrates the steps taken in a rapid HIV test. As the nurses take turns in asking the required questions, the chorus of characters offer their responses. It is fast-paced and funny, and offers an insight into and a recognition of the different answers, prevailing myths and common fears that people hold. The characters' responses depict a diversity of desire, knowledge and gender and sexual orientation. The intention of the director in this scene is clear: to make room for everything. In our interview, Khutsoane emphasized that her intentions in this staging and the change in direction of the play to focus on women's experiences was to provide a space for alterity, seeing the other, as well as illustrating the many different experiences found in South Africa and making such choices known.[39] In doing so, Khutsoane helps maintain a sense of intimacy with her intended audience. Furthermore, I argue that this sense of being complicit, coupled with content that is uncomfortable, but neither didactic nor patronizing, may encourage audience members to be more perceptive of the matter under discussion.

In his analysis of the different forms of aesthetics found in Applied Theatre, White makes reference to Arnold Berleant's *The Aesthetic Field* (1970), which Berleant proposes is created by four components that enable an artistic experience. These include the object, the artist, the perceiver and the performer. Transferring this to an Applied

Theatre-making realm, White draws attention to how Berleant 'gives equal weight to the role of the perceiver in the moment of artistic experience'.[40] Similarly, Machon notes Mike Pearson's emphasis on the audience's need to be percipient and take responsibility for being engaged and responsive to the piece and for exploring what may happen next.[41] In both these productions, the artistic experience, or the moment of sense-making, is heightened and leaves traces behind,[42] because through appropriate invitations the audience is able to be percipient. They are able to be critical and engaged; they have been offered an honest space of possibility in which they can breathe.

Playing with form

Taking a playful approach to the aesthetic form and/or structure is something that suits theatre-making around sex and sexuality. Sex can be playful and if we can be playful with the theatrical conventions, that playfulness will carry through to the audience and the actors, in playing with different levels of intimacy and invitation. For example, *Four Husbands* showed the audience that sex can be playful by moving between multiple narratives in the monologues to songs, short scenes to dances, and interspacing audience interaction with striking images. One example is a scene where a series of young women softly protest and attempt to ward off unwanted attention and attacks from older men, fathers and uncles. As they speak, the men in the cast prowl as hyenas in a stylized manner, circling, taunting, falling back and creeping ever closer. The play opens with men calling out to women in the audience telling them how beautiful they are, which leads to the women in the cast asking the questions that they want to know more about: 'What provokes you to have sex?', 'Why are girls scared of masturbating?' or 'Is it possible that my boyfriend is gay?' The action moves from the cast sharing multiple narratives around the theme of 'I lost my virginity and I didn't feel anything/found L.O.V.E/and I feel happy about it', to scenes that play on stereotypical gender roles, inverting and poking fun at them. Throughout the play there is a continued use of and reference to cake; having a slice of the cake (i.e. having sex or gaining a woman's virginity) is a repeated metaphor, and bread (symbolizing money) is often exchanged for cake in a number of the scenes. Similarly, in *In Your Circle* there are unpredictable, striking moments which cut through the scenes. Specifically it is the use of songs such as Mis-Teeq's 'Scandalous' or Ginuwine's 'Pony' (whose lyrics include 'If you're horny let's do it, Ride it, my pony. My saddle's waiting, Come and jump on it')[43] that break through the narrative, immediately challenging and contradicting the action taking place on stage.

In both productions, a postdramatic form[44] allows a playfulness to emerge which felt intimate. Those moments of intimacy were both exciting and inviting as there were spaces in which we could acknowledge that sex can be both playful and naughty, that different experiences are equally valid and important. All of this is full of possibility and by having these multiple experiences acknowledged in the room it felt that there was a space to talk about these ideas (if not immediately then later, as White asserts, if people wished to do so).

Indeed the multiplicity of narratives found in both *Four Husbands* and *In Your Circle* are a fundamental part of why these two plays successfully create invitations to consider further, or to make sense of, for the different audience members. They both offer an acknowledgement of the importance of choice and the variety of choices. Choice is a problematic concept both in South African and broader African experiences of sex and negotiation. Reproductive health researcher Chi-Chi Undie specifically addresses this idea in her consideration of the notion that while everyone may have the right to choose, a lack of knowledge or awareness of the variety of choices is dangerous. Undie asks 'How much choice do any of us really have when we lack relevant information? The lack of knowledge, which translates into the lack of true/informed choice, gives rise to vulnerability and plays a major role in fuelling the HIV pandemic.'[45] 'True choice' is a loaded concept, particularly within this context, but if we consider Undie's idea as an argument for informed and flexible choice, there exist possibilities and openness. Openness allows for a space to breathe; the spectacular scenes coupled with the multiple narratives and playful forms of both productions is another element that helps to create moments of intimate engagement. The multiple narratives presented offered flexible choices and diverse knowledge; these were invitations to the audience to sense-make in its own way.

Humour and the indignity of sex

The honesty in the fact that sex can be funny, undignified and ridiculous is something that Pieter Dirk Uys has long acknowledged and brought into his ongoing safe sex production *For Facts' Sake*, which he has toured around South Africa at his own cost since 2000.[46,47] In *For Facts' Sake*, Uys is quick to play on the ridiculous and titillating elements of sex when starting the conversation with his young audiences. Watching his productions[48] it is the humour and the acknowledgement of the discomfort of sex that Uys offers that is the invitation into the performance and discussion around sexual health matters. It was wonderful to observe the audiences' engagement, delight, squeamishness and interest as they watched Uys's impersonations of Mandela, Archbishop Desmond Tutu and Tannie Evita encouraging them to practice safe sex. They are hooked and are having fun. There is something delightful, risky and engaging in having an elderly white Afrikaans man doing impressions of revered public figures who are in turn urging mixed audiences of young people to take ownership over their own sexual choices.

The subversion of characters here, as in the messing with the gender roles in *Four Husbands*, is what fixes people's attention; it is engaging and exciting and highly theatrical. In *Four Husbands* there are series of gender reversal scenes ranging from the male cast members performing the traditional all-female reed dance to a tea ceremony which is described in the following manner:

> All the men collect a teacup, saucer and spoon. They come and sit in
> a row at the front of the stage, their legs stretched out in front of them

like women on mats. The women make a tableau at the back, sitting in traditionally masculine positions. A playful movement piece about enjoying a nice hot cup of tea – the men all move in unison with traditionally feminine movements.[49]

This is then followed by the scene entitled 'Husbands for Ma Lindi', where in a reversal of polygamy, Ma Lindi's husbands, with extremely feminized movements, prepare her supper, fight over who is the best cook and generally vie for her attention as she returns from work.

The audience responses to the scenes were vocal and engaged: from shrieks of disbelief to loud endorsement. A shared space of humour and laughter can create a sense of collective intimacy and complicity and this is crucial in terms of discussing sexual health and relationships. We could debate how a reversal of gender does not actually address power structures and yet these scenes recognize that women are oppressed and foreground the problem. While deeply humorous, those scenes demonstrated, albeit temporarily, that alternatives are possible and it was clear that this was exciting for the audience,

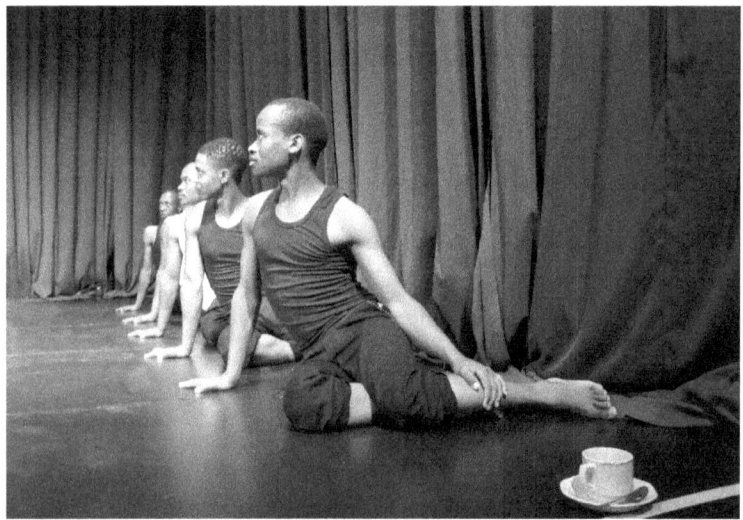

Figure 4: 'Husbands for Ma Lindi'. Photo © Patrick Selemani.

particularly the young women. Commenting on the reaction of the audience, Vaughan noted, 'I also loved how some of the girls would really enjoy the gender reversal scenes; seeing that woman in that position of power was very evocative for them.'[50] In those moments that humour simultaneously brought the spectators in closer to, and distanced them from, the situation, so they were able to appreciate and take pleasure in the ridiculous as well as acknowledge the questions that are unspoken but acknowledged: 'Why can't a woman have four husbands when a man can?' or 'Why can't I negotiate condom use with my boyfriend?' These questions are not answered for the audience, Vaughan and Khutsoane, and I do not think that they should have been. Rather they are ideas to consider further, perhaps for the individual to sense-make for themselves. The fact that there is no right or wrong or a tragic moralistic ending is liberating, it demonstrates flexible choice and possibility.

In this essay, I have brought together some ways in which theatre-making around sexual health can successfully invite and engage its audience to make sense of the topic for themselves. I have offered arguments for the importance of making theatre without dry didacticism, but rather to celebrate the risk-taking, intimacy and exciting links between theatre and sex by focusing on different ways spectators can be invited to explore their own meanings in a space of possibility, a space where they are able to breathe and are not asked to accept blame for their behaviour, which is usually presented as being defective.

Acknowledgements

To the students at Market Lab for generously allowing me to observe their process and practice and answer my questions and to Clara Vaughan, Gareth White and Steve Farrier for all the discussions which helped to develop my thinking in this essay.

6.3 Snapshot – Performing the solution: Cautions and possibilities when using theatre conventions within HIV prevention programmes

Helen Cahill

Theatre is a powerful medium, but it is not necessarily benevolent in its social effect. Theatre-makers seeking to address resistant public health problems, such as the HIV epidemic, face the dual struggle of constructing something that is both good theatre and effective prevention education. Good theatre can potentially be bad health promotion. So 'prevention theatre' should not be assessed by aesthetic standards alone. Rather it must be assessed by the dual standards that pertain to both its socially transformative objectives and its aesthetic objectives.

I encounter three key vulnerabilities of the theatre medium which I believe need particular consideration when using drama-based strategies within HIV prevention initiatives. One entails the tendency towards selection of worst-case scenarios as central subject matter. Worst-case scenarios are readily made into tellable tales and there can be agreement that if they harness audience attention, they must be doing good. But while horror and sympathy can hold audience attention, fear tactics may undermine the health promoting intent of the work.

The logic behind the use of fear tactics within health promotion can be very compelling: if only people understood the risks, they would refrain from their risky sexual practices. The presumption is that once informed, a rational being should avoid such actions. Responding to this urge to warn, theatre-makers may transmit information with a bias towards heightening the negative consequences of 'wrong' choices. However, humans are not strictly rational beings and fear tactics tend to have a null result in relation to behaviour change. Research into effective prevention education shows that the programmes that are effective in reducing risky behaviours do not chiefly rely on knowledge transmission, abstinence messages or fear tactics.[51,52] Along with provision of knowledge or skills, they also have people question and challenge the social norms and material conditions that hold patterns of behaviour in place. They work to generate hope, rather than to transmit fear, and a strong collective sense of the possibility, desirability and permissibility of change.[53]

Use of fear tactics can have a more insidious negative effect than the null result described above. Herein lies a second vulnerability of the theatre medium. This vulnerability pertains to the tendency to use stock characters or stereotypes to distinguish victims from perpetrators, or 'goodies' from 'baddies'. When storylines are constructed around a good–bad binary, they can inadvertently demonize those who pass the infection to others or indeed those who contract the infection as a result of their own 'failure' to be 'good'. This can augment stigma by painting some as contagious and therefore as inherently abhorrent or weak. This can further perpetuate the stigma that holds oppressive practices in place. In order to avoid an inadvertent 'theatre of judgement', it is important to ensure that both the explicit messages and the meta-messages of the theatre piece avoid heightening the individualized narratives of shame and blame which already abound in relation to HIV.[54]

The third challenge I have encountered when using a theatre medium also relates to the choice of subject matter used as the central focus. It presents in relation to the selection of individualized storylines. The capacity to use the singular to capture the general is a strength of the dramatic medium. However, when seeking to raise awareness about how to halt an epidemic, it is important to be able to generate a macro- rather than a micro-view about the actions that are needed. Epidemics, as with most health inequalities, are held in place by a combination of poverty and social practices.[55] Therefore it is insufficient to focus solely on the protective behaviours to be taken by an individual, such as abstinence, condom use, testing or medication adherence. Rather there is an additional need to address the structural and social factors that hold the epidemic in place.[56,57] These factors include poverty, gender inequity, homophobia, acceptance of violence, lack of education, stigma and lack of access to health education, resources and services.[58] These are the social and structural determinants of health that mean that certain groups or subgroups will be more vulnerable than others. If theatre-based initiatives do not recognize these factors, then the meta-message of the theatre piece may be that the entire responsibility lies with the potential victim who should take (or should have taken) the protective actions. There may subsequently be an implicit excusing of governments, institutions and communities, despite that action on their part will be central to preventing new infections.

Despite these cautions about the use of theatre for HIV prevention, there are many possibilities that derive from the versatility of the medium and its capacity to generate critical thought about complex subject matters. To discuss some of these possibilities, I provide below some examples drawn from my own practice in community settings in developing countries in the Asia–Pacific region. In most countries in this region the epidemic is concentrated chiefly among certain sub-population groups, including young people who engage in sex work, those who inject drugs, men who have sex with men, and transgender young people. Thus a focus on destigmatizing is of doubled importance as those most affected are commonly already experiencing forms of marginalization or disadvantage within their community.

I have found that humour is a powerful permission-giving device which can help to disrupt silencing social norms. For example, in a socially conservative religious context, two participants are cast as the characters Mr Abstinence and Mr Condom. Once in role the players must argue about which of them offers the most reliable form of protection from HIV. Located in these roles, the players are able to use the protective shield of humour to engage in explicit talk. They are even able to refer to the issue of desire, which is all too often excluded from discussions about HIV prevention. Mr Abstinence brags that he is 100% cheap and 100% effective against sexual transmission. Mr Condom retaliates that it is good that Abstinence is free, because he would be impossible to market with the consumers having so little desire to use him as a method. Mr Abstinence retorts with the accusation that condoms reduce pleasure, and hence have their own problem with popular demand. When both characters admit that they have a problem with popularity, they begin to examine why – and to brainstorm what can be done about this. They thus enter the territory of social influences and of proactive solution-making.

This use of transgressive humour is activated via the employment of surrealist theatre conventions, whereby the actors play non-human characters. I have found that surrealist conventions are particularly useful in generating a macro-perspective. For example, when the character HI-Virus itself is interviewed about its natural enemies, 'he' confesses to 'his' fear of education, equity, economic progress and explicit talk about the technicalities of safe sex. A dramatization from this standpoint generates very different material from that in the typical human-to-human scene within which the central task may be to transact about condom use. In 'domestic', naturalistic scenarios such as these, any awareness of the structural and social nature of the epidemic can easily be lost.[59]

When the interest is to focus at the relational level, however, drama-based techniques can be used to reveal the way in which social norms work to hold behaviour in place. An enactment of the 'hidden thoughts' of the character can dramatize the internal struggle between conflicting desires. This may, for example, be a struggle between the traditional belief that ignorance protects innocence, and the more modern notion that access to information is both a right and a need. For example, a mother attempts to educate her daughter about sex. The resultant naturalistic dialogue is brief and unhelpful. The daughter not only remains without the knowledge that she needs, but she has also relearnt the message that it is not appropriate to talk openly about matters to do with sex. A subsequent dramatization of the mother's 'hidden' thoughts (use of an alter ego) shows her fear that if she provides information about condom use this may send a signal that sexual activity is permissible, and that she wishes to be a 'good' mother and provide her daughter with the information that she needs to stay safe. This dramatization of the internal scripts caught in the act of shaping behaviour brings forth the way in which gender and cultural norms shape intergenerational educative practices.[60]

From a public health perspective, effective 'prevention theatre' addresses the need for change in the structural and social conditions associated with heightened vulnerability to HIV. This requires: a thought-provoking theatre; a politicizing theatre; a theatre that can diminish the stigma that holds patterns of disadvantage in place; a theatre that not only enhances individual agency, but also mobilizes response at policy and institutional levels.

7

Cancer: Research from the UK, USA and Australia

7.1 Introduction

Katharine Low

Although fundraising for cancer research has now become a multi-billion-pound industry, morbidity is rising and cancer remains one of the main causes of death worldwide. Cancer accounted for 8.2 million deaths in 2012, with an estimated 14 million new cases of cancer reported.[1] Indeed, it is predicted that cases of cancer will increase by 70 per cent by 2035.[2] Despite its worldwide impact and growing burden of disease, cancer was marginalized from the UN's Millennium Development Goals (MDGs)[3] and has not often been a priority in global and country-level health policies.

In terms of fundraising approaches for cancer research, in the public realm there has been a turn to either 'crass materialism',[4] a perception of martyrdom of people living with cancer,[5] or a war-like exhortation that we must 'fight', 'beat' and 'cure' cancer. Indeed, the narratives and languages surrounding cancer are strange and challenging and this is something that Brian Lobel explores in his essay. Lobel, a young adult with cancer, considers recent performances that resist assigning cancer patients to a 'sick' role, but rather engender conversations between cancer patients and diverse audiences.

Furthermore, most cancer prevention programmes lack research into cancer in diverse population groups; while cancer is quite well 'known' in high-income countries, it is a growing concern in low- and middle-income countries.[6] Minority ethnic groups in high-income countries are often under-served and under-diagnosed and, accordingly, can have higher incidences of cancer.[7] Astrid Perry and Lynne Baker consider this situation in their account of a series of theatre projects aimed at addressing the stigma of cancer in diverse communities around Sydney. In their snapshot, Perry and Baker consider the choices made and the impact of the *Alive and Out There* project, run by a local health authority, and make a compelling argument for culture-specific performances that destigmatize cancer and bring it into the public realm for discussion.

7.2 Essay – Proud disclosures and awkward receptions: Between bodies with cancer and their audiences

Brian Lobel

'No one will casually talk to me anymore …', Tig Notaro, 2012

In the 2014 film adaptation of John Green's young-adult novel *The Fault in Our Stars*, the story's two central characters, Hazel Grace and Gus Waters, travel to Amsterdam as part of a Make-A-Wish-Foundation-inspired trip provided to terminally ill children and teenagers.[8] The pair walk to the Anne Frank House, where Hazel Grace – who has weak lungs from treatment – learns that because there is no lifts, she must carry her oxygen tank up multiple steep staircases into the annex. Initially hesitant, Hazel (played by the healthy-looking-other-than-nasal-tubes-and-short-hair Shailene Woodley) bravely (as the music tells us) manages her way up the staircase where, shortly after, she and Gus finally share their first kiss, while the voice of Anne Frank's quote, 'I don't think of all the misery, but the beauty that still remains' plays in the background. The kiss is not a little one: it is long and passionate and deeply fulfilling for viewers who have, for the hour prior, waited for the teenage romance to be consummated. As they pull apart, they are surrounded by Anne Frank House tourists who applaud them as the music swells. Gus bows to their small audience and the scene cuts to the couple having sex for the first time.

In Green's original text, Hazel Grace, the narrator, is significantly more critical of the space and place of their kiss. 'You cannot kiss anyone in the Anne Frank House', she reflects, but then remembers 'that Anne Frank, after all, kissed someone in the Anne Frank House …'[9] By contrast, the film creates a seamless connection between kissing at the Anne Frank House and young (cancer) love. It is in the moment of applause that the self-interestedness of youth comes into direct contact with the expectation that cancer patients will be applauded for anything they do, and be seen as heroic for the cancer they battle.

This essay will consider the tensions and possibilities that exist between the currently distinct medical and social models of disability as they are applied to people living with cancer, and how contemporary artists are using the live space of theatre and performance to challenge, in the immediate, and ultimately reconcile these distinctions. I will employ contemporary examples of live performance-makers, in both the US and UK, whose interplay with the audience highlights the dialogic nature of being a body with cancer in front of an audience, from Los Angeles-based comic Tig Notaro to Cardiff-based performance artist Emily Underwood-Lee. The choice of case studies is intimately related to my own cancer journey – I was treated for testicular cancer in the US, but moved to the UK in pursuit of universal health care and worked artistically with cancer as a subject in the UK where currently based – but there is also significant exchange (both linguistically and visually) between the two national cancer conversations. Through a consideration of Notaro and Underwood-Lee's work, alongside the writing of theorist Audre Lorde and photographer Jo Spence, both working in the 1980s, this essay demonstrates that contemporary performance around cancer resists the more popular medical model of *cure cure cure fundraise fundraise fundraise*, and brings audiences together with cancer patients. Instead of just applauding 'patients' for simply kissing in a public space, audiences and artists together are celebrating a deeper understanding of illness and health.

As a young adult with cancer myself, although never with a terminal diagnosis, I experienced a strange relationship with the non-sick world, particularly as my cancer coincided with (then-unfallen-hero) Lance Armstrong's third Tour de France win in 2002. Casual conversations were filled with words like 'fight' and 'win' and 'beat this' and seemed to include both blanket encouragement – which derived from a socially constructed lexicon of cancer empathy phraseology – and total silence surrounding unfixable or uncomfortable problems, including sadness, diarrhoea, hairlessness and other biological and psychosocial effects of cancer treatment. Although I never tried kissing boys in Amsterdam to see if audiences would applaud me, I was pretty sure, that with my bald head, sunken eyes and post-surgical hunched posture, I could have got away with anything. Critical of these automated applauses, my earliest performance writings about cancer (in *BALL,* 2003, and *Other Funny Stories About Cancer*, 2006) purposefully played with an audience's expectations of how a cancer patient should behave, or really, what a cancer patient can get away with. For example, *BALL* depicts a just-cured twenty-one-year-old Brian wishing the destruction of eight-year-old girls competing against him in a Cancer Survivor Picnic Hula Hoop Contest; *Other Funny Stories About Cancer* focuses on the misogynistic quest of Brian – in a story originally cut from *BALL* – to lose his virginity via any available woman's body.

I did not want to be on the receiving end of people's kindness, nor did I want to be stared at continually out of worry, or because my illness inspired others to live more fully and love more deeply. I just wanted to be in space with other people in the most honest and non-pre-determined manner that I could without, as I called it, pre-praise, or the *a priori* approval and exaltation of all actions of all cancer patients. In this regard, cancer patients are quite distinct from those living with other chronic, serious or invisible illnesses and disabilities – such as HIV/AIDS, mental illness and epilepsy – who may face serious medical interventions in their lives, without either the patronizing sentiment or the financial or emotional support that pre-praise may engender. While this wish to be seen not through a pre-praising lens is relevant for many marginalized identities, very rarely has having cancer – as opposed to being black, being a woman or being disabled – been understood as being a distinct identity in dialogue with audiences who may or may not share commonalities. While film and television have explored cancer as topics or plot devices on selected occasions (*50/50*, *The Big C* and *The Fault in Our Stars* in just the past few years), this distinct relationship between the bodies with cancer and an applauding, caring or tastefully disengaged audience is something that live performance and theatre have been radically refiguring.

The current landscape of cancer is dominated by a number of distinct themes and characteristics including, but not at all limited to: gendered fundraising campaigns for gendered cancers (Movember, Coppafeel, Test One Two and many more); fundraising through physical challenges (Race for the Cure, Light the Night); and a policed positivity around mental attitude and survivorship, as documented by Barbara Ehrenreich's *Bright-Sided: How Positive Thinking is Undermining America* (2009), evidenced by Tara Parker-Pope's *Picture Your Life After Cancer* (2012) and LIVESTRONG, and specifically targeted by recent campaigns by Macmillan and Stupid Cancer. Controversies about cancer abound in the news in both the US and the UK, such as, recently in the US, Susan G. Komen's problematic relationship with branding and political groups seen as anti-women's health and/or corporations whose products are carcinogenic. Pancreatic Cancer UK's recent and deeply unsettling 'I Wish I Had Breast Cancer' Campaign (2014) pitted different cancers, of various 'sexiness' or public profile, against one another in the hope of demonstrating inequality in funding and research.

Each contemporary cancer controversy is met with a firestorm of personal, passionate and often coordinated responses, with a handful of organizations and charities – such as the American Cancer Association or Cancer Research UK – quickly dominating the editorials, the tweets and the viral videos shared with urgency and high emotion. Just as those who participate in Movember or Race for Life often have a specific point of inspiration (an ailing friend, a deceased parent), the response to cancer (which gets played out mostly over social media and popular press) nearly always employs the 'I' or 'my' – the personal connection to illness being the prompt for the emotional or political interjection.

What nearly all of the current controversies and themes around cancer conversations share is the medical model of understanding illness and the need, above all else, to fix what is malignant (or broken) about the body and to get back to a normal – an understanding of the body that is stable, fixed and recognizable as healthy and high functioning. The Cure will find a way to stop the body ever being sick, and Living Strong will allow those with a history of illness to integrate seamlessly back amongst the non-ill majority, for example, a most popular goal that is only recently being reconfigured by organizations like Teenage Cancer Trust who are undertaking significant discussions about post-illness being a space of new normality.[10] The central argument, however, against the application of a purely medical model to understanding cancer is twofold: first, as argued by Siddhartha Mukherjee in *The Emperor of All Maladies* (2010), cancer is a completely normal part of our existence – it grows from our cells and demonstrates cells that have fought against mortality; and second, the goal of *fix and return to normal* is nearly impossible for all cancer patients – bodies are permanently altered, relationships are changed, sexual function is often affected, financial hardships occur, permanent scarring dominates, and many remain on long-term chemotherapy or immunotherapy treatments.

As charted by Lennard Davis, under the medical model, 'people with disabilities were seen variously as poor, destitute creatures in need of the help of the Church or as helpless victims of disease in need of correction offered by modern medical procedures.'[11] Socio-politically, the medical model of disability was popularly seen as repressive and unhelpful, as it promoted the idea that all impairment was an impetus for medical intervention. Contrarily, the social model offered a new perspective, as Davis writes: 'Not plagued by God nor beset by disease, people with disabilities were seen as minority citizens deprived of their rights by a dominant able-ist majority.'[12] Understanding Davis's rubric for the employment of medical or social models of disability, it becomes clear how illness sits uncomfortably next to current disability discourses, especially with regard to his statement, above, about charity. While disability activists have demonstrated a difficult relationship with charity, cancer activists have embraced it and they are running for it,[13] standing up for it,[14] baking for it[15] and even 'motorboating' women's breasts in public for it.[16] Disabled activists eschewing models of charity – evidenced extensively in the writing of both Kuppers and Rosemarie Garland-Thomson and the arts practice of Katherine Araniello (one half of Disabled Avant-Garde) in her performance *Charity Collection Doll* (2013) among others – are at distinct odds with approaches where charity *is* the modus operandi, in terms of both medical funding and ancillary cancer care. While in the UK, disabled activists treat the word 'handicapped' as offensive because of its relationship to the practice of enforced begging for disabled people, cancer patients and those raising money on their behalf seem very comfortable asking for money on the streets, or going door to door.

While the political trajectory of the disability movement – from the Americans with Disabilities Act in the US to the Independent Living Fund in the UK – has embraced a wide range of individuals with a wide range of disabilities, the political trajectory of the cancer community has been splintered, particularly because of the medical model of understanding cancer. In hopes of fixing the problem and returning to 'normal', cancer patients have rarely fought for justice in the same way that individuals with disability have fought for more access and more legal protections. Even among cancer charities during the US's passing of the Affordable Care Act (2010), which greatly benefitted young adults with cancer and cancer histories, few voices were present or passionate. This lack of activism may have many different origins, such as the myopia that cancer (through extensive and exhausting treatments) causes and the lack of language to discuss cancer. It is clear, however, that a dependence on charity and goodwill (and a disinclination to alienate donors through controversial politics) demonstrates that the medical model of understanding disability, as applied to cancer, may – just as it did for disabled people – prevent particular forms of activism. This has not gone unnoticed by those critical of 'awareness'-raising schemes such as pink ribbon campaigns, called out as early as 1998 by Sandy M. Fernandez in the now-defunct *MAMM Magazine*, who focused attention on the relationship between consumerism and fundraising, and the lack of metrics put in place to assess the efficacy of awareness-raising campaigns.[17]

There are a number of clear and passionate outliers who have demonstrated that cancer patients can be ardent activists who are capable of embracing more than Talcott Parson's passive 'sick role', which includes, as described by Arthur W. Frank, a patient's full submission to doctors and their orders.[18] As chronicled in Mukherjee's *The Emperor of All Maladies*, during the 1980s and 1990s, breast cancer activists were particularly emboldened by ACT UP and other HIV/AIDS activists who chanted 'Drugs into bodies; drugs into bodies' to insist upon easier access to chemotherapy and an end to extensive double-blind studies.[19] More than simply a search for a medical cure, these activists spoke passionately about health inequalities, particularly for women, and demanded more critical consideration of health advocacy, funding and treatment.

When a surgeon drew an X on London-based photographer Jo Spence's breast – insisting that she have a mastectomy immediately – Spence leapt (for the first time of many times) out of her 'sick role' and into her position as empowered patient responding to top-down, expertise-laden medical treatment, as documented in her series *The Picture of Health* (1982).[20] Cultural theorist and activist Audre Lorde, in the US, recalled similarly disempowering medical treatment: 'Now that the doctors here have decided I have liver cancer, they insist on reading all their findings as if that were a *fait accompli*. They refuse to look for any other reason for the irregularities in the X-rays, and they're treating my resistance to their diagnosis as a personal affront.'[21] Spence and Lorde both wrote about their personal interventions in these processes – either engaging in alternative therapies or refusing chemotherapy altogether. Both women exemplify the moments of rare and powerful activism that allies them to a social model of understanding disability – reminding their audiences (doctors in the immediate sense and later readers or gallery viewers) that the cure that they sought was part of a much larger tapestry of understanding civil rights: the rights of women, the rights of people of colour and the rights of everyone to determine what happens to their own body. Perhaps the most inspiring revelation of Lorde and Spence's work was this specific breaking of the 'sick role' in which one is conceived of as only sick, only living in sickness and only dealing with sickness, to instead be full people who, despite illness, maintain their political sense of self and their other social identities. Not only were Lorde and Spence not *just* cancer patients, but they did not exist as cancer patients who could be easily applauded for simply being sick with cancer. Keenly aware of the gaze that stared at them, they both employed their work – photography and essay – to devise strategies to stare right back at audiences and those patronizing glances.

Garland-Thomson's *Staring* chronicles the methods and strategies in which a number of people with physical differences and disabilities respond to the look of others, altering the usually oppressive situation of the gaze or the gawk to be something more dialogic, a relationship between 'starer' and 'staree' that is ever-changing and may contain the possibility of equality.[22] Her writing provides an exciting starting point for understanding how cancer patients might also be reconfiguring their relationship to those around them who may be discomforted by their physical and emotional presence in a space. While most media representations deal with cancer as a singular subject, which is medical, needing to be fixed and which warrants pre-praise, both Notaro and Underwood-Lee are using the live body in live theatrical space to reconfigure a passive gaze into a more strategic staring relationship: I see you, seeing me.

Los Angeles-based writer and comedian Notaro's 2012 stand-up set at Largo became an overnight sensation, with viral exposure and instantaneous praise from comics such as Louis C.K..[23] Her bold approach hides nothing from her audiences, walking on stage and starting with:

> Hello. Good evening, hello. I have cancer, how are you? Hi, how are you, is everybody having a good time? I have cancer, how are you? It's a good time. Diagnosed with cancer. It feels good. *Just* diagnosed with cancer. Oh god. Oh my god. It's weird because with humor, the equation is, 'tragedy plus time equals comedy.' I am just at tragedy right now. That's just where I am in the equation …[24]

The audience laughs with a palpable discomfort, seemingly unsure of the truth of Notaro's claims (But why would she lie?), or unsure if they should be laughing or even listening to this supposedly-personal, devastating disclosure. Notaro instantly picks up on the discomfort and plays with it, saying 'Relax, everything's fine, I have cancer.' As she tells the story of her previous week, with familiar cancer plot points of mammograms, biopsies and pains, she returns to talking directly to an audience member: 'Somebody over here just keeps going, "Ooh, ooh, I think she might really have cancer." Who is taking this really bad? Oh, it's ok. It's going to be ok. It might not be ok, but I am just saying "It's ok. You're going to be ok, I don't know what's going on with me."' As the story unfolds, Notaro continually returns to the audience, their reactions to her tale – sometimes they laugh too hard, other times they are too nervous for her. While characters Hazel Grace and Gus took their audience's sympathy as a given, Notaro plays on their interconnection. When she announces that her mother has died (tragically, she adds) just months ago, the audience becomes even more silent, which prompts her to ask 'Should I leave? It's ok, you didn't know her,' and plays on the sympathy of cancer and of people's inability to take in too much tragedy at a given time. Instead of cancer as an isolated, medical issue, Notaro's interaction with her audience extends the frame, realizing the 'cancer patient' identity as one that functions in relation to others. Had her work been the pitch of a fundraiser or profile of a 'cancer patient', the focus of the story would be purely hers, but here Notaro is generous and dialogic: she uses the audience's groans and laughter as the subject of the comedy itself, alerting the audience to understanding that *her* cancer disclosure and *their* audience discomfort are both interconnected and funny. In other words, the humour and the discomfort are mutually reinforcing. As she finishes her set, she notices that the audience has become quieter. 'I really don't mean to bum you out …' she says, and asks 'What if I were just to transition into some silly jokes?' The crowd yells a decisive 'No!' and she parrots right back: 'No, I want to hear more bad news! I'm sorry now that I don't have more bad news to share …'

Embracing the awkwardness of cancer diagnoses, disclosures and speaking about the unspeakable in public, Notaro has moved her audience from passive receptors of her *inspirational* cancer journey to become active allies who are supportive, critical and integral to the process of her coming to terms with this brand new identity. Without demanding a fundraiser or asking even for a cure, Notaro's comedy, and its live engagement with an audience, demonstrates the possibility for performance to move the cancer body from being something that is gawked at to something that is spoken with – and from the cheers and thank yous given from both Notaro and her audience, it appears that this speaking *with* is incredibly powerful and ultimately essential. Despite the fact that Underwood-Lee begins *Titillation* in a hospital gown, her performance remains far away from the medical model of understanding cancer. In the short performance, cancer is barely mentioned in its medical reality, but is instead linked into the process of learning (and unlearning, as she says) to be a woman. Like Notaro, Underwood-Lee is explicitly aware of her audience, playing and teasing them about her breasts and their ultimate revelation.

> As I said I'm here to talk about breasts, I've always thought my own breasts were rather fabulous [*Cup breasts and strike a pose*]. These aren't them though, these are the fake ones. I'll take them off later and show you. I lost the real ones. It's not really like I misplaced them [*Clasp chest – shocked face*]. 'Oh no – where could they be!' I suppose they were more taken away than lost. They've gone anyhow.

The revelation of post-mastectomy breasts or chest has been, and remains, an important trope in art about cancer (beginning with Matuschka's 'Beauty Out of Damage' photograph for the *New York Times*, 1993,[25] and including more recent works such as David Jay's *The Scar Project*, 2011)[26] and in cancer activism, with artists such as Tania Katan defending her right to run topless in breast cancer fundraising marathons (as documented in her book *My One-Night Stand with Cancer*, 2005).[27] Nudity, and the revelation of the nude body with cancer, was a theme repeated extensively after introduced in Margaret Edson's 1999 Pulitzer Prize winning play *Wit*. In my own work, *BALL*, I joked with the audience about forthcoming nudity: 'I can't show you really [what it's like to get a genital ultrasound] because then I'd have to be naked, and I don't want to give away the ending …'[28]

Underwood-Lee's text looks less at her journey through cancer, or its related treatment, and more through the process of becoming a woman, and, as she says 'forgetting how to be a woman'. She achieves this by linking not to the story of her own cancer, but to the story of Patrick Swayze, who died of pancreatic cancer in 2009. By charting her adoration of Swayze, and his heartthrob portrayal of Johnny Knight in *Dirty Dancing* (1987), Underwood-Lee removes the medical questions of cancer and leaves us, instead, with a thoughtful reflection on femininity, feminism and how women's bodies are seen and revealed in public space. The usual coyness around the nude cancer body may be exemplified by the final stage direction of *Wit* which reads, '*The instant she is naked, and beautiful, reaching for the light – Lights out.*'[29] In contrast, at the end of *Titillation*, Underwood-Lee removes her false breasts (with tassels covering the nipples), removes her top and simply stands in front of the audience. At Underwood-Lee's performance at *Fem Fresh* (Queen Mary College, University of London, 2014), the audience remained absolutely still during this final encounter with her body – it didn't demand an audience be sad about her body (and the soundtrack of Depeche Mode's 'Shake the Disease' was distinctly meant to disrupt any kind of sympathetic reading), but the body also did not ease anyone's comfort about her life and future as a woman with cancer. Her final line – 'Patrick never got better and I don't know if I will, but right now, I'm still here' – exemplifies Underwood-Lee's deeply ambiguous ending image, which is more about presence and her changing body than it is about cancer and its treatment. This final image provides audiences with yet another new relationship with cancer bodies, one that bucks the trend of inspiring or cathartic narratives to one that is open, uncomfortable and unendingd. As perhaps a direct parallel to Underwood-Lee's open-ended cancer treatment, her refusing an audience the opportunity to feel wholly happy or wholly sad about her condition provides an unsettling portrayal which, much like Notaro's, tells us that we are all here together. We don't know where this is all going (the performance, the treatment) but we're all here together, and our potential discomfort with her lack of narrative closure, much like Notaro's play on the audience's awkwardness, is itself the aesthetic and political subject of this cancer performance.

The work of Tig Notaro and Emily Underwood-Lee, as well as that of Jo Spence and Audre Lorde, is applauded not out of pre-praise for cancer patients, but owing to their radical stance against the cancer patient being prescribed to their sick role, and their recognition that their experiences are inherently linked to how society views and discusses cancer. By observing their incisive artistic and theoretical outputs, possibilities abound beyond the simplistic models of *cure cure cure fundraise fundraise fundraise*, and a more critical approach can be taken to consider the content created by those experiencing cancer, currently seen as a place beyond criticality. While the social model of understanding disability has catalysed a community of empowered disabled thinkers and artists, the medical model currently burdening the understanding of cancer prevents the majority of patients from feeling that their experiences – outside the inspirational or tragic – deserve space in public discourse. Although young adults with cancer may feel thankful for *The Fault in Our Stars* taking on the subject of teenagers with illness, and many do, performers and thinkers who question the distance between patients and the expectations placed upon them to perform their illness in public space provide examples for not only how to live sick, but for how the sick can live with those who are not – and, ultimately, for us all to live together.

7.3 Snapshot – *Alive and Out There* – Theatre addressing stigma around cancer in diverse communities in Sydney, Australia

Astrid Perry and Lynne Baker

The Multicultural Health Service[30] in Sydney has used Applied Theatre as a health promotion tool, reaching diverse communities. In earlier projects the theatre addressed topics of mental health and domestic violence. The impetus to raise awareness of cancer and stigma through theatre stemmed from the success of a previous project, *Fear and Shame*. Performed in 2008 to 1,600 people over eight performances, this play had explored stigma and mental health in the Macedonian-speaking community in Sydney. The play depicted a young man, Alex Petkovski, developing the symptoms of schizophrenia. Initially his dysfunctional family call in a spiritual healer and a priest who, using 'incantations potions and prayers', fail to change Alex's behaviour.[31] Alex is eventually admitted to a psychiatric ward, but the shame and stigma of this cause his family to become even more dysfunctional. The play then charts the growth of understanding and acceptance by his family and immediate community. Interviews with audience members showed that after viewing *Fear and Shame* they reported increased confidence in seeking help, talking about mental health with others and engaging with the medical system,[32] important factors in overcoming stigma and encouraging timely access to appropriate health care.

The *Alive and Out There* project was led by the Multicultural Health Service, South Eastern Sydney Local Health District and funded by the Cancer Institute NSW. The programme's activities substantiate the case for the use of theatre as a health promotion tool because post-evaluation data shows that audiences understood key messages clearly, the large audience numbers reached and participants who reported enjoyment of the plays.[33] Theatre was chosen by the Multicultural Health Service on its merits as a multisensory educational medium as shown in the *Fear and Shame* evaluations. Theatre has the capacity to address many facets of learning, and interacts with people in a visceral and intellectual way.[34]

Alive and Out There comprised three separate plays targeting cancer-related stigma specifically for the Arabic-, Greek- and Macedonian-speaking communities. These are large communities within the local area, who tend to have lower than average rates of participation in cancer screening programmes[35] and can be hard to reach for health promotion,[36] but who also have a history of participation in community theatre.[37,38]

The cultural authenticity of the plays was important in engaging with the three communities. The development of the plays necessitated identifying the groups' perceptions about cancer through community focus groups so that the theatre pieces were informed by an evolutionary process that allowed for testing of concepts and their use in the plays. Oncology professionals were also consulted regarding the inclusion of clinical themes, such as participation in screening and early intervention. An interactive and collaborative process was adopted to facilitate an informative and culturally appropriate outcome.[39] The plays were individually developed for and with each community, because the style of theatre and the way stigma may be dealt with in each community could be quite different.

Each play focused on one or two types of cancers: prostate, bowel, breast and cancer in general. The methodology for writing the plays varied. The Arabic-speaking group involved two performing artists who wrote and produced the play and hired professional actors for one week to rehearse the play prior to the performances. The Greek group developed their broad storyline with the potential amateur cast in an all-day workshop, with the playwright drafting the script afterwards. The playwright for the Macedonian group developed the script from the content of focus groups and tested it with the amateur theatre group.

The plays were performed up to fifteen times each in theatre or community venues in locations where the communities reside in large numbers. The uniqueness of each play can be seen in the titles and storylines used:

Burra Wa Ba'eed ... Out and Away: Alissar Chidiac and Saleh Saqqaf wrote, directed and produced this play with support from the Urban Theatre Project through the company's SPACE Residency Program.[40] Adapted from a real event, this play told the tale of a woman searching for a missing friend who had admitted herself to hospital for cancer treatment and told her friends and relatives that she was going on holiday. The plot illustrates the extent of stigma in some members of the Arabic-speaking community.

Zoe's Gift: This play was written by Melba Papas, directed by Stavros Economidis, produced by Evelyn Tsavalas and performed by the Hellenic Art Theatre.[41] *Zoe's Gift* was a dramatic comedy about family secrets and explored themes around breast cancer and genetic conditions. To provide additional messages about cancer, the plot incorporated a talkback radio scene depicting a doctor answering a range of questions.

Wrestling the Bear: This play was written by Dushan Ristevski, directed by Stefo Nantsou and performed by the Australian Macedonian Theatre of Sydney.[42] The play revolved around two Macedonian men and their families dealing with cancer, illustrating their struggles to cope with and tell others about their serious illness.

The benefits and impact of *Alive and Out There* were numerous and significant. Audience feedback indicated comprehension of messages about cancer and health services, and the intention to share these messages with families and communities. The actors and playwrights also reported increased knowledge about cancer and a greater appreciation of the health care system. Previous success with using community theatre was also reinforced. The Arabic community were enthusiastic about continuing to use theatre for health promotion, and the Greek group have produced another play targeting mental health. The Macedonian production toured nationally and to Macedonia, and the company has since collaborated with the Arabic group for a new play on community harmony. The collaborative approach used throughout the project encouraged these three communities to interact and get to know each other.

8

Women's Health and Gender Inequity: Experiences from India, Malawi and the Solomon Islands

8.1 Introduction

Veronica Baxter

The World Health Organization (WHO) is very clear on the specific issues that most affect women's health and wellbeing – first among them is the inequality between the sexes, and poverty.[1] In the Global South predominant attitudes towards women's health include viewing it as less important than men's, unless it has to do with sexual reproduction. As a result of inequality, women face unemployment owing to limited education opportunities or because cultural norms require them to be homebound. The cycle of poverty is thus repeated with young girls receiving less education, and then going into poorly paid employment.

An important aspect of gender inequality is the threat of violence against women and girls, including domestic or partner violence and the prevalence of rape in our society. The WHO suggests that 35 per cent of women globally have experienced sexual violence. The prevalence of child marriage, adolescent pregnancies, modern-day slavery and sexual and body-part trafficking of girls and women are all urgent issues, particularly facing the Global South.[2] Women's bodies are increasingly commodified in baby factories for the market in illegal adoptions, as well as for 'womb hire'.[3] Women have many challenges to their health and wellbeing, particularly in the Global South.

In this chapter, these challenges for women and society are discussed through the lens of theatre projects in India, Malawi and the Solomon Islands. Nandita Dinesh examines Darpana Academy of Performing Arts and their process and production of *Shakti*. Dinesh 'reads' the production through Amartya Sen's 'capabilities approach' and 'perception bias'. This throws new light on *Shakti*'s impact and the capacity of theatre to engage with complexity.

Effie Makepeace discusses a Malawian project, instigated by local medical research into the high incidence of burns. Women in the domestic environment mostly deal with burns, and the theatre project demonstrated how to assess burns for severity, and the appropriate treatment, including taking the victim to the hospital if the burns are severe. Makepeace's discussion includes a hopeful account of local women developing their skills, creating employment and providing mutual support for each other.

Finally, Kiara Worth introduces a far-reaching project in the Solomon Islands that aims to empower women through workshops in theatre narrating their experiences of domestic violence. Through an account of seeing a Stages of Change production, and an interview with director Nina Nawalowalo, Worth highlights the urgency for women to have their problem addressed.

Theatre as a means of countering the inequity of wealth and treatment of the sexes, violence against girls and women, and the mental and physical dis-ease amongst women, can have limited impact, despite the urgency for solutions. These writers demonstrate theatre's role in forging a hopeful path forward.

8.2 Essay – The ambiguities of *Shakti*: Performing women's wellbeing in India[4]

Nandita Dinesh

This essay is framed by one principal question around women's health and wellbeing: what are the implications of an Applied Theatre project that focuses on a woman's capabilities rather than her vulnerabilities? Dominant narratives that speak to a woman's wellbeing in India tend to focus on what she does *not* have access to: be it safety, health care services, education or the inheritance of land. However, while these narratives are significant in catalysing awareness of the roadblocks to a woman's wellbeing in the subcontinent, there is considerably less attention paid in these narratives of victimhood to what women's strengths might be; what their capabilities are. With this in mind, this essay focuses on an Applied Theatre project from the repertoire of the Darpana Academy of Performing Arts (Darpana). As an academy that is renowned for its use of Applied Theatre in addressing issues that affect women's health and wellbeing, Darpana creates work precisely with the premise of drawing attention to women's strength. In this essay therefore, one of Darpana's Applied Theatre projects (*Shakti*) is framed by Amartya Sen's ideas on the 'capabilities approach'.[5] This framework examines how gender-based perception biases highlight the ambiguities that surround a woman's wellbeing, focusing on what she does want to accomplish rather than what she cannot.

In contrast to narratives that frame women's wellbeing as being defined by a relative lack of resources, privileges and/or opportunities that are available to men, Sen postulates that judging 'advantage by capabilities focuses directly on a person's ability to do the various things that he or she may wish to do'.[6] In this approach, instead of looking at factors (such as life expectancy and nutrition) that highlight a woman's comparative disadvantages, Sen asks his readers to contemplate the 'complex functionings' that might define a woman's wellbeing in her context.[7] In these complex functionings, Sen includes factors such as 'achieving self-respect, taking part in the life of the community and appearing in public without shame'.[8] Building on this idea, Sen underscores the notion that what women might wish to accomplish vis-à-vis their complex functionings in a context is related to what is perceived as being possible for them to achieve in that context – both by the women themselves and by their communities. It is these intersections between perception biases and capabilities that form the crux of this essay's borrowing from Sen. Furthermore, given that Sen's approach to women's wellbeing is focused on a woman's *shakti*, that is, on her strength and capabilities rather than the lack thereof, Sen's ideas provide a particularly relevant lens through which to analyse Darpana's strategies in their Applied Theatre initiative, *Shakti* (2009).

Darpana articulates the desired impact of *Shakti* by stating that the effects of this initiative will 'be apparent in perhaps a year or two years when we see whether the young girls who are 15 now do in fact postpone the age of marriage; when we see whether some of the women are demanding that their land is transferred to their names'.[9] While Darpana's articulation of *Shakti*'s impact involves the expectations of long-term changes in particular indicators that might signify an improvement in women's wellbeing in the region, what might a Sen-inspired analysis reveal? By using Sen's ideas around the intersections between perception biases and capabilities to frame a reading of *Shakti*, this essay seeks to examine the specific strategies that Darpana utilizes to identify and perform the prejudices that influence women's wellbeing in the Chota Udaipur region of western India. Furthermore, the essay considers the ways in which *Shakti*'s articulation of these biases seeks to question deeply entrenched traditions and to generate a more nuanced understanding of women's capabilities in that context. In so doing, the aim is to put forth the potential of *Shakti* as not necessarily lying in the long-term changes that it might generate but rather in the complexities and ambiguities that the initiative reveals about the influence of perception biases on women's capabilities and wellbeing in the region.

Darpana

From a small dance academy that was founded over six decades ago, Darpana today is a workshop for multiple arts-based programmes.[10] Its departments conduct a range of activities: the creation and performance of professional dance/drama pieces that tour regionally, nationally and internationally; the teaching of various art forms to participants in the city of Ahmedabad; the use of theatre as a tool for development (the focus of this essay); and the production of television, film and other audio-visual material to support the larger goals of the organization.[11] When a number of Darpana's departments began to be contracted by external agencies in the early 1980s for outreach projects related to development issues and agendas, the Darpana for Development programme was officially created 'to spread social awareness/empowerment through the media of performing arts'.[12]

Shakti is a project that emerged from Darpana's Acting Healthy initiative, which sought to address health issues faced by villages in the Chota Udaipur region of Gujarat. By training local actors in the local folk theatre form of *Bhavai* – an aesthetic that is known for its bringing together of satire, social commentary and ritual – a script was written 'based on research done of the understanding, and the tribal customs, which prevented healthy deliveries in the area'.[13] What emerged through the Acting Healthy project was a reflection for Darpana members and actors alike about the gender-related perception biases that lie behind questions surrounding the region's high infant and maternal mortality rates. Upon becoming acutely aware of the various ways in which these biases intersect with notions of women's wellbeing, Darpana created *Shakti* as a sequel to the Acting Healthy initiative. Created as an episodic piece that highlights various issues that affect women in Chota Udaipur – the young age at which girls are expected to get married, to name the most important – *Shakti* uses theatre and song to catalyse a discussion with its spectators. The results of the *Shakti* project, as mentioned in Darpana's documentation about the work, is expected to be seen in the long term with the barometer of *Shakti*'s success being a reduction in the average age at which girls in these villages of Chota Udaipur get married.[14]

I was fortunate enough to be involved with the initial stages of the *Shakti* project, particularly the brainstorming and execution of the initial auditions/workshops that were implemented in order to recruit and train actor-activists from Chota Udaipur. However, this essay also incorporates archival research about the later stages of the project and personal encounters that have nuanced my insights into the group's goals and strategies.

Resonances: Darpana and Amartya Sen

Speaking about a health survey conducted in Singur, a village near the city of Calcutta in the north-eastern region of India, Sen speaks to how illness is understood differently between men and women in that locality. Analysing the responses from the widows and widowers who contributed to the study, Sen presents the startling statistic that 48.5 per cent of the men spoke of having health afflictions, while only 2.5 per cent of the women admitted to being unwell.[15] When further considering responses as to whether 'one was in "indifferent" health, leaving out the category or being "ill" for which some clear-cut medical criteria do exist', Sen states that 45–46 per cent of the men in Singur perceived themselves as being in indifferent health, while not one woman perceived herself as such.[16] Questioning the reasons behind this significant difference in the two groups' articulation of their wellbeing, Sen argues that the disparity in men and women's expression of their wellness, and subsequently their understanding of their capabilities, might be linked to a perception bias – a perception bias that influences women to see themselves as being less disadvantaged even when faced with the same physical circumstances as their male counterparts. While this quality of the women's responses could be presented simply as evidence of their endurance, Sen argues that the non-perception of relative disadvantages 'of a deprived group helps to perpetuate those disadvantages'.[17] Sen states, as a result, that 'perception bias is an important aspect of the problem of the wellbeing of the Indian woman'.[18] Mozaffar Qizilbash underlines the importance of this contribution, that is that Sen's 'arguments about positional objectivity – and women's undervaluation of their own wellbeing and health' is intricately linked to how women's status in a context might be evaluated and understood.[19]

In reiterating the point that 'women may have no clear perception of being deprived of things that men have',[20] Sen draws from another study that he conducted with Jocelyn Kynch. In this study, Sen and Kynch analyse the admissions data from two large public hospitals in Bombay. Sen notes from this investigation that 'it was very striking to find clear evidence that the admitted girls were typically more ill than the boys, suggesting that a girl has to be more stricken and more ill before she is taken to the hospital'.[21] What this finding indicates – like the Singur study – is that a young girl is more likely to be seen as/ to see herself as being healthy, despite embodying the same physical symptoms as a male counterpart; a likelihood that then hinders a nuanced understanding of what it might mean for a woman to be well in that context. Therefore, when dealing with correlations between women's wellbeing and their capabilities, Sen argues that 'there is a need to go beyond the question of the agency of women and to look for a more critical assessment of received values',[22] begging the question that when a girl is told/thinks that she is well even though she might be as physically ill as a male counterpart, how does this impact the girl's understanding of her capabilities?

Once biases in perception have been identified, we begin to see the impact of these biases on how a woman's capabilities are understood both by herself and by those around her. In light of this complexity, Sen suggests that since 'mothers themselves' are not immune from 'the hold of traditional masculinist values', what is necessary is not only 'freedom of action but also freedom of thought – the freedom to question and to scrutinize inherited beliefs and traditional priorities'.[23] When framing *Shakti* with Sen's ideas around capabilities, there are two overarching points: (1) the perception biases that are addressed in *Shakti* and the strategy that Darpana uses to excavate these biases in Chota Udaipur; (2) *Shakti*'s attempts to provoke specific target groups in their audiences to question inherited beliefs and traditions.

Beginning with the perception biases that Darpana highlights, there are multiple instances in *Shakti* where the script takes on women's wellbeing in Chota Udaipur through the use of obvious catchphrases like 'My friend, we need to treat boys and girls equally' and 'If you cheer the birth of a boy, why are you sad when a girl is born?'[24]

However, rather than these more direct instances that tell the audience what to do, how to think and how to act in the face of gender bias, there are other statements in *Shakti* that allude to complex perception biases in Chota Udaipur. For example, by drawing material from the interviews that led to the creation and performance of *Shakti*, a line in the play states, 'They don't believe their women, they doubt them all the time.'[25] A deceptively simple statement, this line points towards a significant perception bias that shapes what women see/are seen as being capable of achieving in Chota Udaipir. The exemplar line implies that not only is women's wellbeing in Chota Udaipur affected by the more obvious inequalities between men and women in their access to education, health care services and/or the ownership of land, but also what is overlooked is that there are less tangible and more complex functionings, like integrity and trustworthiness, that impact on what women are understood as being capable of.

Following this argument, if women are less likely to be trusted than men (generally) in the region, what might be some everyday manifestations of this mistrust? And how might these quotidian indicators subsequently impact on how a woman's capabilities are understood by herself and by those around her? Darpana brings up a common manifestation and repercussion of the mistrust of women by speaking of the suspicion that a woman is faced with if she takes a longer than expected time period to return to her household upon the completion of a chore outside the home. A statement like 'When you went to the well, you took two hours there. Do you have a lover who meets you there?'[26] highlights the mistrust with which women are viewed when carrying out a mundane task. By highlighting this occurrence, Darpana underscores a significant perception bias that impacts on a woman's articulation of what she wants to do (and her capabilities of doing so) in Chota Udaipur. If women are trusted less than men, by both men and women alike, what she sees herself as being capable of doing is irrevocably affected. The consequences of her choices for her life are thus dictated not only by what she wants to do and what she might be allowed to do, but also by what she is *trusted* to do. Inevitably then, the position that trust plays in how women's wellbeing and capabilities are understood in Chota Udaipur begins to interlace with the access that women have to educational opportunities. Therefore, when *Shakti* asks its audiences to educate young women instead of getting them married young, if a woman is seen as being less trustworthy, how will she be allowed to access educational opportunities that could potentially remove her from the controlling gaze of family and friends for extended periods of time? As a character in *Shakti* says, 'If this girl goes out for further education, she will be spoiled!'[27] Therefore, the relatively fewer opportunities in education for women in Chota Udaipur, which in turn links to the young age at which girls are arranged into marriages in the region, are shaped by what women can/cannot be trusted to do (by themselves and by those around them) with that education.

In addition to trust, *Shakti* considers how perception biases around a woman's worth influence her access to education. The questions that families ask, when faced with issues about investing in the education of their girl children, are articulated as, for example: 'She'll need books, clothes, and so much more! I am not going to pay a single penny for that. She'll be educated. And even if she gets a job, what is the benefit to us? She'll go to her in-laws. What do we get?'[28] Since a woman in Chota Udaipur is seen as ultimately benefiting her in-laws' home, her parents are less likely to see her education as being a worthy financial investment for them. Subsequently, once the married woman or girl goes to her in-laws' home, she is not allowed to take on educational opportunities either – because she is not seen as being trustworthy. Seeking to raise the age at which young girls in Chota Udaipur get married is not then about a simplistic advocating for education. Rather, it is about taking into account the ways in which the various stakeholders in a woman's life, and the woman herself, perceive her worth and her integrity.

In contrast with mainstream narratives about violence against women in India, which tend to present simplistic binaries between men and women in the subcontinent, Darpana's approach in *Shakti* presents more nebulous terrain. This unclear territory, which reveals questions related to how women are (not) trusted and (not) considered worthy, forces spectators to encounter perception biases that do not oversimplify the roadblocks to a woman's achievement of her wellbeing. Instead, by scripting and staging perception biases, *Shakti* performs a complexity in discourses surrounding a woman's wellbeing and goes beyond the victim–perpetrator or woman–man binary. While the dimensions added by the presence of these perception biases in *Shakti* warrants discussion in and of itself, it is important to mention the specific strategy that Darpana employs so as to achieve this complexity: an information-gathering–creation–performance–feedback loop:

By using this loop of strategies, Darpana begins their Acting Healthy project with a series of interviews to ascertain the causes behind unhealthy deliveries in the region. This process of interviewing various respondents in Chota Udaipur coincides with workshops to train local actors in theatre techniques, both of which reveal to Darpana the intersections between maternal mortality rates and widely held biases vis-à-vis gender.

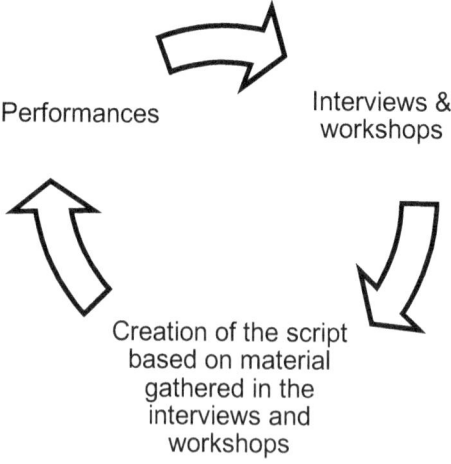

Figure 5: Darpana's creation–performance–feedback loop in *Acting Healthy* & *Shakti*.

The piece that is subsequently created and performed in the Acting Healthy initiative, therefore, includes commentaries about these gender biases – biases that are further discussed with audience members after performances. The outcomes of these post-performance conversations and further interviews then provide fodder for *Shakti*, where again the first round of performances are followed by encounters that reveal how young women themselves define their wellbeing in terms of their marital status. This revelation consequently becomes the primary stimulus for the second round of performances in the *Shakti* initiative, which specifically targets the age at which girls get married in Chota Udaipur and the related roadblocks to a woman's access to educational opportunities. By using this consistent feedback loop between information-gathering, script creation and performance, Darpana seeks to constantly excavate the complexities surrounding how women are perceived in Chota Udaipur.

Shakti is centred on inspiring a freedom to question and scrutinize beliefs. This objective is further explained by Darpana as the desire to create a project 'that would provide a sketch of the prevalence' of gender-biased attitudes and 'track changes' in these mindsets 'over time'.[29] In addition to using the information-gathering–creation–performance loop to present the complexities caused by perception biases, *Shakti* seeks to address women's wellbeing by asking their audiences to question whether girls in Chota Udaipur should get married at a young age. From the surveys that provide the content for the prequel to *Shakti*, in other words the Acting Healthy project, Darpana showcases interviews in which respondents make a number of statements that reveal deeply entrenched attitudes surrounding women, marriage and child-bearing. For instance, one woman speaks of her husband's desire to try for a boy despite the health risks that arise from her having a descended womb. Other respondents in the documentary speak of the importance of a boy child to maintain family lineage by inheriting property; others (men and women alike) speak of the necessity of a boy child to ensure the parents' wellbeing when they get older.[30] The perception biases that these statements indicate are clear: the inability to bear a boy child could lead to a woman's health being discounted. Furthermore, Darpana's documentary highlights statements made by young women who express their desire to get married young.[31] If only a married woman (who then bears male children) is seen as being well and successful in this cultural context, then the health risks from adolescent pregnancies will be viewed as secondary to the 'wellness and success' of adolescent marriage. The incapability of young girls to deal with the complications of marriage and motherhood are perhaps even irrelevant challenges. How does one question such strongly entrenched beliefs?

Shakti utilizes a message-based approach to inspire such a spirit of questioning in its spectators and these messages present an interesting multidimensionality that targets different members in their audience. For instance:

> You love this henna but soon it will lose its colour. You love this sari but soon it will lose its colour. You feel great wearing that necklace? In two or three days it will weigh you down.[32]

It doesn't mean that a girl should marry at a young age. She isn't mature enough. She won't know how to do the work. When she goes to her in-laws, she won't know how to behave. She's unable to handle the responsibilities of the family. It will go well for a few days. But after that, the fighting will begin.[33]

In both these examples, in order to address the perception bias towards marriage and the age of girls when they get married, the institution of marriage is questioned. By implicating the institution of marriage in women's wellbeing, *Shakti* presents two messages at the same time, for two different target groups in the audience: girls should be wary of marriage and get married later in their lives, when they are better equipped (possibly) to deal with spouses and new families. In the first example, *Shakti* presents a cognisance that it is not only a family's opinions that shape what a girl can/cannot or does/doesn't do; what is central is how the girl perceives marriage herself. *Shakti* therefore asks young girls to be wary about what they might be getting themselves into and in so doing, forces them to critically consider their perceptions of an event that is considered to be a woman's traditional priority in many parts of the Indian subcontinent.

With regard to the second example, *Shakti* reframes the discussion around a woman's access to education by focusing on the benefit of this expansion of her capabilities to her in-laws and children. Since a woman's wellbeing in Chota Udaipur is defined by those she benefits outside of herself, if *Shakti* were to speak of the importance of education for the woman herself – as an individual – the idea would be less likely to resonate. Therefore, *Shakti* speaks of the way in which an educated woman might benefit those around her, with the implication that a woman needs to be educated so as to be a better wife/daughter-in-law/ mother being possible evidence of Darpana's subversion. While asking girls to be wary of marriage could become potentially inflammatory in the context of Chota Udaipur, asking her to be wary of marriage with the qualification that if she is better educated and older she will make a better wife/daughter-in-law/mother seems to render the message more palatable. It might be said, then, that in order to provoke the freedom of thought that Sen deems necessary in battling perception biases, Darpana could not simply disagree with the perception bias in question. Rather, Darpana reframed the discussion in *Shakti* and positioned diversely framed statements to target particular subsections within the spectators about their perceptions of marriage.

By presenting the importance of education in benefiting a woman's in-laws while simultaneously asking young women to be wary of marriage, *Shakti* uses contextually relevant perceptions around marriage to reach two different target groups in their audience. In interviews that are recorded with spectators after the performances of *Shakti*, it becomes obvious that the particularity of this message resonates with spectators. For example, spectators to *Shakti* say the following: 'Girls should get married at 20 or 22. By doing that, they will make their child's life better'; 'It [the girl child's education] will benefit her and her in-laws.'[34] This interpretation of educating a girl child, while contentious, seems to stick with audiences precisely because *Shakti* presents education as being important to how women contribute to their homes: a possibly subversive tactic that seeks to catalyse a change in women's educational opportunities and marital ages, but within a framework that is relevant for their spectators.

As mentioned earlier, I place *Shakti* in conversation with Sen so as to consider the perception biases that *Shakti* addresses and to examine Darpana's approach in catalysing a freedom to question inherited beliefs. Going back to Sen's capabilities-based approach, where a woman's wellbeing is articulated in terms of what she wants to do and the capabilities that she might possess to achieve those goals, there are three primary aspects to flag from this analysis of *Shakti*. First, the perception biases that shape how a woman is (not) trusted influences the opportunities that she has access to, and as a result, how she frames what she might want to accomplish. Second, biases that influence perceptions of a woman's worth become significant in determining the age at which she gets married and the educational opportunities that become available to her. And finally, the biases that surround the deeply entrenched link between marriage and the perceptions of a woman's wellbeing impact on that which she seeks to become capable of achieving with her life.

Although *Shakti*'s script includes its fair share of clichés, catch-phrases and slogans, looking at this project through Sen's lenses presents a potentially rich resource with which to excavate nuances surrounding women's health and wellbeing. Sen's ideas might indeed allow Applied Theatre projects that target women's health and wellbeing to uncover the complexities that surround gender-based differences without simplifying them into binaries such as victim–perpetrator and oppressor–oppressed. Although this approach might present relatively more ambiguities when compared with a straightforward articulation of desired long-term changes – like a measurable increase in the average age at which girls get married in a particular locality – in the words of Sen, 'if an underlying idea has an essential ambiguity, a precise formulation of that idea must try to capture that ambiguity rather than attempt to lose it'.[35] It is this capturing of ambiguity and complexity, therefore, towards a larger goal of the precise formulation of what makes women well, that reveals potential when Applied Theatre projects that address women's wellbeing are framed by the intersections between Sen's approach to capabilities and perception biases.

8.3 Snapshot – Women's drama group in Malawi targets mothers and children for burns prevention

Effie Makepeace

In 2010, Nanzikambe Arts Development Organisation,[36] a Theatre for Development NGO in Blantyre, Malawi, was approached by a team of doctors from Scotland and the local hospital, Queen Elizabeth Central. They had received funding from UKAid to develop a much-needed paediatric burn-prevention strategy in Malawi.[37] The Reduction of Burns and Scalds in Children in Malawi (ReBaS) project focused on improving patient outcomes in the Blantyre burn unit and prevention at home, which Nanzikambe was commissioned to spearhead.

The project was unusual because of the close working connection with the hospital and the opportunity to employ a group of local young women. The group consisted of twenty women who had been identified as vulnerable and had attended weekly drama workshops with Nanzikambe for two years. They had drama skills, experience performing to large groups and a close community of support, trust and creativity.

Using data collected from patients admitted to the burn unit, ReBaS were able to determine common, recurring patterns of accident that led to burns and scalds in children similar to patterns seen across sub-Saharan Africa.[38,39] They also identified inappropriate or ineffective first-aid management of burns or scalds in the community, such as using traditional first-aid treatments that can cause infection.[40]

This information fed into the group's devising process enriched with personal experiences. It is recognized that women and girls are at a higher risk of burns, owing to the time spent near common heat sources in the home when cooking and heating water, and that targeting mothers is key to preventing child injury.[41,42,43] As mothers themselves, the group had direct experience of the issue, evident from their own scars and stories; one of the group members had lost a child due to burn injuries. Group members were paid for work on the project, and a savings cooperative was started within the group, with some starting small businesses.

The resulting performance of six short sketches highlighted key risks, with local songs rewritten with relevant lyrics. The sketches were high-energy, clearly drawn and entertaining. Fire was brought to life through props or through a group of singing, masked performers with red and yellow material tied to their limbs. At the point of crisis (a burns injury), a performer would 'freeze' the action to engage the audience in conversation about the events onstage. The conversations were informal and conversational in style – allowing the women to share experiences from the audience and advice from performers about what they had learnt from the doctors. Performances were strategically arranged to target mothers and children at pre- and post-natal clinics and primary schools. The reach of the performance was extended beyond a one-off by adding longer-lasting materials such as murals and take-home flyers for children to share with their parents.

Research was embedded in the project; admissions data were collected and analysed from the hospital, pre- and post-performance questionnaires, transect walks and focus group discussions with audience members up to six months after. Over three years there were fifty performances in Blantyre, reaching approximately 33,800 people, and more in a rural project extension in three districts. During the project, there was a decrease in the number of admissions to the burn unit and an increase in the correct use of first aid, with a reduction of inappropriate first aid applied.[44]

By using data on the aetiology of burn injuries and employing performers who have similar experiences to the audiences, the performance was deeply relevant to audiences and engaged them in the opportunity to share experiences with peers and form a shared understanding of practical solutions recommended by doctors which in turn positively impacted admissions at the burn unit.

8.4 Snapshot – *Stages of Change*: Using theatre to address domestic violence in the Solomon Islands

Kiara Worth

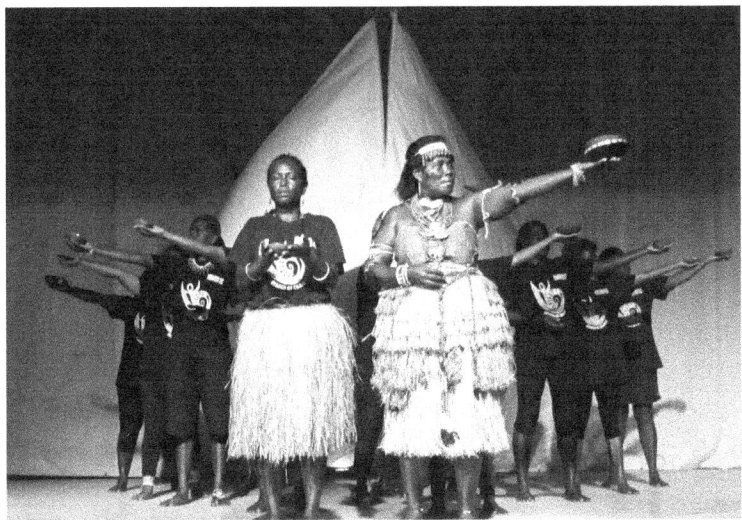

Figure 6: Women performing in *Stages of Change*, a theatre piece discussing domestic violence in the Solomon Islands. Photo © Kiara Worth.

The stage is dark, simply set with a series of white screens. One by one, candlelight appears behind each of the screens, silhouetting a woman within its frame; one is sweeping the floor, another stirring a pot, another rocking back and forth. The lights go out and there is the sound of skin slapping skin, a stifled groan and a gasp for breath. A black screen rolls across the stage, clearing the montage, wiping away the activities and the signs of violence hidden behind them.

This is the opening scene from *Stages of Change*, a socially reflective performance piece at the Melanesian Arts and Cultural Festival in Papua New Guinea in July 2014. The performance is part of a two-year theatre workshop project that uses theatre as a vehicle for discussing violence against women in the Solomon Islands. Run in collaboration with the Solomon Islands Planned Parenthood Association, the British Council and the Conch Theatre Company, New Zealand, the initiative is the first of its kind in the country and is creating a powerful platform for discussing sensitive issues.

Domestic and gender-based violence is a serious, widespread issue in Pacific nations. The World Development Report on Gender Equality and Development documents that approximately 64 per cent of women in the Solomon Islands experience domestic violence, generally perpetrated by intimate partners.[45] Violence against women has been the subject of constant denial, and until recently, political leaders have been slow in developing a relevant response.[46] The first nationwide study determining the extent of domestic violence was only conducted between 2007 and 2012, which led to the first national policy on eliminating violence against women.[47] The study determined that domestic violence has serious impacts on the income and non-income dimensions of wellbeing; women experience escalated health problems and high legal and household costs, causing negative socio economic repercussions for the country at large.[48] While not determined as yet for the Solomon Islands, the cost of domestic violence to the Fijian economy was estimated at 6.6 per cent of GDP.[49]

The main drivers of social change have been local non-governmental and faith-based organizations. Over the years they have taken an active role in establishing safe havens and engaging with local communities to discuss sensitive issues. Typically these engagements have taken the form of talks and flyers, and while effective in raising awareness, they have not effected behavioural change.[50] Unless motivation for behaviour change comes from within both individuals and communities, efforts to promote change will not be sustainable.[51]

Stages of Change started in 2013, and their key focus has been on working with abused women to share stories around domestic violence. The programme does not work directly with men, but aims to empower women and initiate a dialogue with the broader public.[52] The programme is divided into six ten-week blocks over two years, with each block culminating in a production performed in different communities to encourage a dialogue between participants and audience. Each block begins by training a group of survivors of violence with basic performance techniques that help to build a platform for creative discussion. An important precursor for this level of collaborative activity is the establishment of a 'safe space' where participants feel comfortable to learn new skills and face the conflict central to their creative discussion.[53] The women share their personal stories, building a sense of camaraderie and trust,[54] finding refuge in both their own narrative and in the shared experience of others. Talking about domestic violence is still considered taboo and the simple act of sharing narratives through theatre helps to make the discussion more accessible.

Creating personal narrative is an effective means of healing and has particular application in cases of domestic violence.[55] Indeed, 'a battered woman's words carry no weight whatsoever when used to confront the perpetrator of violence and in fact his power lies in his ability to keep her silent'.[56] A survivor's narrative literally and figuratively becomes their key to empowerment and freedom from abuse, serving as 'an act of transformation' that begins a journey toward emotional safety.[57] The act of storytelling is creative with a new narrative of a better life: 'to tell our stories is to recreate ourselves'.[58] *Stages of Change* works with established women's organizations and NGOs to ensure that women have access to shelters to promote their emotional and physical safety.

Stages of Change theatre director Nina Nawalowalo explains that the first step in this narrative process is 'unburdening the shame'.[59] Many abused women feel responsible for their own abuse and isolated in their plight against overcoming it. Indeed, domestic violence has become a social norm to the extent that 73% of women believe there are situations where men have good reason to beat their wives.[60] By using the creative arts, women are able to draw on their cultural performance heritage to foster dialogue around a traditionally sensitive topic.

As the narratives of women are shared, they participate in a theatre workshop process that relies on role playing and exploring symbols that represent the role of women in society and their challenges.[61] A performance piece organically emerges and Nawalowalo crafts the narrative into a theatrical production to have impact for a broader audience.[62] Careful attention is paid to the ethics of representing true-life experiences, in particular to maintain the privacy and dignity of the individuals, as well as to protect them against further abuse. As such, there are two aspects of the performance work – the private and process-driven work of the women, and the public advocacy work that makes use of their theatrical pieces. Nawalowalo explains that *Stages of Change* uses the power of suggestion and symbolic theatre that has greater potential for dialogue.[63] As a result, theatre helps to involve the community in identifying areas of concern and reflect on current conditions and causes of a situation, thereby identifying points of change and analysing the impact that may have.

Stages of Change has been being well received by the women, local communities and government of the Solomon Islands. The women involved explain that the process has given them the 'gift of confidence' and 'personal transformation' of how they value themselves and their role in society.[64] Six pieces have been performed to audiences of over 300 people at one time, and these performances have led to extensive and meaningful discussions with local communities and the Pacific region at large. The Solomon Islands government recognized the impact of the programme and there are suggestions that *Stages of Change* could initiate a national theatre company in the Solomon Islands.[65]

In the final scene of the play, the women stand together, each holding a small candle in the shell of a coconut. They lift the candles up as sign of their hope and determination, and the glowing red lights are a reminder of their collective experience, their struggle, their transformation and their triumph.

9

Mental Health: Perspectives from South Africa, the UK and Brazil

9.1 Introduction

Veronica Baxter

Any book addressing health would be remiss to leave out the significant component of mental health, wellbeing and emotional resilience. The difficulty here is the space to cover this meaningfully, and to provide some global perspective on differing cultural perceptions of mental health. The obvious route to take would be to include dramatherapy scholarship, but dramatherapy is well represented in critical writing, tends to be exclusively process-oriented and has a wide scope beyond this book's brief. In order to diversify case studies on mental health from multiple perspectives, this chapter focuses on mental health performance practices in southern Africa, the United Kingdom and Brazil.

Mental health and wellbeing is a highly contested arena, with the dominance of the Western-oriented *Diagnostic and Statistical Manual of Mental Disorders* (DSM)[1] often pitted against culture-specific understandings of mental health. For example, Augustine Nwoye[2] argues that the so-called 'biopsychosocial' (BPS) model that most psychologists view as an integrated approach to diagnosis and treatment does not take into consideration a fourth element: the spiritualist element. When faced with inexplicable behaviour, African elders would tend to look 'beyond the external manifestations of the illness, to determine "who" is speaking through such illnesses and what the relatives or family members are expected to do on behalf of the sick individual to effect healing'.³ Nwoye uses Victor Turner's concept of 'social drama' (with phases of 'breach', 'crisis' and 'redress') to explain this approach to reading social dramas and psychopathology. He also refers to the diagnostic process and the treatment as 'rituals of questioning misfortune'.⁴ This is where Sinethemba Makanya begins her account of traditional healers' functioning in southern African society, and addresses the specific question 'How would a traditional healer treat depression?' She situates the processes within performance, closing the gap between the spiritualist and BPS model.

Caoimhe McAvinchey explores the impact of Bobby Baker's *Mad Gyms and Kitchens*, which was performed as part of London's Cultural Olympiad in 2012. Baker underwent serious physical and mental illness, and while recounting her experiences with the medical fraternity, also asks of her audiences what their coping strategies are. Designed to some extent as conventional performance on a stage, Bobby Baker seeks the engagement of her audiences in a unique way. As with Makanya, the boundaries are blurred between notions of performance and theatre applied to mental health contexts.

Vitor Pordeus, a Brazilian transcultural psychiatrist from the Madness Hotel and Spa, argues that 'Health is a Performance – Disease is a Performance'. Using the allegory of *The Bacchae*,⁵ and the symbolic contest between bacchic Dionysus and rigid Pentheus, he discusses the importance of revelry, public rituals and dancing in sustaining health. He advocates the arts as a means towards mental health, as a way to release the imagination and know yourself.

9.2 Essay – Between the 'traditional' and the theatrical: Forms and performances of healing depression in South Africa

Sinethemba Makanya

South Africa is a country rich with diverse races, cultures and traditions. It has a range of problematic social issues resulting from a history of colonization and displacement. These issues are said to have 'contributed to poverty, violence, lower social economic levels, the rise of HIV infections and disturbed social relations'.[6] Although everybody in South Africa has been affected by these, black South Africans have been the most affected, and consequently being black in South Africa may 'increase risk factors associated with mental illnesses'.[7] Sorsdahl, Stein and Lund maintain that South African morbidity data indicate that mental disorders are the third highest contributor to the local burden of disease, and although these are more 'disabling than physical disorders, they are 10 times less likely to be treated'.[8] South Africa's diversity 'poses significant challenges when adapting western diagnostic conventions, research tools and psychosocial interventions'.[9] Hence, it is difficult to have a single unifying model since 'cultural manifestations of distress or illness may not fit in with dominant depressive discourse'.[10] In necessarily scaling up mental health care services, 'it is vital that interventions are socially and culturally appropriate'.[11] Although traditional African beliefs 'are more prevalent in rural and under-developed areas of the country',[12] many African people living in urban areas and townships are able 'to hold hybridized explanatory systems that allow for the incorporation of both Western and traditional African premises'.[13]

In light of the above statement, I suggest that the understanding of traditional medicine can play an important role in helping to address the mental health care needs in South Africa by offering culturally appropriate treatment. I draw this impulse from my own position within two traditions. As a drama therapist, I was trained in role theory and method, which informs my understanding of mental health and the practice of drama therapy. I am also an initiate of traditional healing, learning the practices of *iNyanga* (herbalist), *umThandazi* (faith healer) and *iSangoma* (diviner and ancestral guide), discussed later in the essay.[14] As such, I would like to frame the intervention of traditional healing within the concept of 'performance' and argue that the performativity of this practice makes it a viable option for healing. In examining traditional healing through this lens, it is 'necessary to rethink performance in non-Eurocentric ways'[15] and necessarily broaden definitions of it. I suggest that traditional healing, particularly the performative aspects of it, can be effective in treating depression and can inform strategies to help communities build resilience against it. This will be a brief study due to space, and is therefore concerned with 'descriptions of experiences not explanations or analyses'.[16]

Performance is understood as the 'embodied processes that produce and consume culture, performance makes things and does things',[17] it 'engages human attention through patterned activities'.[18] It is seen as 'including much more than theatre, but [runs] along an entire spectrum, which ranges from everyday life to rituals and art'.[19] Performance can be placed on a continuum between 'the polarities of play and ritual, with some performances involving mostly emotional release and … social fun, while others are more on social or religious efficacy'.[20] Performance can be seen as a kind of cognitive play, the foundation of which is 'the ability to simulate alternative, imaginary and future worlds'.[21] The idea that ancient forms of healing are seen as the beginnings of modern-day theatre is an idea expressed by many theorists.[22,23,24] Drama and healing are seen as influential dual forces that have 'provided a gateway to the effective therapeutic encounter'.[25] Phil Jones maintains that ritual space is analogous to dramatic space because ritual activity is dramatic. It calls for the subject to create a representational world through symbolic means and it relies upon the belief that events can be changed by mimetic action.[26] Ritual exhibits similar characteristics to performance because it 'takes place in special, often sequestered places, the very act of entering the sacred space has an impact on participants'.[27] In this space, participants are confronted by a heightened reality and state of being that transports people into an imaginary, dramatic reality. In this liminality, people can become selves other than their daily selves; they temporarily become or enact another, and perform actions different from what they do ordinarily. As such, traditional healers and drama therapists alike work from the assumption that 'dramatization allows an experience to exist by giving it a place in time, thus making it present'.[28]

Cultural performances, social or individual, can be characterized by 'a limited time span, an organized program of activity, set of performers, an audience, a place and occasion, they are created by cultural specialists, people who are especially recruited, trained, paid and motivated to engage in performances'.[29] Furthermore, Alexander suggests that performances contain the means of symbolic production and *mise-en-scène* where 'social actors engage in dramatic social action, entering into and projecting the ensemble of physical and verbal gesture'.[30] Within these performances individuals can 'rehearse situations of danger, stress, pain and occasional death to enable humans to process traumatic experiences in their lives that have no logical or probable explanation or outcome'.[31] The performance of rituals in this way serves not just as 'mirrors but active agents of change, they provide moments to enact, comment on, critique and evaluate the norms and values of a culture'[32] or an individual. Individuals and communities can thus relive and transform experiences from traumatic to pleasant, through performative acts.

Traditional medicine is the use of 'plant, animal and/or mineral based medicines, spiritual therapies, manual techniques and exercises to maintain well-being, as well as to treat, diagnose or prevent illnesses'.[33] Traditional healers are often 'called' to this path by their ancestors 'through dreams and other significant experiences'.[34] The initiation process generally takes six months to one year. The duration varies depending on finances and the speed at which the initiate learns and reaches each milestone. There are various classes of traditional healers in South Africa. Traditionally, these figures were seen as separate in terms of their practices. In a modern-day South Africa, however, one healer can use various modalities. The choice of which modality to use is often dictated by the needs of the patient. The *Sangoma* 'operates within a traditional religious context as accepted medium with the ancestral shades'.[35] They act as diviner/diagnostician, priest and healer within the community, using her knowledge of rituals and mediation with the ancestors to heal. Although the *Sangoma* may have knowledge of herbal medicine, traditionally she would refer a patient to *iNyanga* for this type of treatment. The *Nyanga* is a traditional doctor, 'who specializes in herbal medicine'.³⁶ The *Nyanga* is not a diviner, though they may use the counsel of the ancestors to diagnose and administer medication to their patients. The calling of *iNyanga* is usually less intense than that of *iSangoma*, the latter often experiencing physically and emotionally debilitating experiences. However, the skill of *iNyanga* has often been learned and passed down from someone in the family. *UmThandazi* (or *umProfethi*) emerged from the rise of the African independent church movement which broke away from the more Western-oriented missionary churches. Many of the roles of *iSangoma* 'have been taken over by *umThandazi* within a modern supernatural religious and urban setting'.³⁷ In modern-day South Africa, the healer employs, applies and recommends the 'appropriate action in the form of counselling, prescribing medicines and/or instructing on ritual ceremonies'.³⁸ In this approach 'humans and spirits are not seen as separate but are all within the world, and with the use [of] medicines, influence these forces on the physical, psychological and spiritual/transpersonal levels'.³⁹ The system of diagnosis and treatment is not based on intuition and divining alone, but is also based on 'testing such plant therapies for observed and replicable effects for many generations'.⁴⁰

Traditional healing is based within a paradigm that views the health of an individual 'not only as consisting of a healthy body, but as a healthy situation of everything that concerns [them]. Good health means the harmonious working of the Universe and everything existing within it.'⁴¹ Health does not only exist within a medical framework, primarily based on biology, but has aspects of the social and spiritual as well. As such, mental health cannot be separated from physical and spiritual health. As spirituality is an everyday reality, 'it is understood that there is constant dialogue and interaction between present reality and the spirit world'.⁴² Health is dependent on community and the relationships of the individual within the community. The philosophy of *Ubuntu* (humanness) 'reflects in people's relationships with each other'.⁴³

Depression is understood as a condition with the 'presence of sad, empty or irritable mood, accompanied by somatic and cognitive changes that significantly affect the individual's capacity to function'.[44] The depressive state is characterized by loss of interest in daily life, withdrawal from activity and people, loss of energy, and feelings of hopelessness and guilt.[45] In the most extreme cases it is associated with impaired concentration, inability to function and suicidal ideation. Depression is understood to be a complex condition where 'biological, psychological, and social factors all play a causal role'.[46] African perspectives on disease are manifold and interrelated. Disease in traditional healing is often looked at in terms of causation and not symptoms. Illnesses can occur from either natural or unnatural causes.[47] Natural causation manifests in biological conditions caused by natural factors like viruses. Unnatural causes are those that are linked to illnesses given by ancestors or spirits influenced by other people. These may further be divided into three categories: mystical, animistic and magical.[48,49,50,51] Mystical causes are cited when one is seen to be in a state of 'pollution' due to circumstances such as bereavement or witnessing a violent crime; this state is when the individual is more vulnerable or exposed. Animistic causes are cited when one has 'displeased the ancestors',[52] either by not observing certain rituals correctly or a failure to uphold the moral values of their community. Magical causation 'tends to be associated with witchcraft'.[53]

Depression within African perspectives is best described using local languages. Although this essay is written about the South African context, I have borrowed from other studies of depression based elsewhere in Africa. There are no direct translations of the word depression; similar concepts are *umzwangedwa*, a Zulu word describing an 'overwhelming sense of loneliness such that a person is no longer able to control the hurt'.[54] A study by Ventevogel, Jordans, Reis and De Jong showed that understandings of depression differ as seen in languages across Africa. For example, in Luo (South Sudan), *wehie arenjo/arir* describes a destroyed or abnormal mind; this is seen as a temporary condition ending as suddenly as it began. *Nger yec*, meaning cramped stomach, describes constant fatigue and diarrhoea. In Kakwa (South Sudan), *yeyeesi* describes people whose minds are always busy with thoughts. Within the Congo in Kinande, *amutwe alluhire* describes someone with a 'tired' head. In Burundi, *ibonge* or *akabonge* describes a state of sorrow in which a person is not able to function normally.[55] These terms are used to describe feelings of sadness, lack of appetite, passivity, suicidal ideation and the irregular sleeping patterns that come with depression. Within this perspective, depression is more likely to 'be ascribed to social or spiritual problems, poverty, social issues, major life events' and 'thinking too much',[56,57] because common mental disorders are viewed as the result of everyday life challenges rather than as treatable conditions.

iSangoma Mandla Ngwane maintains that the physiological consequences of thinking too much affect the heart and causes the veins to slowly constrict; this constriction of the veins causes tension in the body, for example in the head and shoulders, as not enough blood flows to the brain.[58] Monique Starkowitz maintains that sadness is a basic human emotion; however, traditional healers see a similar concept to depression as 'the more severe and at times more dangerous experience of sadness, which requires more intensive treatment'.[59] In this sense, depression is seen as 'consequential of sadness not being dealt with'.[60] Although factors such as unemployment and poverty are identifiable as natural causes of depression, factors related to bereavement, child birth and witnessing gruesome events can be classified under unnatural causes. These are the mystical causes also described as *ifu elimnyama* (dark cloud) in Zulu and speak of a withdrawal of God and the ancestors, or a state of vulnerability. Depression can also be viewed as a 'potential experience for growth'.[61] The sadness that comes with depression can be seen as 'necessitated by the individual needing to heal [or learn] something on a spiritual level'.[62]

In integrating the cultural understandings of depression, I suggest that depression as a concept can be viewed as occupying a continuum. At one extreme is a chronic mental condition that requires ongoing, close monitoring from a traditional healer or therapist. At the other is depression expressed as general feeling of sadness caused by both internal and external factors, and that when dealt with reconstitutes the healthy emotional functioning of an individual. Various factors may contribute to an individual moving from one extreme to another, and using techniques from traditional medicine with individuals and communities may build resilience and maintain wellbeing.

The performance continuum

Traditional healers are also seen as counsellors for their patients,[63,64] as they offer patients an opportunity to talk through their problems. In the performance of rituals, the healer encourages a space for the patient to take responsibility for his/her problems, giving them a sense of agency often lacking during a depressive episode. According to Sorsdahl and others, during treatment the patient is encouraged to live with the traditional healer or visit them on a regular basis to ensure adherence to treatment and that 'someone is always there to take care of the patient'.[65] Medicinal plants are used for both physical and spiritual uses. For numerous plants that are administered internally for spiritual healing purposes, there are physical and psychological therapeutic effects. Through rituals such as *ukuphalaza* (vomiting), *ukuchatha* (taking enemas), *ukugcatshwa* (small cuts in the skin) and *ukufutha* (steaming), the herbs are taken into the body. They cleanse the body by releasing toxins through diarrhoea, vomiting and sweating. These water rituals operate in the same way as hydrotherapy, which Mooventhan and Nivethetha define as the external or internal use of water (water, ice, steam) for health promotion or treatment of various diseases. The benefits of hydrotherapy are relaxation, detox through sweating, regulation and stimulation of blood flow and skin hydration improving elasticity. These help in combating the symptoms of depression on a physiological level as they help in serotonin synthesis, and the improvement in physical appearance can help boost the self-esteem of a depressed person.[66] This first stage of treatment also 'loosens' the body, giving the individual greater motivation to carry on with treatment.

Furthermore, the performances of these rituals are beneficial on a psychological and spiritual level. Roger Grainger maintains that things need to be lived out through performance, not simply thought through. There is a need to act out ideas and emotions in an embodied way, and to interact with other people.[67] Performance can help the individual access alternative states of being because the space is 'fluid and temporal, presents alternative experiential insights, is not bound by tradition, requires repetition and importantly places emphasis on outcomes, that of the reinvention of the self, rather than the art product'.[68] In these cleansing rituals, time is taken by the healer and the client to set up the ritual space. Candles and *impepho* (incense) are used to invoke the ancestors and ask them to bless the ritual. Candles 'light' the way for clients, with the belief that different colours invoke specific ancestors and evoke certain qualities during the ritual.[69] With the space prepared, the client is enrolled into the role of the 'dirty one', and through the symbolic act of cleansing the body, dark energy is washed away, making the client more accessible to the ancestors and vice versa. The repetition of these rituals enforces the progress to the 'clean one', and in embodying this role, the client is able to move past the depressive state to a more functional state. The choice of which types of medicines to use for these cleansing rituals is dependent on the 'energy' of the medicine. Energy in this sense is conceived of in terms of colour. Black/red medicines are potent medicines and are utilized early in the process to expel negative energy. White medicine is used at the end of the process to work off the effect of the black/red medicine and to restore the client to health.[70] The ritual of *ukulahlwa* (to be thrown away) also utilizes blood sacrifices. The sacrificial act is not only to appease the ancestors and offer the animal as a scapegoat, but also symbolizes a covenant between person and ancestors that will further solidify the person's commitment to remain clean.

The ritual of *ukuqiniswa* (strengthening) employs the technique of *ukugcaba*: this is when 'small incisions are usually made around the joints and medicines are applied in the incision to serve as a protective measure. Joints are said to be vulnerable points through which evil elements can enter the body.⁷¹ The performance of this ritual places the client in the role of the 'weak one' and through the action it moves the client from this role to that of the 'strong one'. The materials utilized further enforce qualities of strength and courage as animal fats, such as that of a lion, make up the medicines. In this dramatic reality, the patient is encouraged to act out certain aspects or desired qualities such as strength and rebirth. Such rituals bring feelings of lightness and relief and can also help remove impairments and blockages in the patient's thinking.

Depression often causes a person to withdraw socially and is further perpetuated by the feeling of aloneness that comes with this withdrawal. Traditional healers may attempt to influence the socioeconomic status of the individual by finding them a job or money, increasing psycho-social support, breaking through social withdrawal and strengthening social cohesion.[72,73] *Umsebenzi* is a ceremony where the patient or the family of the patient offers a ritual sacrifice to the ancestors. These ceremonies have both a spiritual and social purpose. They break through social withdrawal as they place the patient in the centre of a social drama, with much singing and dancing, where emotions are highly charged and expressed symbolically. The patient is made to 'feel important and the object of social concern, but the ritual also relates what is happening to [his]/her wider cosmological concerns'.[74] Such ceremonies are important for community engagement. They empower 'natural' social support systems already in place at local levels and strengthen social cohesion and social capital within communities.[75] The singing, dancing and drum playing are beneficial as the physical activity encourages motor activity, which increases 'the firing rates of serotonin neurons. This results in increased release and synthesis of serotonin',[76] implicated in the treatment of depression.

Treatment in the spiritual domain is further determined by the nature of the cause of the depression. In the instance of mystical causation, individuals 'are required to observe certain taboos and to perform a variety of rituals to protect themselves and others from the effects of their pollution'.[77] Many of these rituals have been discussed above as cleansing rituals and *ukuqiniswa*. When animistic causation is cited, appeasing the ancestors through the sacrificing of an animal or the observance of a ritual or rite of passage 'is viewed as a potential mechanism for overcoming misfortune and avoidance of future harm. There are often strict rules about the actors and places of performance of such rituals.' When magical causation is suspected, 'the cure involves being "un-bewitched" by an herbalist or healer'.[78] The process of being 'un-bewitched' entails rituals of cleansing and sacrifice through *ukulahlwa* mentioned above. Prayer is an essential component in the treatment of depression on a spiritual level. Prayer offers 'communication with ancestry'[79] who guide the process of recovery. Praying is dramatic and can transport the individual into a new reality where communication with a higher power is possible. In praying, the client strengthens their relationship with God and the ancestors.

Conclusion

In necessarily widening the definition of 'performance', this essay suggests that the performativity of ritual in traditional healing facilitates the process of alleviating the symptoms of depression. The performance of cleansing and protective rituals, as well as the medicines used, is established within a ritual space. This enables the client to symbolically embody and perform the undesirable qualities in order to transform them to the desired qualities of strength, courage and resilience, allowing for clarity of mind, body and soul. The social performance (*umsebenzi*) further strengthens *Ubuntu* (humanity) within a person and community, allowing connections to be made and support systems to be established within the community.

The spiritual domain is the main driver of treatment within traditional healing. Diagnosed through primarily spiritual means, it is the ancestors who guide the process of recovery. Although the client has taken responsibility, there is relief in knowing that recovery is guided by something stronger than us. This belief is inherently dramatic as much faith needs to be exercised, and one needs to perform in accordance with the rules of the performance as set by God or the ancestors, occurring in the space in between the physical and spiritual. Furthermore, physiologically, the cleansing of the body helps rid itself of toxins. The aspect of self-care facilitates relaxation and helps clear up blocked aspects of the mind and soul. The performance of these rituals facilitates a better mind, body and soul interaction and in this way is therapeutic.

9.3 Snapshot – *Mad Gyms and Kitchens*, Bobby Baker and Daily Life Ltd

Caoimhe McAvinchey

Introduction

> Our work at Daily Life Ltd challenges the well-intentioned trend of the wellbeing agenda that strives towards the homogeneous delivery of arts for health as an alternative to medical treatment for illness and disorder: with artists seen merely as field workers and the talent, individuality and potential of participants underestimated and overlooked. There is the risk that the arts in health is no more than modern-day basket weaving.[80]

Bobby Baker is a British performance artist whose work has, since the mid-1970s, playfully and rigorously critiqued the cultural politics of everyday life – what is publicly visible, discussed and valued. Originally trained as a painter, Baker found the medium of her body, in direct engagement with live audiences, to be the most compelling form for her practice. Her work is underpinned by humour – from self-parody through to fierce observation of the absurd in daily life – engaging audiences in a shared interrogation of personally or socially complex subject matter as evidenced in the politics of motherhood (*Drawing on a Mother's Experience*, 1988*)*, childhood (*Grown Up School*, 1999) and mental illness (*How to Live*, 2007).[81] Baker's work has been presented in major cultural institutions and more intimate spaces, including women's refuges and Baker's own kitchen. While the stage persona of Bobby Baker has remained reassuringly familiar over the past four decades, the scale, form, content and site of her practice has been mercurial, reflecting Baker's continued commitment to engage audiences in a shared examination of daily life.

In the mid-1990s, Baker's life was disrupted by a prolonged period of physical and mental ill health. 'In 1997 I officially had a breakdown. I received a psychiatric diagnosis but I think that breakdown explains it much more efficiently. I became, through experience, an expert of the mental health system.'[82] This experience of illness, recovery and the negotiation of expertise within the mental health system has shaped the trajectory of much of the work that Baker has made since and, in particular, informs the positioning of her company, Daily Life Ltd, as an arts and mental health charity. *Pull Yourself Together* (2000), *How to Live* (2007) and *Give Peas A Chance* (2008) have, in very different ways, addressed the treatment and representation of mental distress while also grappling with the economic and ethical terrain of the pharmacological and therapeutic industries built upon this. However, it has been the exhibition and publication of Baker's *Diary Drawings* (Wellcome Collection, London, 2009), 158 drawings and water colours illustrating the anguish, despair and duration of Baker's mental and physical illness and recovery between 1997 and 2008, that has given wider public attention to her articulation of and commitment to address the stigmatization of those who experience mental health issues.[83]

Mad Gyms and Kitchens

> I felt more and more, from my personal experience of being on the receiving end of projects, that it was a top-down approach: people within the mental health system were being delivered to rather than having any say in what they wanted or needed ... I wondered, how do people with personal experience of mental health issues come up with ingenious ways of enjoying daily life? How are these strategies overlooked, or underestimated by health professionals, or people themselves?[84]

This snapshot focuses on *Mad Gyms and Kitchens* (2012), Baker's show commissioned as part of Unlimited, a £3 million Cultural Olympiad programme celebrating the arts and cultural work of over 800 disabled and deaf artists as part of the London 2012 Olympics.[85] This extract from Baker's successful funding application details her 'unlimited' vision:

> *Mad Gyms and Kitchens* is a large-scale touring project based on Bobby Baker's (BB) experience of recovery from serious mental and physical illness. Ostensibly investigating the benefits of exercise and nutrition in pursuit for health and 'wellbeing', the show burgeons into Bobby's 'visionary crusade' on behalf of autonomy and personal choice. By celebrating and critiquing some of the advice she has received as a result of her disabilities, BB aims to elevate the experiences of day-to-day survival onto the platform offered by the London 2012 Olympics – and a world-class stage …[86]

With *Mad Gyms and Kitchens*, Baker wanted to create a 'small, exquisitely formed show that would reach the parts that others don't reach, that would meet people where they are: in community and health living centres, church halls, village halls as well as designated cultural venues'.[87] As well as a more general public audience, Baker explicitly wanted to engage with people who were experts in issues of mental health through lived experience and professional practice. Within the academy, Baker's work is more often considered in relation to live art, feminist performance and increasingly disability performance practice rather than Applied Theatre.[88] *Mad Gyms and Kitchens*, however, in both its invitation to and participation of the audiences in the creation of communities of expertise, helpfully blurs some of the disciplinary boundaries that may otherwise interrupt fruitful examination.

The performance

Baker always begins her shows by introducing herself (her name, her age and the fact that she is a woman, not a man) and is usually wearing a white overall. Her stage persona is a playful acknowledgement of Baker as a white, middle-class woman from the South-East of England.

Her style of engagement with the audience is one of direct address and, while appearing to be informal, Baker crafts a series of carefully curated moments that give insight into complex experiences in daily life that, while being rooted in biography, are not confessional; rather, they are springboards for the audiences' consideration of their own lives. *Mad Gyms and Kitchens* makes this idea joyously explicit as Baker 'talks' to the audience for the first 50 minutes of the show before then inviting them into dialogue with each other.

At the beginning of *Mad Gyms and Kitchens*, the stage is set with five large, mysterious looking flight cases, of different sizes, positioned across the breadth of the playing area. After Baker welcomes the audiences and introduces herself, she reveals an almost life-size drawing outlining her body and detailing the various illnesses and surgeries that she has negotiated.

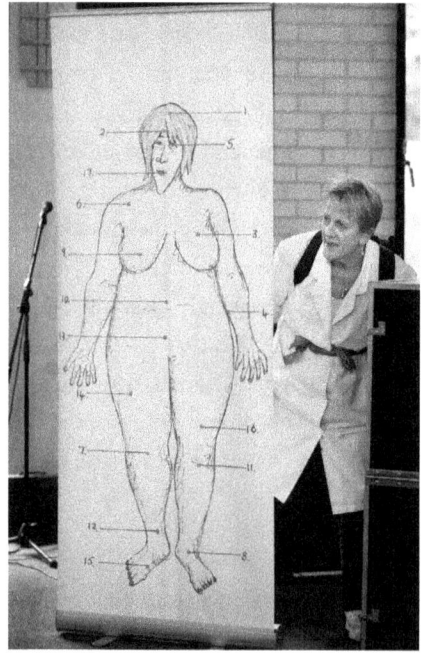

Figure 7: *Mad Gyms and Kitchens*, Bobby Baker. Photo © Tim Smith 2012.

She then guides the audience through each of her strategies for wellness, introducing us to the contents of each flight case that, together, make up her 'recovery apparatus': a gym, a kitchen, a bed and her living room. These are revealed to us as each of the beautifully and differently designed flight cases are opened with a delighted flourish. The 'rooms' were developed in collaboration with the sculptor Charlie Whittuck, who is also Baker's son. She models her strategies for wellbeing – exercise (pedalling on her bike), eating well (frying garlic in her kitchen and eating fruit with yogurt and porridge oats before washing everything up with running water), rest (snuggling into her welcoming bed with a gloriously yellow blanket) and pleasure (reading and listening to music in a pink armchair surrounded by objects from people she loves). Throughout the modelling of each strategy, Baker talks about specific moments in her odyssey of revelation and self-care. With a playful nod to the Olympics, she dons a series of 'medals' (including a water bottle from the gym, a bulb of garlic from the kitchen) to reward herself for taking care of a body that is less publicly acknowledged but equally as extraordinary as the bodies that are celebrated and televized in Olympic stadia around the UK.

As the show unfolds, and with it the contents of each flight case, the stage is transformed into a gallery of sculptural invention. Within the audience there is a growing sense of anticipation as Baker approaches the fifth case that is positioned centre stage. There is audible delight as Baker unlatches the final flight case to reveal the Art Kart: a glorious construction that is a table, a tea trolley and a cupboard filled with art-making materials. As the steam rises from the huge pots of tea, the china mugs chink as they are set alongside the plates of biscuits. This is the moment when the already porous boundary between Baker, as performer, and the audience of anonymous individuals dissolves. Bobby, along with two assistants, invites the audience to join her in having tea and to consider, through reflection and conversation with others in the audience, their expertise in wellbeing: what do you do to *be* well? To *keep* well? Around the room, there are pockets of chatter and moments of intense focus as the audience illustrate their 'Top Tips'.

These are shared with people in the room in real time and, through an online digital scrapbook, to others who may come to this work and dialogue at another time, in another place.[89] The scrapbook reveals a playful, thoughtful articulation in both words and images of an eclectic range of strategies for wellbeing: 'a good cry and a good laugh: sometimes at the same time'; 'feeding the wild birds every morning', and 'prescription medication and eccentric children', along with an abstract collage of materials including a bourbon biscuit and brightly colourful card, encouraging both the artists and the viewer, 'when you look, remember to see'.[90]

Behind the scenes

In the eighteen months between January 2011 and September 2012 during the Cultural Olympiad, Baker's *Mad Gyms and Kitchens* culminated in 32 performances in a range of health, education, community and cultural venues across England. Over 1,600 members of the public attended the show, including National Health Service (NHS) volunteers, nurses, service users, carers, psychologists, psychiatrists, occupational therapists, art therapists, GPs, NHS Health Commissioners and chaplains. In order to engage less traditional theatre audiences, *Mad Gyms and Kitchens* used a dialogic and labour-intensive approach to develop relationships with cultural centres, health services, survivor networks and voluntary organizations working to support people with experience of mental ill health. This included the exhibition of a mini-version of the *Diary Drawings* in health care contexts, public talks and creative training workshops for local mental health community workers. *Mad Gyms and Kitchens* in its form, audience and ambitions addresses social rather than individual change while extending the spectrum of practices that may be identified as arts in health.[91] In *Mad Gyms and Kitchens,* Baker created a shift in thinking about the audiences' collective capacities and strategies for wellbeing: 'Mental illness is commonly seen as a deficit and a weakness, I want to show otherwise: that we have much to contribute and teach. That society has much to learn from us.'[92] For

Baker, this collaborative reconsideration of 'the expert' fuels both the political ambition and radical playfulness of *Mad Gyms and Kitchens*.

9.4 Interview – Dionysus and ritual ecstasy: Madness and medicine

Vitor Pordeus (VP) is interviewed by Katharine Low, London, 10 May 2014

Can you tell us a little about how The Madness Hotel started, and its founding ideas?[93]

VP: The Madness Hotel and Spa, along with the DyoNises Theatre, are spaces for confirmation of the Shakespearian maxim:

> All the world's a stage,
> And all the men and women merely players.[94]

We are reactivating Brazilian psychiatrist Nise da Silveira's ideas.[95] She worked in our hospital from the 1940s to her death in 1999. She was researching expressive tools as occupational therapy for her psychiatric patients, at a time when others used lobotomies, electroconvulsive therapy and (from the '70s onwards) over-prescription of drugs. We are confirming her findings and theories and proposing new models for a culture of care.

One of the most interesting aspects is your definition of madness, which is different to how we may describe it in the UK. So to begin, could you tell us how you define madness?

VP: Madness for me is a terrain of human existence. So, madness is everywhere. Madness is shaping culture … This can be related to what Jung called the collective unconscious. I think that this word [madness] is too loaded with prejudice, surrounded by ignorance. It would be better if we could talk about it in a more clear, direct and light way; with humour, criticism and intelligence. So, everywhere we go, we see madness.

I think your use of the term 'lightness' to describe how we talk about mental health is interesting – it suggests an alternative way of addressing the topic.

VP: Bertolt Brecht was the practitioner who first opened my understanding to this particular kind of theatre, with his description of an epic and dialectic theatre with humour and intelligence. A theatre that is thinking. A theatre that is alive, with permanent and responsive dialogue … After research [we] came to the idea that we are dealing with a psychic healing tradition, an expansion of consciousness, collective organization and pedagogy.

After reading a lot of stuff – for sure the most important play was *Life of Galileo* – I started training in street theatre with Amir Haddad in Rio.[96] He was a practitioner who in the past thirty-five years refounded a theatrical tradition – which is those Dionysian pageants, public performances with poetry and singing poets, circular dances in open public spaces, democratic spaces. Both of these influences (Brecht and Haddad), coupled with the collective nature of theatre, are important to my practice.

Theatre is a collective tradition of Western society. If we do not make theatre in a lively manner – make it healthy and healing, communitarian and territorial – we have a public, collective, health emergency. We already have pandemics of mental illness and anxiety – because there is no ritual. There is no deep understanding of our collective and communitarian challenges. Madness Hotel's main challenge is health. Without health it does not matter if you have money.

This modern mental illness pandemic has links with the myth of Dionysus and Pentheus in *The Bacchae* by Euripides. When Dionysus (or Bacchus, god of wine, revelry, ritual madness and theatre) arrives in Thebes, he finds a sick city – a city that is under the oppressive rule of Pentheus, who has forbidden all the public rituals such as dancing rites and the Bacchic. The tragedy that comes reminds everyone that the Gods are eternal powers and must always be observed through rituals.

Could you share with us how the audience responds to the Madness Hotel's performances?

VP: For example, what happened in the Dragon Café in London, one of the most magical moments I have had in my work. Here I am, doing my theatre that I believe is restorative, and suddenly a woman in the audience – a chronic psychotic, sixty+ years old woman, in an apparent condition of suffering and isolation, rises up and recites Act Three, Scene Two, the speech of Hamlet to the actors. She told me afterwards, 'Hamlet is so personal to me – and I saw the actor struggling – and I had to do it.' She got up and performed the speech, and it was amazing – and something miraculous happened. People change and people see things they weren't seeing before. And this to me is therapeutic. The best responses of the audience are to participate, dance together and sing together. This is when the dialogue is effective, when the real healing takes place.

When you talk about your work at the Madness Hotel, do you describe it as therapy or therapeutic?

VP: I don't know how to differentiate theatre from medicine. Theatre and medicine are very much the same: health is a performance, disease is a performance … it's the dramaturgy that works with memory and image, self-image. Medicine and theatre deal with identity in a very intricate way.

Do you perform back to the patients what they're sharing with you or do you create a performance with them?

VP: Dialoguing all the time, and we work a lot with music, dance, poetry, singing and mythological images. The first rule is the acknowledgement that anything can happen; improvisation is the basis of theatre; dialogue is the basis of theatre. After that, poetry, myth, archetypical characters emerge. One of the key difficulties is to have a cultural repertoire broad enough to allow the recognition of those patterns, discourses. In the case of Brazilian culture, and particularly in Rio de Janeiro, the archetypes I observe in our presentations and workshops are related to African and indigenous culture. At the hospital, the Museum of Images of the Unconscious[97] plays a key role as an experimental archive of artistic images [of archetypes] that prove the 'collective unconscious' concept.

You take quite well-known archetypes of mental health to start those interactions/conversations?

VP: Yes, and they mobilize the actors, patients and non-patients alike. And the actors manifest themselves in the performances, so patterns emerge and open new avenues of work. My professor of theatre in Brazil, Amir Haddad, says 'theatre is not about representation; it's about manifestation'. This is very similar to Brazilian-African religions, which (in the Nigerian traditions I studied in Rio) say the same, that Orixá, the Yoruba term for God, is a manifestation of nature.

How would you define the difference between manifestation and representation in theatre?

VP: Manifestation is the content that is presented. Each person carries his or her ancestors, stories, myths and songs. When you are doing the theatrical ritual, you have to be able to allow those manifestations to happen/emerge. If you come with your ego and give no space, you can play only yourself as an actor. But if you are attentive and sensitive, you can manifest yourself. Representation, in the way it's being done in our times, is the realistic representation – the idea that you have to make real pictures and real images, like mimicking explosions and violence and guns: this is literally a tragedy because what frees [us] is poetry, fantasy, the opportunity to imagine and dream.

How do your fellow psychiatrists view the work of the Madness Hotel?

VP: The main cooperative psychiatrist and artist we have is Dr Lula Wanderley, who worked with Nise da Silveira, the founder of the Museum of the Images of the Unconscious. We also work with the brilliant Brazilian artist Lygia Clark, internationally famous for her relational objects.[98] I also have other psychiatrists who send patients who are artists to our site. The psychiatric mainstream ... I'm not even interested in listening to them, because they are slaves of the pharmaceutical industry.

It's a science that 'fixes' but doesn't support the patient?
VP: The practice of medicine is an art; it's one of the oldest arts of humankind. Science is biology. If you want a science, go to biology. Go study the animals, the plants, the waters – go see the healthy behaviour of nature ...

In proposing that 'medicine is an art', you argue that medicine is one of the oldest art forms. How? Why do you describe it that way?
VP: Because as an artist, and as a physician, you have to be attentive, you have to be sensitive, you have to listen, and you have to be able to identify traditions and identify cultural lineages, identities, stories.

A lot of people say, I want liberty, I want health, I want life – but their cultural and symbolic practice is authoritarian; they don't dialogue with anyone. So, this is a challenge to find our own coherence and understand it better.

How does the Public Health Office of Rio de Janeiro Municipality support your work?
VP: A sensitive Public Health Authority officer at [the] time, [the] end of 2008, Dr Hans Fernando Dohmann, invited me to open the Centre for Culture, Science and Health. Through this [we have been] working with the possibility of change, of creation; so it's been five years of political, scientific and artistic negotiation inside the office. We mapped competencies in Rio de Janeiro's territory – Dr Nise da Silveira, the Tá Na Rua Institute for street performances about citizenship and education, the Botanic Garden with fifty years of experience, and their collection of medicinal plants. We went on exchanging methods, and exchanging ways of doing and it just made the work much easier.

10

Snapshots of Practice: Environmental Health, Medical Dramaturgy, Addiction and Ebola

10.1 Introduction

Veronica Baxter

For some years the theme of 'uncertainty' or 'precarity' has become part of the academic lexicon.[1,2,3] Although many would trace this development back to 11 September 2001 or the 2008 economic meltdown, for others it has been a constant state of anxiety for decades. However research has shown that a socioeconomic crisis has an impact on health and wellbeing that is far reaching.[4]

This chapter examines a range of snapshots of performance practice that are responsive to crises in health: performance activism about food security, video film performances about the Ebola virus, addicts moving towards recovery through dance, and an experimental performance about epilepsy. In all cases, the snapshots reveal a move away from the medicalization of health and towards a humanizing effect through the arts.

Lisa Woynarski's discussion of Violeta Luna's work in Mexico specifically relate her performances to protesting against genetically modified foods, in this case maize or corn. Luna demonstrates a recolonized body, a site of appropriation for monopoly corporations that undermine local traditional Latin American corn-growing. Nick Hamer and Alex Sutherland show the damage that Westernized consumption patterns, climate change and HIV/AIDS have done to food security in the Eastern Cape, South Africa. Their theatre is framed as a means of reporting research findings back to the communities in which the research was conducted, an approach that is termed Ecohealth.

On an individual basis there are few things as destabilizing to the individual as living with epilepsy, when seizures happen mostly without warning. Deirdre McLaughlin and Joanne Scott have pursued an intermedial performance form that they term 'medical dramaturgy' where they aim to bring their audiences closer to understanding the experience of epilepsy.

Zoe Zontou recounts working with addicts through dance, linked to the company Fallen Angels. This work lifts addicts out of the medicalization of their condition and into the realm of physical and psychological recovery through dance.

Lastly, what do you do if live performance is not possible, because to perform could expose actors to a deadly disease? Gloria Ernest-Samuel analyses a video film called *Ebola Doctors*, which 'performed' in West Africa. Comically dispelling myths about prevention of Ebola, the video film allows information to be disseminated in a popular Nollywood form.[5] The West African outbreak of Ebola in 2014–15 demonstrated the ill-prepared health systems in the region.[6]

While these snapshots are unrelated to each other, they nevertheless present additions to the focus of the book that reflect on broader practices of performance in health and social wellbeing.

10.2 Snapshot – Ecological health in Violeta Luna's *NK603: Action for Performer & e-Maiz*

Lisa Woynarski

As philosopher David Abram suggests, in Navajo cosmology 'the health, balance, and well-being of each person is inseparable from the health and well-being of the enveloping earthly terrain', a concept prevalent in many Indigenous worldviews.[7] Mexican performance artist Violeta Luna enacts this inextricable link in the context of globalization in her work *NK603: Action for Performer & e-Maiz* (2014). Through her body, she connects maize (corn) growing, the impact of genetically modified (GM) crops and land health on the identity of an Indigenous culture. Historically, Indigenous Latin American cultures have harvested maize and it remains a staple of their diet, with over sixty indigenous species grown. Culturally and spiritually, maize is foundational to creation stories; it is considered the flesh and blood of the Maya people for example.[8] Monsanto, the multinational biotech corporation and the largest producer of GM seeds, has been distributing a strain of GM maize (known as NK603) in Mexico since 2009, which is currently only allowed to be grown in an experimental form, although there is lobbying for full legalization. NK603 is a maize hybrid that is resistant to the herbicide Round Up (also produced by Monsanto), which means that maize crops can be sprayed with the herbicide and will not die.[9] According to the protestors against this GM maize (many of whom are Mexican farmers), the introduction of Monsanto and GM crops into maize agriculture will not only result in a loss of biodiversity potentially making 'native' varieties extinct, but will have a profound impact on Indigenous peoples and their cultures.[10] In her performance, Luna locates this contested ecological site on her body; it is the site of memory, culture and capitalist intervention. The wellbeing of her body is inextricably connected to the land and its ecology.

Through affective imagery drawn from *campesinos*,[11] anti-GM protests, Latin American Indigenous rituals, the previous resistance movements and biotechnology experimentation, Luna examines and comments on how GM crops have affected the health of the land in Mexico. At once disturbing and compelling, she performs the manipulation of GM maize crops on her body, connecting the maize plant to the manipulation of her body and wellbeing. Luna's piece has toured festivals around the world since 2009, including Colombia, Serbia, the USA, Peru, Spain, New Zealand and Mexico, bringing the GM maize conflict to a global audience.

232 Applied Theatre: Performing Health and Wellbeing

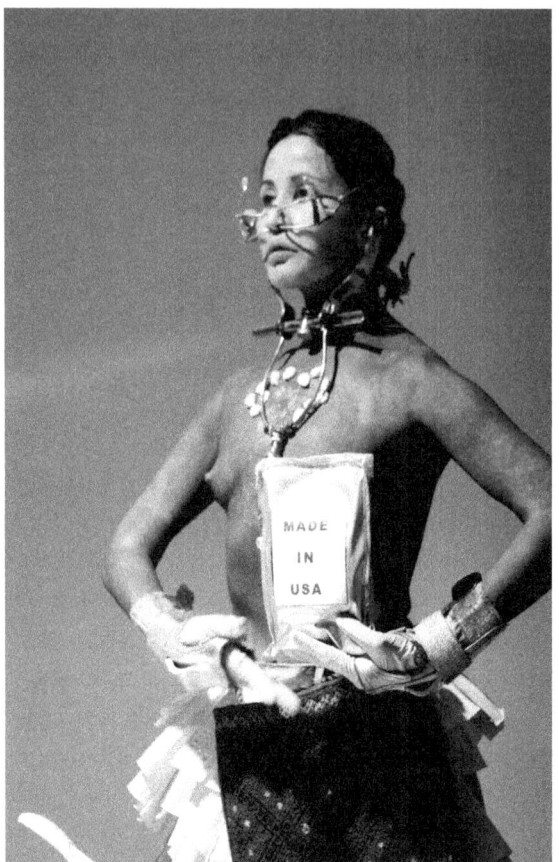

Figure 8: Violeta Luna – *NK603: Action for Performer & e-Maiz*. Photo © Greg Craig.

The performance begins with Luna entering a dimly lit theatre in a skirt made out of dried maize husks, a grey *chal* (shawl) and a straw hat with two long black plaits, brandishing a machete. Black-and-white images of *campesinos,* protests, scientific testing and maize plants are projected on a white sheet behind her with a sound track of news reports and corporate videos about the safety of GM foods. Her upper body is painted a deep purple, representing the heart and sacredness in Indigenous Latin American cultures,[12] with seeds stuck to her chest forming the shape of a blossoming plant. She has a maize plant painted on her back, symbolizing the inseparability of Indigenous cultures, corporeality and maize. The maize is a source of food and sustenance, making the health of the crop intimately connected with the health of the body. Its cultural significance means that is it also closely connected with Indigenous peoples and the continued survival of their epistemologies, traditions and stories.

In the performance, Luna puts on white medical gloves and tightly ties her long black plaits into a gag around her mouth. She uses medical instruments to contort and prod her body as she takes surgical pliers and rips off the seeds stuck to her chest. A scientist in a lab coat tightly binds her torso in duct tape. She puts on a metal corset with sharp nails projecting from it and injects her arm with a needle. She puts on a wired headpiece that forces her mouth open. As Luna is poked and prodded, bruised and bloodied, the physical health of her body parallels the loss of biodiversity and genetic manipulation of the maize plants. Her body is implicated in the interventions into the land, in the globalization of rural Mexico and in the loss of heritage and culture associated with maize. If the health of the crops is degraded or made extinct, her body and identity as an Indigenous person is also made vulnerable to extinction.

The manic video collages and electronic music (by collaborators Roberto Varea and David Molina)[13] violently intervene in the action. Near the end of the performance, the scientist cuts off the tape binding her torso and reveals that the painting of the maize on her back has transferred to the duct tape bonds. The rich tradition of growing maize has now been transferred to multinational corporate interests and the happy myth of progress. She then takes a red scarf, ties it around her nose and mouth, and stares defiantly out at the audience, a clear allusion to the Zapatista movement of the 1990s, in which Indigenous peoples and *campesinos* staged a revolution for agricultural and social reforms in Chiapas, Mexico.[14]

Luna embodies the struggle of the maize plants themselves as well as the land and farmers. Her ecological body is implicated in the interventions into the land, in the globalization of rural Mexico, in the loss of biodiversity, heritage and culture associated with maize. This work is also rooted in environmental justice, an activist gesture in response to the systemized inequity of neoliberal capitalism, oppression of the culture and heritage of Indigenous peoples, their ongoing resilience and resistance, and the use of GM crops as monoculture. The performance does not represent land health; rather it illustrates the inseparability of ecological conditions and human wellbeing. Luna cites Indigenous cosmologies in which the environment is not an abstract 'other' but is intertwined with the life and health of each person.

10.3 Snapshot – Storying climate change adaptation: Theatre as a research tool in an Ecohealth research process in the Eastern Cape, South Africa

Nicholas Hamer and Alexandra Sutherland

Because of its ability to communicate research findings in an emotive and embodied manner, theatre holds particular potential for health research, which often engages in complex questions of the human condition.[15]

August 2013

A team of actors and researchers climb into small buses to travel the bumpy road to an *imbizo* (important meeting). The hall where they will perform their play *Vukani!* (meaning 'Awake!' in Xhosa) gradually fills with a diverse group from children to traditional leaders to a local pastor. The six actors, four from these villages, use Xhosa performance forms (a 'poor theatre'[16] approach incorporating physical theatre, mime, song, dance, storytelling, chorus work and vignettes) to show life in the past when more wild foods were harvested and there was no option of reliance on the state for survival. The heightened performance style uses stock characters such as the nosy and busy villagers who tell us about life in the present, a life filled with crime, poverty, alcohol and an overreliance on shop-bought foods and state grants; the narrator gives us glimpses of the futures that await us, reminding us to work collectively to build on assets and adaptive strategies that are part of our capacity and strengths.

Background to *Vukani!*

Vukani! was a theatre piece commissioned to engage communities with research themes from a four-year Ecohealth research project in two rural Eastern Cape sites, involving researchers from South Africa and Canada. The project explored the vulnerabilities and stressors that rural communities face within the context of HIV/AIDS and climate change, as well as the adaptation and coping strategies that are currently taking place in the communities. This project undertook various strategies to avoid a one-way dissemination of knowledge from scientists to communities. Susan Cox[17] names 'research-based theatre' as a way for (social) scientists and theatre-makers to communicate complex research knowledge and findings. The theatre piece discussed here was another opportunity (in the project) to create dialogue about local adaptations to climate change within the context of vulnerabilities associated with the AIDS epidemic, food security, poverty and crime.

As Cox argues,[18] there will always be tensions in research-based theatre between aesthetics and the 'accurate' presentation of research findings. What this example highlights is theatre's ability to engage with 'complex questions of the human condition', which facilitates ownership and identification with research stories and themes brought back to the community. Performed in local theatrical forms, the audience were able to see their everyday struggles and triumphs as visible, meaningful and recognized. These local forms are non-naturalistic and episodic in style, contesting 'the linear, naturalistic form of traditional textual renderings of research findings particularly from qualitative research'.[19]

The International Development Research Centre (IDRC) defines Ecohealth as an approach that recognizes 'that there are inextricable links between humans and their biophysical, social, and economic environments, and that these links are reflected in a population's state of health'.[20] *Vukani!* attempted to create an aesthetic, embodied realization of these Ecohealth links, brought about through a theatre workshopping process that engaged community voices with the research project's findings. The research and theatre piece highlighted the strength of traditional practices as an effective means of adaptation to the challenges in environmental and human health. The character of *uMakhulu* (old woman) reflects on this in the play:

> I do not have money to buy the things I need, not even the basics … I struggle to buy seeds. It was easier when I was growing up. Things were better for us all in our community … When I grew up my parents farmed; we never starved. Harvest was always good. There was milk, meat. There was no unemployment … Life was so good. We were healthy, fat sometimes but very happy, my dear. Today I ask people for help. I am a beggar, today.

The play was not trying to romanticize a rural idyll – a past that under apartheid destroyed rural families, communities and the environment.[21] Rather, the research project highlighted existing community-based assets derived from indigenous knowledge systems that can generate adaptation strategies within the current context. These include the harvesting of wild food sources, more farming, less reliance on government, and an asset-based approach that pools resources existing within community structures.

Initial meetings between the theatre-makers and scientists were challenging and surfaced some of the tensions faced in the question of how knowledge can be shared. The research team tended to want to present a clear message of *how* to adapt to change and vulnerabilities. The theatre team wanted to find ways of highlighting different perspectives and show the complexity of conflict, resilience and agency in the research examples. Academic research findings can convey important messages to policymakers (this was an outcome of this project), but these 'truth' statements do not necessarily resonate with communities.

In addition, simply reporting to communities the problems they face does not assist in building capacity. It was important to make visible the agency and institutions that exist in communities as well as the tensions and possibilities within different coping strategies. One of the ways of doing this was to examine the overall concept of change and adaptation in the past, the present and what can be learnt for the future when changing weather patterns will alter the physical, social and political landscape. An example can be found in the following extract between an older woman, who believes in harvesting wild foods, and younger people who have started a gardening group to share knowledge and work collectively. The extract also highlights the problems of always relying on government departments for support such as social grants or food aid, which is not always practical or sustainable.

> **MaNgwanya**: You are all idiots for planting on the wrong season! Why not plant cabbages, spinaches and onions? That's what I call 'All Seasons'!
> **Nondaba**: Listen here MaNgwanya, the Department of Agriculture is the one who gives us the wrong seeds in the wrong season!
> **MamaCirha**: Hey MaNgwanya, since you have all this knowledge about the SEASONS, why are you still sitting down on your bottom? Why not stand up and come to our Garden Group and join us?
> **MaNgwanya**: HAVE YOU EVER CALLED ME? Never!
> **Mamtolo**: MaNgwanya, people join! You must bring some money and join.
> **MaNgwanya**: What? With my social grant money? I'd rather go to the bushes and collect *amakhowa* [mushrooms]. Then walk to the sea and catch me some fish and I shall eat for free!

Observation of audience reactions, a post-show discussion, as well as follow-up interviews with performers and audience members indicated that the show was well received and appeared to be an effective tool for engaging stakeholders in discussions about their serious challenges in dealing with food security in the context of climate change and HIV/AIDS. Pumelela Nqelenga, who facilitated interviews with audience members, noted that older people felt more comfortable in discussions after the theatre piece, because they were not being presented with one unchallengeable truth – in contrast to when a university researcher made a presentation.

Although it is clear that *Vukani!* succeeded on a number of different levels, it remains an ongoing challenge to integrate theatre into developmentally centred research processes, as it requires time, resources and openness on behalf of researchers and theatre-makers to find negotiation between messages and dialogue, aesthetics and research findings.

10.4 Snapshot – Generating a medical dramaturgy: Live intersections between intermediality and health

Deirdre McLaughlin and Joanne Scott

This snapshot introduces our intermedial practice as research (PaR), exploring the intersections between live media practice, disability and health. As part of this collaborative work, we are seeking to discover new ways of formulating and expressing Deirdre's autobiographical and phenomenological experience of temporal lobe epilepsy through improvised events, created using the tools of Jo's live media practice. In such events, Deirdre's lived experience of the condition and its treatment emerges through combinations of text, movement, sound and image, generating a 'medical dramaturgy' which reflects, refracts and responds to the real-time experience of living with disability.

In December 2012, the first of a series of PaR experiments took place at the Royal Central School of Speech and Drama, in the form of a three-hour sharing of collaborative practice. Jo was positioned in one area of a black box space, along with a set of technologies, enabling the live creation and mixing of sound and images on a large screen opposite. Deirdre positioned herself between this 'technical area' and the screen, moving within the space, both to prompt and to respond to the images and sounds generated by Jo. The audience was seated to one side and invited to witness the interactions through which the intermedial space was generated.

The event that prompted this first experiment was Deirdre undergoing a 24-hour ambulatory EEG, as part of a series of tests to monitor her neurological activity. At the time of this test, Deirdre had been diagnosed as epileptic for roughly eight years, but was undergoing a new series of tests in response to an increased period of both simple and complex partial seizures. Our focus was to explore the possibilities of positioning PaR within the larger medical event of the diagnostic test. We were specifically interested in how Jo's live media practice – the improvised mixing of image, sound, object and body – could intersect with Deirdre's experience of the test, to express the altered state of consciousness associated with temporal lobe epilepsy.

What this particular approach offered was a way of creatively engaging with a real-time medical event, through generating a series of intermedial exchanges that mirrored, refracted and responded to the conditions of the test in ways that a retrospective performance *about* that experience never could. This kind of 'active aesthetic'[22] places emphasis on 'the act of doing as the generator of meaning',[23] specifically in this case 'our process in the act of performing'[24] as opposed to the product of that process. In this sense, we were not performing or activating a seizure per se, but rather exploring Deirdre's subjective experience of her seizures in relation to her ongoing diagnostic testing.

In adopting this approach, we are signalling a move away from a narrative retelling of a medical event or diagnostic experience towards an improvised exploration within the structures of that experience. We are proposing the term 'medical dramaturgy' to account for this type of approach, which on a micro level explores the relationship between Deirdre and her health as mediated through the experience of an actual diagnostic test. On a macro level, the dramaturgy expands to explore Deirdre's lived experience, as it intersects with Jo's intermedial practice. This intersection is significant in that the improvised practice offers the means to open up and explore the conditions of the test in the moment of its occurrence. In this sense, it encompasses both the medical and performance events, emerging through a series of interactions between Deirdre, Jo and the intermedial spaces that are created.

In generating this particular medical dramaturgy, we were interested in how the materials and the medical environment, including the time allotted for a specific test and the shape of the data collected, could become active within the performance event. This meant gathering materials, including official paperwork related to the procedure and instructions to the patient, diverse images of the affected area of the brain, facts related to temporal lobe epilepsy as well as historical accounts of the condition and more abstract and evocative images, sounds and texts which related to Deirdre's experience of her seizures.

These materials were activated live through a range of technologies, including a live feed camera, sound sampler, synthesizer, microphone and loop pedal. This resulted in texts being spoken, written and sung, while images were created, mixed and shifted in relation to Deirdre's body in the space, creating a series of exchanges between the live media artist (Jo) and the performer (Deirdre).

From these exchanges, an intimacy and vulnerability emerged between us, which was at the forefront of the experience, as the condition of temporal lobe epilepsy became visible through Deirdre's body, her spoken narrative and the intermedial space which was generated around and in response to it. A marked example of this was a moment when Deirdre was describing a particularly personal account of the experience of a seizure, while a large image of Jo's hands, projected live from the webcam, encircled and seemed to offer both protection and illumination through the light this generated.

Another example was a conversation related again to Deirdre's experience of seizures, which was conducted between us through live voice (Deirdre) and live writing (Jo), typed up onto the screen. In both cases, something about the dispersal and dislocation of our interaction seemed to offer a conversely closer connection between us than bodily touch or an unmediated conversation. Furthermore, this exchange also appeared to reveal more about the nature of Deirdre's condition as both coming and going, simultaneously in the present and the past, resulting in an altered, and sometimes fractured, sensorial experience, reminiscent of temporal lobe epilepsy itself.

Crucially, these intermedial exchanges were emergent properties of the intersections between the medical test itself and the live intermedial space we generated around and in relation to it. In this sense, the event created was an *'active framework … non-linear, changeable, and unstable'*.[25] Through its improvised co-creation, a medical dramaturgy was formulated, where components were 'softly assembled'[26] through 'complex interrelations of time, substance and processes',[27] allowing the states, connections and exchanges described above to emerge.

We continue to develop and explore our practice through live experiments, where materials related to Deirdre's condition and its treatment become active within the framework of the performance event. At this point in our practice, we contend that this 'medical dramaturgy' functions most effectively when expressed in an active doing, emerging from the intersections of a live intermedial space and Deirdre's lived experience of temporal lobe epilepsy.

10.5 Snapshot – 'Dance lifts us up in the world': Socially engaged theatre with people in recovery from addiction

Zoe Zontou

The research project Staging Addiction Recovery (SAR) is a four-year programme (2012–16) conducted at Liverpool Hope University. The project seeks to investigate the role of socially engaged theatre in supporting problem drug users towards their journey to recovery. It aims to advance the findings of my previous research[28] and to examine critically the relationship between participatory theatre, recovery from addiction to alcohol and other drugs and notions of wellness. In doing so, the project explores the work of Fallen Angels Dance Theatre

Company[29] (henceforth Fallen Angels). Fallen Angels works with addicts, people in recovery and the wider community to inspire and support them to make positive choices. Their recent creative project, *Dance Lifts Us Up*, was funded by Awards from All (Big Lottery Fund). The aim was to deliver a dance theatre project working with people in recovery from addiction in Liverpool. Ten people participated in the project, both male and female, aged between twenty-five and sixty years old. The project enabled the group to meet weekly for twelve months in 2013–14. The focus of SAR was to examine the process of creating a dance theatre performance based on the participants' personal narratives of recovery.

Recovery from addiction to alcohol and other drugs is a long and complex process. It requires the individual to find ways to detach from their 'cellular relationship with the drug'[30] and to construct a completely new lifestyle. This can lead to a number of multifaceted issues in terms of sustaining recovery that are largely associated with the social stigma attached to drug users and the medicalization of addiction treatment. Moreover, the term 'recovery' itself is deeply problematic,[31] but when discussed in association with addiction tends to refer to psychological, mental and social wellbeing. Historically, wellbeing in this context has been regarded as a spiritual process, which includes a deep exploration of the embodied experience of addiction that can lead to a form of self-recognition and thus perform as therapy. Many self-help treatment programmes such as Alcoholics Anonymous and others have employed narrative therapy, symbolism and spirituality as important factors in the treatment of addiction. As Srdjan Sremac asserts 'by spirituality [in the treatment of addiction we] refer to transpersonal processes that transcendence [sic] ordinary material existence and its characterizing the quest for meaning'.[32]

Exploring the plurality of addiction experiences through dance theatre techniques is embedded in Fallen Angels' creative process, which is approached as a spiritual journey. Similar to Sremac's understanding of spirituality, Fallen Angels regard dance as a transcendent process. In the project *Dance Lifts Us Up*, the creative activities were framed on themes surrounding the process of recovery and designed to create a platform for the participants to express themselves, better understand their emotions and share their mutual experiences. Its purpose was to allow the participants to reconfigure their past experiences by finding alternative and imaginative ways of exploring them.

In the first workshop, the facilitator Paul Bayes Kitcher asked the participants to bring in a personal photograph that represents their journey to recovery. The participants were asked to share with the other members, reflect on them and come up with keywords that described their journey to recovery. They brought images ranging from family photos, landscapes and objects to more abstract forms. For instance, one participant brought an image of her foot taking a step which she described as symbolizing her first step to recovery. The narrative telling and sharing of personal memories was a fundamental aspect of the creative process as it urged the participants to convey new meanings to their stories and add a symbolic dimension. On the secondary level of the creative process, participants were encouraged to further demonstrate the symbolism of their stories by using a combination of movement, physical images and creative writing, which were then developed into individual and group dance routines. The materials produced during the workshops were choreographed and formulated into the final piece entitled *Letting It Go*. This was performed at the Lowry Theatre in Manchester, Salford Quays and the Royal Opera House and toured in other venues and festivals in the UK. This experience allowed the participants to reflect upon their mutual experiences, renegotiating in this way the issues of addiction recovery, stigma and acceptance. Dancing their stories was a spiritual and empowering experience, as it provided an alternative framework to conceptualize their past experiences and give them a new form and meaning. Furthermore, performing to a public audience has allowed the participants not only to bridge the gap between recovery services and the wider community but also to elucidate issues of social exclusion and acceptance.

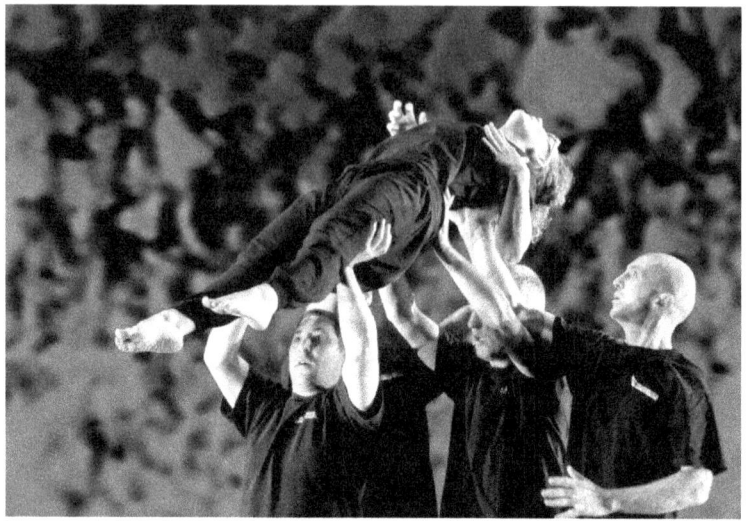

Figure 9: *Letting it Go*, Recipe for Life, West Yorkshire Playhouse. Photo © Kevin Hickson, Space2, http://www.space2.org.uk.

The evaluation of the project foregrounds these issues as it provided evidence that involvement in the dance activities has been a significant means for the participants to engage with their communities. In 2013–14, Fallen Angels reached approximately 1,500 audience members in more than six performances and open workshops. To this end, the group operated as a supportive creative network that aimed to ensure the participants' wellbeing and sense of belonging. Within the first intake in 2012, six out of eight members are now employed and two members moved into further education. All of the participants are engaging with the arts through frequent theatre visits and have taken voluntary roles in various local organizations. During a reflective discussion in June 2014, a participant responded that the project has helped them to 'feel connected with the world', and another member mentioned that 'I feel so much more in touch with the body – extreme feeling of "wellness" – optimistic about my next moment, the project helped me to feel motivated, inspirational, energized, connected, and creative.'[33]

Considering the participants' responses, alongside the project's evaluation and the findings of similar research projects[34,35] that have been conducted in the field of arts and addiction recovery, all are in agreement that participation in socially engaged theatre has a positive impact on the participants' wellbeing. My argument is that theatre can be a key component of individual and collective recovery, and that meaningful artistic and cultural production around addiction and recovery can help the individuals to gain control over their representation. It can provide a focal point within which the individual is being supported to grow, reconstruct their social identity and reorient focus on physical, mental and social wellbeing. Finally, performing personal stories of addiction to a public audience is a powerful strategy to increase the visibility of the recovery communities and promote advocacy.

10.6 Snapshot – The performance of Ebola: A critical analysis of *Ebola Doctors*

Gloria Ernest-Samuel

On 20 July 2014, Nigerians woke up to the news that a Liberian diplomat, Mr Sawyer, was diagnosed with the Ebola Virus Disease (EVD) in a Lagos hospital. Ebola was a relatively unknown disease to the majority of Nigerians and this, coupled with Ebola's high mortality rate in neighbouring Liberia and Sierra Leone, compelled the Nigerian government and non-governmental organizations (NGOs) to embark on a series of nationwide social and behaviour change communication (SBCC) campaigns that detailed the deadly disease.[36]

The mode of infection of Ebola was of great concern, since the virus is passed on through contact with bodily fluids of an infected person, and various cultural norms including burial rituals in West African society contributed to the spread.[37] Live performance was not possible as a means to educate people about the virus, but film-makers in Nollywood responded to entertain more than 150 million Nigerians. Using films to address Ebola was not a new phenomenon; indeed, Jonathan Haynes observes that Nollywood films do not 'wear high seriousness on [their] sleeve, yet the videos constantly address the problems of the Nigerian society'.[38] In Nigeria, videoed performances (as a form of public awareness) are often highly stylized and, at times, brutally comedic. In this snapshot, I will consider the impact of a comedic film created to address Ebola.

In response to the emergence of Ebola in Nigeria, film-maker Evans Orji created a comic video film called *Ebola Doctors*,[39] which was distributed in Video CDs (VCDs) at open markets across the country. The confusion and myths surrounding the Ebola virus made this video film production an instant success.[40] *Ebola Doctors* was not just the re-enactment of the Sawyer–Nigerian experience; it also exposed the prevailing myths in Nigeria that emerged during the Ebola outbreak, including the myths that certain local concoctions like drinking and bathing with salt water, as well as chewing bitter kola nut, could prevent Ebola infection.[41]

The opening scenes of the film introduce a couple of local tenants in a public yard, who were ignorant of Ebola. A sick Mr Swaner (the film name of Mr Sawyer), a Liberian visitor, is introduced with blood dropping from his nostrils. Leroy and Roquet note that 'Human Ebola virus (EBOV) infection causes haemorrhagic fever and death within a few days.'[42] With reference to this, and the transcript of Sawyer's fate in Nigeria, Mr Swaner collapses at the hotel, and the unsuspecting driver rushes him to the hospital, where he dies a couple of days later, also infecting a doctor and a nurse. The rest of the largely comical drama revolves around the uninformed and uneducated tenants and their schemes to survive the Ebola crisis through purchasing the now very exorbitantly priced bitter kola and bags of salt – scarce commodities in the world of the film.

The sequel, *Malaria Ebola*, continued to reveal public ignorance of key Ebola issues that allowed fake health workers to exploit ordinary people. The sequel allows the film-maker to tighten loose ends from the storyline of *Ebola Doctors*. For instance, the surviving nurses at the hospital where Swaner died were quarantined, but there were no efforts to trace the driver who brought Swaner to the hospital.

The Ebola virus was represented in both videos as an invincible disease, more deadly than AIDS, and preventable only by avoiding physical contact or by wearing protective shields, gloves, helmets and protective boots. To drive home this message, the characters were dressed in exaggerated costumes such as raincoats. The physical symbols of Ebola were overstated: for example, gory boils on the faces and bodies of the infected patients. Mr Swaner, the infected doctor and the nurse all bore these sores. Chief, a well-to-do character in the film, who had purchased 2,000 bags of salt (which he baptized 'warfare against Ebola'), died of an overdose of salt intake. This reinforced the dangers of belief in superstition.

Another important aspect of the film was the music created to educate the masses on the nature of Ebola. The background music in the film has lyrics that reinforced the comedic portrayal of the panic surrounding Ebola:

> Ooh! See how everybody dey fear, dey scatter, just because of Ebola. This lifewey we dey live, everybody dey fear, just because of Ebola. Ebola na dangerous disease, e dey spread like wildfire. Make you no catch Ebola, make you no spread Ebola, make you no see Ebola. If you catch Ebola, your own don kpaa …

The music used at critical moments in the video film illustrates the very real public fear of Ebola. The comic nature of the video film demands exaggerated actions to implant the advocacy message and scare tactics. The instruction, 'if you catch Ebola, your own don kpaa' suggests that any person who is infected with Ebola is doomed, although some people did survive. One of the characters, Jekwu, whose fiancée worked as a nurse in the hospital, stubbornly refused her access to his home, but instead he invites the police to take her away for monitoring. This comically presented action, although seemingly cruel, drives home the need for people to be cautious with people exposed to Ebola.

Ebola Doctors may be highly farcical in nature, but it did fill a need for public education through the farce. Orji, the film-maker, saw the war on the Ebola epidemic in Nigeria as crucial. He adopted a comic or farcical form to reach the grassroots audiences, who follow comedies featuring star actors like Chiwetalu Agu and Dede One Day. Yet it is also important to consider the broader ramifications of the comic framing of people's genuine fears and instinctive responses. Despite the fact that comedy can be used to mock and ridicule powerful people and fears, I wonder if by making the behaviour farcical (such as the satiric focus on the fake cures or the lack of knowledge), Orji ran the risk of promoting these behaviours. Although Orji's decision to mock particular behaviours was to raise awareness, I would argue that in fact he was further stigmatizing Ebola and making the victims and their family members even greater objects of fear. Indeed, I think that the comedic focus and structure of *Ebola Doctors* demonstrates one of the major problems in using performance for health education – that tension between bringing critical attention to risky behaviours and unintentionally endorsing that which you seek to critique.

Afterword

Veronica Baxter and Katharine Low

The scope of *Applied Theatre: Performing Health and Wellbeing* represents our desire to reflect multivalent and global voices in Applied Theatre and performance, in and for health and wellbeing. From its inception, we were determined to engage in dialogue across continents and borders, and foreground experiences and scholarship from the Global South as well as from the Global North. The range of research essays, snapshots and interviews is wide in geopolitical regions and subject matter, bringing together an astounding spectrum of practices under the banner of Applied Theatre. In addition, the book as a whole addresses many concerns reflected in the Millennium Development Goals, and will continue to be relevant to the Sustainable Development Goals (SDGs) released in 2015. Despite the best efforts of the United Nations, however, the critique of the SDGs is instructive for a new generation of those who would seek to work in the field of arts in health and arts for health. While the overall focus on poverty eradication is welcome, there are some fundamental contradictions inherent in the SDGs. For example, Jason Hickel argues that the solutions presented to many of the challenges '[rely] precisely on the old model of industrial growth – ever-increasing levels of extraction, production, and consumption'.[1] The same may be said for approaching health through the biomedical model, embracing the 'silver bullet' of developing medication to cure illness, rather than socioeconomic change to prevent it. The biomedical approach also privileges the 'gold standards' of research in this area, namely randomized-controlled trials and systematic reviews,[2] rather than understanding or appreciating a more participatory, individual and qualitative account of impacts emerging from the practice.

Throughout the editing and writing process, we have remained acutely aware of the Commission on Social Determinants of Health's call to action to both governments and NGOs and civil society to respond to global health crises.[3] Accordingly, the health concerns that have been addressed in this book are ones we felt were essential to discuss, either because they are concerns that have significant global impact or because they are not often considered or addressed on a global stage. Throughout the book there is an interlinking between certain chapters that focus on more of a biomedical framework of health compared to others that engage with the socio-cultural perspectives of health and wellbeing. In all of this we are conscious of the relationships between the global move towards neoliberal values and agendas and the structural constraints on health provision in the Global South. We are also aware of the tension between the experience of art-making or involvement in the arts compared with advocacy through the arts, which can lead to significant frustration and misunderstandings across different contexts; frustration in the inability to change the circumstances of dysfunctional health care provision where the theatre and performance takes up the cudgels in the absence of the political will to fulfil the World Health Organization's mandate.

In addition, this book challenges notions of wellbeing in part due to their close associations with political agendas and social organizations, such as the Happiness Index[4] or Action for Happiness.[5] These arguably displace attention from the structural causes of unhappiness and ill health. A person's perception of their wellbeing might be influenced by their optimism; but optimism in itself is a cultural construct, and exists in a socioeconomic context. Additionally, while we have not addressed, other than tangentially, the role of spirituality in the context of wellbeing, the glib calls for happiness, as in Augusto Boal's 1997 campaign, 'have the courage to be happy',[6] should be weighed against the real structural and social determinants of health. And, indeed, the contributors to this edited collection have not fallen into simple 'solutions' to address the health issues they consider. Rather, the work is provocative, challenging and exciting, offering alternative ways of addressing and understanding health and wellbeing. Underlying each practice lies a deep commitment to activism, beautiful theatre-making and exploring and understanding health issues globally and across all generations. Furthermore, echoing John Ashton's view, the practices discussed fundamentally recognize that 'Arts and culture are a part of every human's makeup and potential, assets that should be explored and developed – not commodities that can be separated from the essence of the person and exploited.'[7]

As a result, this book is responsive to many challenges in Applied and performance and reactive to particular health crises. However, we were not able to consider all significant health challenges facing the global population. For example, we have not adequately looked at health issues facing children and youth, especially considering the statistics:

> There are about 1.8 billion young people between the ages of 10 and 24 – the largest youth population ever. Many of them are concentrated in developing countries. In fact, in the world's 48 least developed countries, children or adolescents make up a majority of the population.[8]

Other than briefly considering domestic violence in a snapshot, we have not addressed violence, constituting 'interpersonal violence, namely child maltreatment, youth violence, intimate partner and sexual violence, and elder abuse',[9] as a health issue. The violent upheavals of war are studied in *Applied Theatre: Resettlement*.[10] Nor has there been enough focus on maternal health considering that 'for every 100,000 babies born in sub-Saharan Africa, 510 women die from maternal causes. Globally, some 800 women die every day from causes related to pregnancy.'[11] We note these absences not to undermine the breadth of topics discussed in this book, nor to suggest that Applied theatre is a panacea for all contexts. Rather we wish to draw attention and encourage an increased focus on these health challenges. Alongside this, while focus on major problems may feel glossed over owing to the snapshots' brevity, it felt imperative to note growing trends, such as environmental health and intermediality in health contexts, at the very least in brief.

In conclusion, we hope that the reader has found the inspirations and provocations promised in the introduction. We close by looking forward to the future developments and further research in theatre and performance in wellbeing and health, where we work alongside each other, critiquing and celebrating making art in and for health together.

Notes

Introduction

1 Richard Horton, 'GBD 2010: understanding disease, injury, and risk', *The Lancet* 380 (2012): 2053.
2 Mohsen Naghavi et al., 'Global, regional, and national age-sex specific all-cause and cause-specific mortality for 240 causes of death, 1990–2013: a systematic analysis for the Global Burden of Disease Study 2013', *The Lancet* 385 (2015): 117.
3 Ibid., pp. 142, 128.
4 WHO, *Closing the Gap: Policy into Practice on Social Determinants of Health – Discussion Paper*, World Health Organization, Department of Ethics, Equity, Trade and Human Rights (Geneva: WHO, 2011).
5 Dean T. Jamison et al., 'Global health 2035: a world converging within a generation', *The Lancet* 382 (2013): 1899.
6 Commission on Social Determinants of Health, *Closing the Gap in a Generation: Health Equity Through Aaction on the Social Determinants of Health: Commission on Social Determinants of Health Final Report* (Geneva: WHO, 2008), p. 18.
7 Peter Bazalgette, 'Use the arts to boost the nation's health', *Guardian*, 28 December 2014, http://www.theguardian.com/commentisfree/2014/dec/28/arts-boost-nations-health-nhs-funding-arts-council (accessed 5 January 2015).
8 For more information on the APPG for Arts, Health and Wellbeing, see: http://www.artshealthandwellbeing.org.uk/APPG (accessed 5 January 2015).
9 John Ashton, 'Let's Invest in Real Health', in Arts Council England, *Create: A Journal of Perspectives on the Value of Art & Culture* (Manchester: Arts Council England, 2014), p. 95.
10 See: Helen Nicholson, *Applied Drama: The Gift of Theatre* (Basingstoke: Palgrave Macmillan, 2005).

11 James Thompson, *Applied Theatre: Bewilderment and Beyond* (Oxford: Peter Lang, 2006).
12 Gareth White, *Applied Theatre: Aesthetics* (London: Bloomsbury Methuen Drama, 2015).
13 Tom Barone and Elliot W Eisner, *Arts-Based Research* (London: Sage Publications, 2012).
14 Alain de Botton and John Armstrong, *Art as Therapy* (Oxford: Phaidon Press, 2013).
15 Emma Brodzinski, *Theatre in Health and Care* (Basingstoke: Palgrave Macmillan, 2010), p. 15.
16 François Matarasso, *Regular Marvels: A handbook for Animateurs, Practitioners and Development Workers in Dance, Mime, Music and Literature* (Leicester: Community Dance and Mime Foundation, 1994), pp. 3–4.
17 An HDI rating is a combined measure of indicators that record levels of 'life expectancy, educational attainment and command over the resources needed for a decent living'. UNDP, *Human Development Report 2013: The Rise of the South: Human Progress in a Diverse World* (New York: United Nations Development Programme, 2013), p. 1, http://www.undp.org/content/undp/en/home/librarypage/hdr/human-development-report-2013/ (accessed 16 July 2014).
18 Tony Payne, '"The Rise of the South" – or the Disappearance of the South?', *HDialogue blog*, 14 June 2013, http://hdr.undp.org/en/content/%E2%80%98-rise-south%E2%80%99-%E2%80%93-or-disappearance-south (accessed 24 July 2014).
19 World Bank, *Gini Index (World Bank Estimate)* (2016), http://data.worldbank.org/indicator/SI.POV.GINI (accessed 14 March 2016).

Chapter 1

1 We have chosen the spelling of 'wellbeing', but maintained authors' original spelling in quotations.
2 Karelisa V. Hartigan, *Performance and Cure: Drama and Healing in Ancient Greece and Contemporary America* (London: Duckworth, 2009), pp. vii–viii.

3   Edwin Heathcote, 'Architecture and Health', in Charles Jencks and Edwin Heathcote (eds.), *The Architecture of Hope: Maggie's Cancer Caring Centres* (London: Frances Lincoln Ltd, 2010), p. 56.
4   Hartigan, pp. 14–15.
5   Heathcote, pp. 55–6.
6   Ibid., p. 56.
7   Eleonora Belfiore, 'The arts and healing: The power of an idea', in Stephen Clift and Paul M. Camic (eds), *Oxford Textbook of Creative Arts, Health, and Wellbeing: International Perspectives on Practice, Policy and Research* (Oxford: Oxford University Press, 2015), p 13.
8   Ibid., pp. 13–14.
9   Susan Sontag. *Illness as Metaphor and AIDS as Its Metaphors* (London: Penguin Classics, 1991).
10 Marilyn Bordwell. 'Dancing with Death: Performativity and "undiscussable" bodies in still/here', *Text and Performance Quarterly* 18:4 (1998): 375.
11 Friedrich Nietzsche, *The Gay Science* (New York: Vantage Books, 1974), pp. 176–7.
12 François Matarasso, '"No appealing solution": evaluating the outcomes of arts and health initiatives', in Martyn Evans and Ilora G. Finlay (eds), *Medical Humanities* (London: BMJ Books, 2001), p. 39.
13 K. M. Boyd, 'Disease, illness, sickness, health, healing and wholeness: exploring some elusive concepts', *Medical Humanities* 26 (2000): 9–12.
14 Ibid., p. 17.
15 George Canguilhem (1991), p. 196f, cited in Boyd, 'Disease, illness, sickness, health, healing and wholeness: exploring some elusive concepts', p. 14.
16 Malcolm MacLachlan, *Culture and Health: A Critical Perspective Towards Global Health*, 2nd edn (Chichester: John Wiley & Sons, 2006), p. 20.
17 Alan Blum, *The Grey Zone of Health and Illness* (Bristol: Intellect, 2011), p. 13.
18 MacLachlan, *Culture and Health*, p. 21.
19 Blum, *The Grey Zone of Health and Illness*, p. 13.
20 Ibid., p. 13.
21 Ibid., pp. 13–14.
22 Marian Pitts and Keith Phillips, *The Psychology of Health: An Introduction* (London: Routledge, 1998), pp. 6–7.

23 WHO (1946), Preamble to the Constitution of the World Health Organization as adopted by the International Health Conference, New York, 19–22 June, 1946; signed on 22 July 1946 by the representatives of 61 States (*Official Records of the World Health Organization*, no. 2, p. 100) and entered into force on 7 April 1948.
24 Richard Doll, 'Health and the environment in the 1990's', *American Journal of Public Health* 82, no. 7 (1992): 933.
25 Rodolfo Saracci, 'The World Health Organization needs to reconsider its definition of health', *British Medical Journal* 314 (1997): 1409.
26 Department of Health, South Africa, *Vision & Mission* (2016), http://www.health.gov.za/index.php/shortcodes/vision-mission (accessed 2 January 2016).
27 National Department of Health, Papua New Guinea, *Health is Everybody's Business*, 2015, http://www.health.gov.pg/ (accessed 2 January 2016).
28 Ministry of Health, Singapore, *Vision, Mission, Values*, 2016, https://www.moh.gov.sg/content/moh_web/home/about-us/vision-mission-values.html (accessed 2 January 2016).
29 Saracci, p. 1409.
30 Niyi Awofeso (2005), 'Re-defining "Health"', comment on Bedirhan T. Üstün and Robert Jakob's 'Calling a spade a spade: Meaningful definitions of health conditions', *Bulletin of the World Health Organization* 83, no. 11 (2005): 802–3, http://www.who.int/bulletin/bulletin_board/83/ustun11051/en/ (accessed 4 February 2013).
31 National Aboriginal Community Controlled Health Organisation, *Constitution for the National Aboriginal Community Controlled Health Organisation*, 2011, pp. 5–6, http://www.naccho.org.au/download/naccho-governance/NACCHO%20CONSTITUTION%20Ratified%20Ver%2015111%20for%20ASIC%20.pdf (accessed 4 February 2013).
32 Richard Horton (2003), p. 505, cited in Mike White, *Arts Development in Community Health: A Social Tonic* (Oxford: Radcliffe Publishing, 2009), p. 55.
33 Mike White, *Arts Development in Community Health: A Social Tonic* (Oxford: Radcliffe Publishing, 2009), p. 54.
34 WHO, *Closing the Gap: Policy into Practice on Social Determinants of Health – Discussion Paper* (Geneva: World Health Organization, Department of Ethics, Equity, Trade and Human Rights, 2011), p. 8.

35 David Cameron cited in 'Money can't buy happiness – or can it?', *The Economist*, 30 November 2010, http://www.economist.com/blogs/theworldin2011/2010/11/happiness_and_gdp (accessed 2 January 2016).
36 Allegra Stratton, 'David Cameron aims to make happiness the new GDP', *The Guardian*, 14 November 2010, http://www.theguardian.com/politics/2010/nov/14/david-cameron-wellbeing-inquiry (accessed 21 November 2014).
37 White, *Arts Development*, p. 50.
38 Marc Pilkington, 'Well-Being, Happiness and the Structural Crisis of Neoliberalism – An Interdisciplinary Analysis Through the Lenses of Emotions', *Mind & Society* (2015): 5–7, DOI: 10.1007/s11299-015-0181-0.
39 William Davies, 'Spirits of neoliberalism: "Competitiveness" and "wellbeing" indicators as rival orders of worth', in Richard Rottenberg, Sally E. Merry, Sung-Joon Park and Johanna Mugler (eds), *The World of Indicators: The Making of Governmental Knowledge through Quantification* (Cambridge: Cambridge University Press, 2015), pp. 301–2.
40 Atul Gawande, *The Reith Lectures 2014: The Future of Medicine: Lecture 4: The Idea of Wellbeing*, http://www.bbc.co.uk/programmes/b04v380z (accessed 21 December 2014).
41 Jean M. Twenge cited in Daniel Dorling, *Injustice: Why Social Inequality Persists* (Bristol: Policy Press, 2011), pp. 277–8.
42 Ray Pahl, 'Society, community, well-being', in Martyn Evans and Ilora G. Finlay (eds), *Medical Humanities* (London: BMJ Books, 2001), p. 29.
43 Richard Eckersley, 'Culture health and well-being'. In Richard Eckersley, Jane Dixon and Bob Douglas (eds), *The Social Origins of Health and Well-Being* (Cambridge: Cambridge University Press, 2002), pp. 51–70.
44 Ibid., pp. 56–62.
45 Ibid., p. 61.
46 Richard Ings, Nikki Crane and Marsaili Cameron, *Be Creative Be Well: Arts, Wellbeing and Local Communities: An Evaluation* (London: Arts Council England, 2012). The Be Creative Be Well programme was a three-and-a-half year project which funded over 100 artistic and cultural projects in twenty London boroughs aimed at improving health and wellbeing and increasing community engagement in impoverished

communities: http://www.welllondon.org.uk/31/be-creative-be-well.html (accessed 12 January 2013).
47 Ibid., p. 27.
48 New Economics Forum, *Five Ways to Wellbeing* (London: New Economics Forum, 2008), p. 17, http://www.neweconomics.org/publications/entry/five-ways-to-well-being-the-evidence (accessed 12 January 2013).
49 Felice Yuen et al., '"You Might as well Call it Planet of the Sioux": Indigenous Youth, Imagination, and Decolonization', *Pimatisiwin: A Journal of Aboriginal and Indigenous Community Health* 11:2 (2013): 269–81.
50 MacLachlan, pp. 21–3.
51 Ibid., p. 30.
52 Emma Brodzinski, *Theatre in Health and Care* (Basingstoke: Palgrave Macmillan, 2010), p. 15.
53 White (2014), p. 5.
54 Ibid.
55 Ibid.
56 Ibid., p. 6.
57 Stephen Clift, 'Creative arts as a public health resource: Moving from practice-based research to evidence-based practice', *Perspectives in Public Health* 132: 123, cited by Belfiore (2015), p. 16.
58 Belfiore (2015), p. 16.
59 Deirdre Heddon, 'Perspectives on the impact agenda from inside', presented at When the Writing is On the Wall: A Discussion of the Ecology of Research, Creativity, Impact and Value, TaPRA Applied and Social Theatre Working Group Interim Event, 9 May 2015, Royal Central School of Speech and Drama, London.
60 Eleonora Belfiore and Oliver Bennett, *The Social Impact of the Arts: An Intellectual History* (Basingstoke: Palgrave Macmillan, 2008), p. 106. Emphasis in original.
61 Ibid.
62 Ibid., p. 194.
63 Ings et al., p. 2.
64 Peter Baelz, 'Philosophy of Health Education', in Ian Sutherland (ed.), *Health Education: Perspectives and Choices* (London: Allen and Unwin,

1979), p. 32, cited in Mike White, *Arts Development in Community Health: A Social Tonic* (Oxford: Radcliffe Publishing, 2009), p. 43. Emphasis in original.
65   White (2009), p. 43.
66   WHO, *About WHO: Leadership Priorities*, 2014, http://www.who.int/workforcealliance/members_partners/member_list/who/en/ (accessed 5 July 2014).
67   MacLachlan, p. 21.
68   Glenn Laverack, *Health Promotion Practice: Power and Empowerment* (London: SAGE Publications, 2005), p. 2.
69   E. Ashworth Underwood. 'Rudolf Virchow', Encyclopædia Britannica, 2016, http://www.britannica.com/biography/Rudolf-Virchow (accessed 17 March 2016).
70   Laverack (2005), pp. 1–2.
71   Daniel Pridan, 'Rudolf Virchow and Social Medicine in Historical Perspective', *Medical History* 8 (1964): 274–8.
72   Rudolf Virchow cited in Daniel Pridan, 'Rudolf Virchow and Social Medicine in Historical Perspective', *Medical History* 8 (1964): 278.
73   WHO, *World Health Organisation: Member Profile*, 2014, http://www.who.int/about/agenda/en/ (accessed 5 July 2014).
74   Full details of the development and history of the MDGs can be found at http://www.un.org/millenniumgoals/ (accessed 5 July 2014).
75   UN, *Conferences, Meetings and Events: Millennium Summit (6–8 September 2000)*, 2014, http://www.un.org/en/events/pastevents/millennium_summit.shtml (accessed 5 July 2014).
76   UN Millennium Project, *Investing in Development: A Practical Plan to Achieve the Millennium Development Goals* (New York: United Nations Development Programme, 2005), p. 4.
77   The concern with global security was particularly heightened following the 9/11 attacks in the US, with the Secretary-General, Kofi Annan, emphasizing 'the vital importance of multilateral efforts to maintain international peace and security'. *Report of the Secretary-General*, 2002, p. 3, http://www.un.org/millenniumgoals/sgreport2002.pdf?OpenElement (accessed 7 July 2014).
78   Matthew Clarke and Simon Feeny, *Millennium Development Goals beyond 2015* (Abingdon, Oxford: Routledge, 2013), p. 2.

79 For example, in 2002, Kofi Annan informed UN member states that '[a] much larger effort is needed from all actors, working together in a true global partnership in which all partners have mutual responsibilities and commitments and accept mutual accountability'. *Report of the Secretary-General*, 2002, p. 3, http://www.un.org/millenniumgoals/sgreport2002.pdf?OpenElement (accessed 7 July 2014).
80 DfID, DfID: Annual Report and Accounts 2012–2013, https://www.gov.uk/government/uploads/system/uploads/attachment_data/file/208445/annual-report-accounts2013-13.pdf (accessed 7 July 2014).
81 Ibid., pp. 23–7.
82 c.f. Radelet 2004, cited by Clarke and Feeny (2013), p. 4.
83 Malcolm Langford, Andy Sumner and Alicia Ely Yamin (eds), *Millennium Development Goals and Human Rights* (New York: Cambridge University Press, 2013), pp. 2–4.
84 Jan Vandermoortele, 'A fresh look at the MDGs', in Matthew Clarke and Simon Feeny, *Millennium Development Goals beyond 2015* (Abingdon, Oxford: Routledge, 2013), pp. 14–16.
85 Ibid., pp. 15–16.
86 DfID, p. 19.
87 Langford, Sumner and Ely Yamin (2013), p. 7.
88 WHO, *Social Determinants of Health: Key Concepts*, 2016, http://www.who.int/social_determinants/thecommission/finalreport/key_concepts/en/ (accessed 2 January 2016).
89 Marmot Review, *Fair Society – Health Lives: Strategic Review of Health Inequalities in England Post 2010* (London: Marmot Review Team, 2010), p. 3.
90 Paul Farmer, *Pathologies of Power: Health, Human Rights, and the New War on the Poor* (Berkley: University of California Press, 2005), p. xvi.
91 Ibid., p. 8.
92 Ibid., p. 40.
93 Ibid., p. 50.
94 Ibid., p. 41.
95 Hereafter, 'the Commission'.
96 Commission on Social Determinants of Health, *Closing the Gap in a Generation: Health Equity Through Action on the Social Determinants of Health: Commission on Social Determinants of Health Final Report* (Geneva: WHO, 2008), p. 18.

97 Ibid.
98 Paul Heritage and Silvia Ramos, 'Talking about a revolution: Arts, health and wellbeing on Avenida Brasil', in Stephen Clift and Paul M. Camic (eds), *Oxford Textbook of Creative Arts, Health, and Wellbeing: International Perspectives on Practice, Policy and Research* (Oxford: Oxford University Press, 2015), p. 180.
99 Ibid., p. 184.
100 Daniel Dorling, *Injustice: Why Social Inequality Persists* (Bristol: Policy Press, 2011), pp. 288–90.
101 Commission on Social Determinants of Health, pp. 18–19.
102 Funded by the Bill and Melinda Gates Foundation, the 2010 GBD study was a global investigation incorporating research and analysis from 486 researchers from more than fifty countries over a five-year period. It is unique in that it attempted to develop a systematic, scientific approach to analyse and understand the differing trends in health issues. In 2013 an updated GBD study was undertaken. Full details can be found at: http://www.thelancet.com/global-burden-of-disease (accessed 7 July 2014).
103 Richard Horton, 'GBD 2010: understanding disease, injury, and risk', *The Lancet* 380, no. 9859 (2012): 2053.
104 Ibid., p. 2054.
105 When considering the burden of disease on the global population, health researchers employ a measurement called disability-adjusted life years (DALYs). This measurement is one way of comparing and understanding the impact of ill-health on the world's population and, crucially, a way of comparing and cross-examining different health crises. The WHO describes DALYs as follows: 'One DALY can be thought of as one lost year of "healthy" life. The sum of these DALYs across the population, or the burden of disease, can be thought of as a measurement of the gap between current health status and an ideal health situation where the entire population lives to an advanced age, free of disease and disability', WHO, 2014, http://www.who.int/healthinfo/global_burden_disease/metrics_daly/en/ (accessed 5 July 2014).
106 Christopher J. Murray et al., 'Disability-adjusted life years (DALYs) for 291 diseases and injuries in 21 regions, 1990–2010: A systematic analysis

for the Global Burden of Disease Study 2010', *The Lancet* 380, no. 9859 (2012): 2198.
107 Ibid.
108 Ibid., p. 2218.
109 Sarah Boseley, 'UK child death rate among worst in western Europe, say experts', *The Guardian*, 3 May 2014, http://www.theguardian.com/society/2014/may/02/uk-child-death-rate-western-europe-health (accessed 30 May 2014).
110 Ingrid Wolfe et al., *Why Children Die: Death in Infants, Children and Young People in the UK Part A* (London: Royal College of Paediatrics and Child Health, 2014), p. 18.
111 Boseley (2014).
112 Dorling, *Injustice: Why Social Inequality Persists*, pp. 288–90.
113 Matthew Connolly, *Fatal Misconception: The Struggle to Control World Population* (Cambridge, MA: Harvard University Press, 2008), p. 29, cited in Dorling, *Injustice: Why Social Inequality Persists*, p. 291.
114 Dorling, *Injustice: Why Social Inequality Persists*, pp. 288–91.
115 Michael Marmot, 'Social determinants of health inequalities', *The Lancet* 365, no. 9464 (2005): 1100–2.
116 Ibid., p. 1103.
117 Marmot Review, p. 1099.
118 Denise Roland, 'Experts Critize World Health Organization's "Slow" Ebola Outbreak Response', *Wall Street Journal*, 12 May 2015, http://www.wsj.com/articles/experts-criticize-world-health-organizations-slow-ebola-outbreak-response-1431344306 (accessed 30 May 2015).
119 Commission on Social Determinants of Health, p. 1.
120 Vandermoortele, p. 17.
121 Thomas Pogge, 'Poverty, Hunger, and Cosmetic Progress', in Malcolm Langford, Andy Sumner and Alicia Ely Yamin (eds), *Millennium Development Goals and Human Rights* (New York: Cambridge University Press, 2013), pp. 210–12.
122 David Buck, 'Tackling Health Inequalities: We Need a National Conversation', *The King's Fund Blog*, 24 February 2014, http://www.kingsfund.org.uk/blog/2014/02/tackling-health-inequalities-we-need-national-conversation (accessed 12 May 2014). In his discussion, Buck points to the 2010 Marmot Review, which concluded that there was

disparity between the poorest and richest communities in the UK, equivalent to a difference of seven years in life expectancy and seventeen years in disability-free life expectancy, and questions why Public Health England has neglected to develop a strategy or analyse the situation. This situation, when coupled with the increasing cuts to the NHS, has resulted in a difficult situation for the general population, particularly the poorer population.
123 Gabriel Scally, 'Have we lost the battle to improve health inequalities?', *The King's Fund: Think Differently Blog*, 24 January 2013, http://www.kingsfund.org.uk/time-to-think-differently/blog/have-we-lost-battle-improve-health-inequalities (accessed 12 May 2014).

Chapter 2

1 There are many other terms, including Theatre of the Oppressed, Popular Theatre for Social Change, Travelling Theatre and Community Theatre. For analysis of the nuances between these terms, see Tim Prentki, *Applied Theatre: Development* (London: Methuen Bloomsbury, 2015).
2 See Tim Prentki for a discussion of the terminology around 'applied' theatre and performance, and the term 'development'.
3 WHO. Factsheet on Alcohol (WHO, 2015), http://www.who.int/mediacentre/factsheets/fs349/en/ (accessed 13 April 2016).
4 Ibid.
5 Peter O'Connor and Michael Anderson, *Applied Theatre Research: Radical Departures* (London: Methuen Bloomsbury, 2015, Kindle edn).
6 Jane Plastow, 'Domestication or transformation? The ideology of Theatre for Development in Africa', *Applied Theatre Research* 2:2 (2014): 107–18.
7 L. Dale Byam, *Community in Motion: Theatre for Development in Africa* (Westport, CT: Greenwood Publishing Group, 1999).
8 Kees Epskamp, *Theatre for Development: Introduction to Context, Applications and Training* (Chicago: Chicago University Press/Zed Books, 2006).
9 Here the reference to drama specifically includes classroom or

process drama, or the realm of work that was once known as drama-in-education.
10 James Thompson, *Performance Affects: Applied Theatre and the End of Effect* (London: Palgrave Macmillan, 2009), pp. 136–59.
11 Gareth White, *Applied Theatre: Aesthetics* (London: Bloomsbury Methuen Drama, 2015).
12 Thompson, p. 6.
13 Jacques Rancière, *The Emancipated Spectator*, trans. Gregory Elliott (London: Verso, 2009), p. 14.
14 George Bernard Shaw, 'Maxims for Revolutionaries', *Collected Works of George Bernard Shaw: Plays, Novels, Articles, Letters, Essays* (e-artnow, 2015, Kindle edn).
15 Brad Haseman and Joe Winston, '"Why be interested?" Aesthetics, applied theatre and drama education', *Research in Drama Education: The Journal of Applied Theatre and Performance* 15:4 (2010): 465–75, DOI: 10.1080/13569783.2010.512182.
16 Ibid., p. 470.
17 Anthony Jackson, *Theatre, Education and the Makings of Meanings* (Manchester: Manchester University Press, 2007).
18 Robert Landy, *Drama Therapy: Concepts, Theories and Practices* (Springfield, IL: Charles C. Thomas, 1994).
19 Michelle Sleed, Kevin Durrheim, Anita Kriel, Vernon Solomon and Veronica Baxter, 'The effectiveness of the vignette methodology: A comparison of written and video vignettes in eliciting responses about date rape', *South African Journal of Psychology* 32 (3 December 2002): 21–8.
20 Ibid., p. 25.
21 Prentki, *Applied Theatre*, pp. 27–9.
22 Zakes Mda, *When People Play People – Development Communication Through Theatre* (Johannesburg: Wits University Press, 1993), pp. 115–63.
23 Paulo Freire, *Pedagogy of the Oppressed*, trans. Myra Bergman Ramos (London: Penguin, 1996).
24 These terms are most frequently used on the international website for The Communication Initiative, http://www.comminit.com (accessed 17 March 2016).

25 Mda, *When People Play People*, pp. 162–3.
26 Ibid., pp. 160–1.
27 Prentki, *Applied Theatre*, pp. 27–9.
28 Henry A. Giroux, *On Critical Pedagogy. Critical Pedagogy Today Series* (New York: Continuum Books, 2011), ePublication.
29 David Kerr, '"You just made the blueprint to suit yourselves" – a theatre-based health research project in Lungwena, Malawi', in Tim Prentki and Sheila Preston (eds), *The Applied Theatre Reader* (London: Routledge, 2009), pp. 100–7.
30 Ibid., p. 102.
31 United Nations, Universal Declaration of Human Rights, http://www.un.org/en/universal-declaration-human-rights/ (accessed 17 March 2016).
32 This was also an indicator in DramAidE's 1992–9 work, where the intervention culminated in a community festival where other performances by participants were presented.
33 P. Siriwardhana, A. H. Dawson and R. Abeyasinge, *Alcohol and Alcoholism* 48:2 (2013): 250–6 (254), DOI:10.1093/alcalc/ags116.
34 Ibid., p. 254.
35 John Gill, 'Does rudeness have a place in academia?', *Times Higher Education*, 7 November 2013. Sayre's Law was coined by Wallace Sayre, Columbia University, who argued that 'academic politics are so vicious precisely because the stakes are so small'.
36 Francois Matarasso, 'Smoke and mirrors: a response to Paola Merli's "evaluating the Social impact of participation in Arts activities"', *International Journal of Cultural Policy* Vol. 9, No. 3 (2003): 337–46, DOI: 10.1080/1028663032000161759.
37 Mike White, *Arts Development in Community Health: A Social Tonic* (Oxon: Radcliffe Books, 2009).
38 Ibid., p. 203.
39 Ibid., pp. 203–4.
40 https://twitter.com/alaindebotton/status/394021414816075776 (accessed 17 March 2016).
41 Eugene van Erven, *Community Theatre – Global Perspectives* (London: Routledge, 2001), p. 9.
42 Claire Bishop. *Artificial Hells: Participatory Art and the Politics of Spectatorship* (London: Verso, 2012), p. 242.

43 Irit Rogoff, 'Turning', *e-flux journal* (November 2008), www.e-flux.com. (accessed 22 December 2015).
44 Ibid., p. 274.
45 Soori E. Nnko, Susan R. Whyte, Wenzel P. Geissler and Jens Aagaard-Hansen, 'Scepticism towards insecticide treated mosquito nets for malaria control in rural community in north-western Tanzania', *Tanzania Journal of Health Research Volume* 14:2 (April 2012): 8, DOI: http://dx.doi.org/10.4314/thrb.v14i2.2.
46 Kim L. Niewolny and Arthur L. Wilson, ' "Social Learning" for/in Adult Education? A Discursive Review of What it Means for Learning to be "Social" ', Adult Education Research Conference proceedings, 2009, http://www.adulterc.org/proceedings/2009/proceedings/niewolny_wilson.pdf (accessed 19 January 2016).
47 Augusto Boal, *Theatre of the Oppressed* (London: Pluto Press, 1979).
48 Veronica Baxter, 'Forum theatre: Learning to live with Limitations', *South African Theatre Journal* 19 (2005): 130–42.
49 Thompson, *Performance Affects*, pp. 60–5.
50 Ibid., p. 46.
51 Ibid., pp. 47–8.
52 Ibid., p. 49.
53 Elektra Tselikas, 'Social Theatre', in Sue Jennings (ed.), *Dramatherapy and Social Theatre* (London: Routledge, 2009), pp.15–29.
54 Ibid., p. 20.
55 Bertolt Brecht and John Willett, *Brecht on Theatre: The Development of an Aesthetic* (London: Methuen, 1964).
56 Arvind Singhal, Michael J. Cody, Everett M. Rogers and Miguel Sabido, *Entertainment-Education and Social Change: History, Research, and Practice* (Mahwah, NJ: Laurence Erlbaum, 2008).
57 Arvind Singhal and Everett M. Rogers, *Entertainment-Education: A Communication Strategy for Social Change* (Mahwah, NJ: Lawrence Erlbaum Associates, 1999). p. 9.
58 A. Bandura, 'Social cognitive theory for personal and social change by enabling media', in A. Singhal, M. J. Cody, E. M. Rogers and M. Sabido (eds), *Entertainment-Education and Social Change: History, Research, and Practice* (Abingdon: Taylor and Francis eLibrary, 2008), pp. 75–96.

59 Ibid., p. 77.
60 Ibid., p. 78.
61 Ibid., Chapter 20: 'Entertainment-Education Through Participatory Theatre: Freirean Strategies for Empowering the Oppressed'.
62 Lynn Dalrymple, 'Has it made a difference? Understanding and measuring the impact of applied theatre with young people in the South African contex', *Research in Drama Education (RIDE)* 11:2 (June 2006): 201–18.
63 Despite the critique above of Bandura's theories, an exceptional success story for health and performance is the television series *Soul City*, http://www.soulcity.org.za/ (accessed 2 May 2016).
64 S. Vatan and D. Lester, 'The internal consistency and concurrent validity of the Hopelessness, Helplessness, and Haplessness Scale in a Turkish clinical sample', *Psychological Reports* 103 (2008): 701–2.
65 Genevieve Minota Stander, 'Class, Race and Locus of Control in Democratic South Africa', unpublished thesis (University of Stellenbosch, 2014).
66 Rotter (1990), in Stander, 'Class, Race and Locus of Control', pp. 84–5.
67 Pertti J. Pelto and Rajendra Singh, 'Community Street Theatre as a Tool for Interventions on Alcohol Use and Other Behaviors Related to HIV Risks', *AIDS Behavior* 14 (2010): 147–57, DOI: 10.1007/s10461-010-9726-8.
68 Ibid., p. 151.
69 Ibid., p. 156.
70 Ibid., p. 155.
71 Beth Osnes, *Theatre for Women's Participation in Sustainable Development* (London: Routledge, 2014).
72 Ibid., p. 18.
73 http://www.starfish-impact.org (accessed 21 February 2016).
74 Ibid., p. 83.
75 Ibid., p. 86.
76 Ibid., p. 95.
77 Dan J Stein, 2009. 'The Psychobiology of Resilience', *CNS Spectr* 14:2 (Suppl. 3): 41–7.
78 Ibid., p. 44.
79 Shelley E. Taylor and Jonathon D. Brown, 'Positive illusions

and well-being revisited: Separating fact from fiction', *Psychological Bulletin* 116:1 (July 1994): 21–7, DOI: http://dx.doi.org/10.1037/0033-2909.116.1.21.

80   Martin Seligman, *Flourish: A New Understanding of Happiness and Wellbeing and How to Achieve Them* (London: Nicolas Brealey Publishing, 2011, Kindle edn), p. 167.

81   Ibid., pp. 197–200.

82   Ibid., p. 193.

83   Theatre-making workshops were conducted with a company of inmates and parolees over a year, a collaboration between Help I Am Free and the University of Cape Town Drama department. http://www.helpiamfree.com/ (accessed 2 May 2016).

84   Mark E. Koltko-Rivera, 'Rediscovering the later version of Maslow's hierarchy of needs: Self-transcendence and opportunities for theory, research, and unification', *Review of General Psychology* 10:4 (December 2006): 302–17, http://dx.doi.org/10.1037/1089-2680.10.4.302.

85   http://www.singforyourlife.org.uk/ (accessed 13 March 2016).

86   Ann Skingley and Hilary Bungay, 'The Silver Song Club Project: singing to promote the health of older people', *British Journal of Community Nursing* 15:3 (March 2010): 135–40.

87   Ross Prior (ed.), *Journal of the Applied Arts in Health* (Intellect Books), http://www.intellectbooks.co.uk/journals/view-Journal,id=169/ (accessed 17 March 2016).

88   Paul Camic, Stephen Clift and Norma Daykin (eds), *Arts in Health – An International Journal for Research, Policy, and Practice* (Taylor and Francis), http://www.tandfonline.com/action/journalInformation?show=editorialBoard&journalCode=rahe20#.VuxEIfl97IU (accessed 17 March 2016).

89   Geoffrey Crossick and Patrycja Kaszynska, *Understanding the Value of Arts & Culture: The AHRC Cultural Value Project* (Arts and Humanities Research Council, 2016), pp. 100–12.

90   Ibid., p. 107.

91   Francois Matarasso, *Use or Ornament? The Social Impact of Participation in the Arts* (Stroud: Comedia, 1997).

92   Francois Matarasso, 'Smoke and mirrors: a response to Paola Merli's

"evaluating the Social impact of participation in Arts activities"', *International Journal of Cultural Policy* 9:3 (2003): 337–46, DOI: 10.1080/1028663032000161759.

93 Matthew Jennings and Andrea Baldwin, '"Filling out the Forms was a Nightmare": Project Evaluation and the Reflective Practitioner in Community Theatre in Contemporary Northern Ireland', *Music and Arts in Action* 2:2 (2010), http://musicandartsinaction.net/index.php/maia/article/view/communitytheatre (accessed 17 March 2016).

94 Christopher Odhiambo Joseph. 'Theatre for development in Kenya: interrogating the ethics of practice', *Research in Drama Education* 10:2 (June 2005): 189–99, DOI: 10.1080/13569780500103836.

95 Ibid., p. 195.

96 M. Okioma. 'Law needed to check errant NGOs', *Daily Nation*, 30 August 2004, p. 7.

97 Augusto Boal, *Rainbow of Desire: The Boal Method of Theatre and Therapy* (London: Routledge 1995), p. xix.

98 Peter Abbs, *The Educational Imperative – A Defence of Socratic and Aesthetic Learning* (London: Falmer Press, 1994), p. 17.

99 Augusto Boal, *Games for Actors and Non-Actors* (London: Routledge, 1992), p. 234.

100 Claudia Orenstein, *Festive Revolutions: The Politics of Popular Theatre and the San Francisco Mime Troupe* (Jackson: University Press of Mississippi, 1998), p. 16.

101 Ibid., p. 14.

102 Space does not allow further engagement here, but the work of Clowns without Borders, South Africa, is instructive in developing a more optimistic outlook, and therefore contributes to resilient wellbeing. www.cwbsa.org (accessed 2 May 2016).

103 Keyan Tomaselli, 'Action Research, Participatory Communication: Why Governments Don't Listen', *Africa Media Review* 11:1: 1–9.

Chapter 3

1 WHO, *World Report on Ageing and Health* (Geneva: World Health Organization, 2015), p. 3.

2   Until recently, most of the impact of dementia has been seen in developing nations. However, the 2015 World Alzheimer Report noted that this has now shifted and most of the increase in dementia figures anticipated by 2050 will be seen/experienced in low- to middle-income countries. Alzheimer's Disease International, *World Alzheimer Report 2015: The Global Impact of Dementia: An analysis of Prevalence, Incidence, Cost and Trends* (London: Alzheimer's Disease International, 2015), p. 22.
3   UN, *World Population Ageing 2013*, Department of Economic and Social Affairs Population Division (New York: United Nations, 2013), p. xii.
4   David Oliver, 'Ageing Well: Whose Responsibility is it?', *The Guardian* (online), 6 August 2014, http://www.theguardian.com/society/2014/aug/06/ageing-well-whose-responsibility (accessed 11 October 2015).
5   Ibid.
6   Bradford Dementia Group, Handouts on issues raised by the film *Ex Memoria* (Bradford: Bradford Dementia Group, 2007), www.brad.ac.uk/acad/health/bdg (accessed 3 March 2012).
7   WHO, *Report on Ageing and Health*, pp. 15–17.
8   Allan Kellehear, 'A Social History of Dying', in Sarah Earle, Carol Komaromy and Caroline Bartholomew (eds), *Death and Dying: A Reader* (London: SAGE Publications, 2009), pp. 61–2.
9   Ibid., p. 64.
10 Ibid., p. 62
11 Seymour Fisher, 'Motionless Body', in Sarah Earle, Carol Komaromy and Caroline Bartholomew (eds), *Death and Dying: A Reader* (London: SAGE Publications, 2009), pp. 7–9.
12 See David Cutler, *Aging Artfully: Older People and Professional Participatory Arts in the UK*, http://baringfoundation.org.uk/wp-content/uploads/2009/08/AgeingArtfully.pdf (accessed 13 November 2014).
13 Caoimhe McAvinchey, 'Coming of Age: Arts Practice with Older People in Private and Domestic Spaces', *Research in Drama Education: The Journal of Applied Theatre Research* 18:4 (2013): 361.
14 Ibid..
15 An overview of the different types of dementia can be found on the

Alzheimer's Society website: http://alzheimers.org.uk/Facts_about_dementia/What_is_dementia (accessed 17 November 2014).
16 See http://www.alzheimers.org.uk/statistics (accessed 17 November 2014).
17 See http://www.alzheimers.net/resources/alzheimers-statistics (accessed 17 November 2014).
18 See 'An Evidence Review of the Impact of the Arts on Older People', http://www.mentalhealth.org.uk (accessed 14 November 2014).
19 See http://www.artscouncil.org.uk (accessed 3 December 2014).
20 Michael Mangan, *Staging Ageing* (Bristol: Intellect, 2013), p. 154.
21 Baz Kershaw, 'Building an Unstable Pyramid: The Fragmentation of Alternative Theatre', *New Theatre Quarterly* 9:36 (1993): 345.
22 Mangan, *Staging Ageing*, p. 155.
23 Pam Schweitzer, *Reminiscence Theatre* (London: Jessica Kingsley, 2007), p. 239.
24 Helen Nicholson, 'Making home work: theatre-making with older adults in residential care', *NJ Drama Australia* 35:1 (2011): 50.
25 Ibid., p. 80.
26 Ibid., p. 88.
27 Ibid.
28 Nicola Hatton, 'Theatre and Dementia in North America', Winston Churchill Memorial Trust, 2013, p. 9, http://www.wcmt.org.uk/fellows/reports (accessed 3 December 2014).
29 Clayton Drinko, *Theatrical Improvisation, Consciousness and Cognition* (New York: Palgrave Macmillan, 2013), p. 29.
30 Mary Crilly O'Hara interviewed by Nancy Maes in *Forget Your Lines*, Chicago Health Online, http://chicagohealthonline.com/forget-your-lines/ (accessed 3 December 2014).
31 Bethan Harries, 'The Storybox Project: Examining the role of a theatre and arts-based intervention for people with dementia', 2013, p. 15, http://www.ihs.manchester.ac.uk/events/pastworkshops/2013/MICRA_Storybox_19-03-13/Storybox_Project.pdf (accessed 3 December 2014).
32 Ibid.
33 Ibid., p.19.
34 See, for example, Age Exchange's RADIQL study: http://www.age-exchange.org.uk/wp-content/uploads/2015/01/Reminiscence-Arts-Dementia-Impact-on-Quality-of-Life.pdf (accessed 5 December 2014).

35 Andrea Gilroy, *Art Therapy, Research and Evidence-Based Practice* (London: Sage Publications, 2006), p. 10.
36 Jenny Hughes, Jenny Kidd and Catherine McNamara, 'The Usefulness of Mess: Artistry, Improvisation and Decomposition in the Practice of Research in Applied Theatre', in Helen Nicholson and Baz Kershaw (eds), *Research Methods in Theatre and Performance* (Edinburgh: Edinburgh University Press, 2011), p.188.
37 Ibid.
38 Audience feedback: *Kicking the Bucket* Festival, 2012, http://www.kickingthebucket.co.uk (accessed 14 June 2014).
39 http://www.kickingthebucket.co.uk (accessed 14 June 2014).
40 A chance for those of all faiths or none to be buried amid nature and contribute to the creation of a beautiful woodland which will be enjoyed by generations to come, http://www.woodlandburialwestmill.co.uk (accessed 21 September.2014).
41 Nell Dunn, *Home Death* (London: Nick Hern Books, 2011).
42 'Kicking the Bucket' is a euphemism for dying, originating from the practice of standing on a bucket, which was then kicked away, when being hung, or hanging oneself. Despite the violence of the origin of the term, it is now widely used as a euphemism for any kind of death.
43 http://www.theguardian.com/lifeandstyle/2015/may/18/few-britons-discuss-dying-and-plans-after-their-death-finds-survey (accessed 20 May 2015).
44 Audience feedback from the 2012 Festival, http://www.kickingthebucket.co.uk (accessed 14 June 2014).
45 Atul Gawande, *Being Mortal: Illness, Medicine and What Matters in the End* (London: Profile Books in association with the Wellcome Foundation, 2014), p. 7.
46 Ibid., p. 28.
47 Stephen Jenkinson, quoted in 'Bringing death back into our lives', *Therapy Today* 25:8 (British Association for Counselling and Psychotherapy) (October 2014): 8.
48 http://www.playoflighttheatre.co.uk (accessed 20 May 2015).
49 Nicola Shaughnessy, *Applying Performance: Live Art: Socially Engaged Theatre and Affective Practice* (London: Palgrave Macmillan, 2012), p. xiv.

Chapter 4

1. Daniele Lantagne et al., 'The Cholera Outbreak in Haiti: Where and how did it begin?' *Current Topics in Microbiology and Immunology* 379 (2013): 145–64.
2. GBD 2013, 'Mortality and Causes of Death Collaborators. Global, regional, and national age–sex specific all-cause and cause-specific mortality for 240 causes of death, 1990–2013: a systematic analysis for the Global Burden of Disease Study 2013', *The Lancet*, 2014, DOI: http://dx.doi.org/10.1016/S0140-6736(14)61682-2.
3. WHO, *Tuberculosis: Fact Sheet*, 2015, http://www.who.int/mediacentre/factsheets/fs104/en/ (accessed 3 January 2016).
4. Ibid.
5. WHO, *Zika Virus*, 2016, http://www.who.int/mediacentre/factsheets/zika/en/ (accessed 24 January 2016).
6. Julia Belluz et al., 'Zika virus, explained in 6 charts and maps', *Vox: Science & Health* (2016), http://www.vox.com/2016/1/20/10795562/zika-virus-cdc-mosquitoes-birth-defects (accessed 24 January 2016).
7. Jo Atkinson et al., 'A qualitative study on the acceptability and preference of three types of long-lasting insecticide-treated bed nets in Solomon Islands: implications for malaria elimination', *Malaria Journal* 8, no. 119 (2009), DOI: 10.1186/1475-2875-8-119.
8. Soori E. Nnko et al., 'Scepticism towards insecticide treated mosquito nets for malaria control in rural community in north-western Tanzania', *Tanzania Journal of Health Research* 14:2 (2012), DOI: http://dx.doi.org/10.4314/thrb.v14i2.2.
9. Christopher W Koehler, 'Consumption the great killer', *Modern Drug Discovery: From Concept to Development* 5:2 (2002), http://pubs.acs.org/subscribe/archive/mdd/v05/i02/html/02timeline.html (accessed 20 May 2015).
10. Ibid.
11. 1907, Göteberg Museum of Art.
12. 1900, Munch Museum.
13. 1879, Musée d'Orsay.
14. Clark Lawlor, *Consumption and Literature: The Making of the Romantic Disease* (London: Palgrave Macmillan, 2007), p. 5.

15 Ibid., p. 43.
16 Guiseppe Verdi, *La Traviata*, premiered 1853, Venice, Italy.
17 Giacomo Puccini, *La Bohème*, premiered 1896, Turin, Italy.
18 Baz Luhrman, *Moulin Rouge* (Twentieth Century Fox, 2001).
19 Anna Richards, 'Consumption and Literature: The Making of the Romantic Disease' (review), *Bulletin of the History of Medicine* 82:3 (Fall 2008): 725–6, DOI: 10.1353/bhm.0.0077..
20 Lawlor, *Consumption and Literature*, p. 6.
21 Ibid., p. 187.
22 Ibid., p. 186.
23 Centers for Disease Control and Communication, 'Tuberculosis Data and Statistics', 2014, http://www.cdc.gov/tb/statistics/ (accessed 5 December, 2015).
24 Jonathan Larson, *Rent*, premiered 1996, New York.
25 Chris Columbus, *Rent*, film adaptation (2005).
26 Guy Lodge, 'The "U-Carmen eKhayelitsha" team returns for another Africanized opera makeover, this time with less dynamic results', *Variety*, 9 February 2015, http://variety.com/2015/film/festivals/berlin-film-review-breathe-umphefumlo-1201427629/ (accessed 5 December 2015).
27 Jonathan Romney, 'Breathe Umphefumlo', *Screen Daily*, 9 February 2015, http://www.screendaily.com/reviews/the-latest/breathe-umphefumlo/5083031.article (accessed 5 December 2015).
28 These cramped conditions emphasize the poverty of the characters as well as one of the main causes of TB – i.e. poor ventilation and cramped living conditions.
29 Mary Edginton, 'TB: Past, Present and Future', editorial, *HST UPDATE* 56 (Health Systems Trust, October 2000), http://www.hst.org.za/sites/default/files/upd56.pdf. (accessed 27 August 2015).
30 Richard E. Chaisson and Neil A. Martinson, 'Tuberculosis in Africa – Combating an HIV-Driven Crisis', *New England Journal of Medicine* 358 (2008): 1089–92, DOI: 10.1056/NEJMp0800809.
31 Edginton, 'TB: Past, Present and Future', p. 4
32 Medicine sans frontiers, 'South Africa: Drug shortages threaten progress made in the world's largest HIV programme', 2015, http://www.msf.org/article/south-africa-drug-shortages-threaten-progress-made-world%E2%80%99s-largest-hiv-programme (accessed 5 December 2015).

33 Chaisson and Martinson, 'Tuberculosis in Africa'.
34 The African potato, part of the lily family, *Hypoxis hemerocallidea*, is widely used as a medicine, or 'muthi', in the southern regions of Africa, http://www.healthline.com/health/african-wild-potato (accessed 5 December 2015).
35 Manto Shabalala-Msimang was Health Minister from 1999 to 2008, serving in Thabo Mbeki's presidency. Both were infamous for their HIV/AIDS denialism.
36 Tuberculosis is a notifiable infection in South Africa; however, many infections may not be reported.
37 Michele Tameris, Executive Summary, *Carina's Choice* Wellcome Trust proposal (14 March 2012), unpublished document.
38 http://www.satvi.uct.ac.za/ (accessed 25 April 2015).
39 Tameris, Executive Summary.
40 *Carina's Choice*, produced by SATVI and the Global Partnership to Stop TB (WHO, 2010).
41 Jason Jacobs, Koleka Putuma, Kathleen Stephens and Krystle Marrier d'Unienville worked on performer training and workshopping. Matthew Burn, with assistance from Leigh Bishop and Maggie Gericke, designed costume and set.
42 The collaboration has received another Wellcome Trust grant to further this work, through street theatre and visual arts.
43 Bey-Marrié Schmidt, Amber Abrams and Michele Tameris, 'Engaging adolescents in tuberculosis and clinical trial research through drama', *Trials* 17 (2016): 1, DOI: 10.1186/s13063-016-1291-7.
44 BCG is only effective in preventing tuberculosis meningitis, and protecting children from pulmonary tuberculosis, until about the age of ten.
45 This term means a process of devising, usually through collective input.
46 This style is attributed to Peter Zadek and Wilfried Minks and the Bremen theatre style, with an empty stage but using large Pop Art images on the cyclorama. See Marvin Carlson, *Theatre is More Beautiful than War: German Stage Directing in the Late Twentieth Century* (Iowa City: University of Iowa Press, 2009), p. 30.
47 National TB management Guidelines, Department of Health, Pretoria, South Africa.

48 Irmhild Horn, 'Learner-centredness: an analytical critique', *South African Journal of Education* 29 (2009): 511–25.
49 Ibid., p. 2.
50 'Skoolbank – Worcester Senior Sekondêr', *Worcester Standard*, 12 September 2013, p. 16, http://www.issuu.com/worcesterstandard/docs/worcester_standard_12-09-2013 (accessed 5 December 2015).
51 Personal communication with actors Eurika van Wyk and Mary-Ellen Martin, September 2013.
52 Department of Health, South Africa, National Tuberculosis Management Guidelines, 2014. TB medicines are currently provided free and involve an intensive period of two months treatment that are followed by four months continuation, to ensure no relapse, http://www.sahivsoc.org/upload/documents/NTCP_Adult_TB%20Guidelines%2027.5.2014.pdf (accessed 17 December, 2015).
53 Mara Kardas-Nelson, 'Anger over drug access in TB trial', *Mail and Guardian*, 5 July 2013, http://www.mg.co.za/article/2013-07-05-00-anger-over-drug-access-in-tb-trial (accessed 5 December 2015).
54 Katherine Childs, 'TAC takes on big pharmaceutical firms for cutting TB vaccine production', *Times Live*, 4 December 2015, http://www.timeslive.co.za/local/2015/12/04/TAC-takes-on-big-pharmaceutical-firms-for-cutting-TB-vaccine-production (accessed 6 December, 2015).
55 http://www.livelihoods.org.za/projects/delft-youth-theatre, 2013 (accessed 15 December 2015).
56 In 2015, I conducted research on uses of TfD by local Malawian NGOs for my PhD research at the University of Leeds.
57 Jane Plastow, 'Domestication or transformation? The Ideology of Theatre for Development in Africa', *Applied Theatre Research* 2:2, (2014): 107–18.
58 Augusto Boal, *Theatre of the Oppressed* (London: Pluto Press, 1979).
59 As above in note 1.
60 Patrick Mangeni, 'Negotiating Space: Challenges for Applied-Theatre Praxis with Local Non-Governmental/Community Based Organisations in HIV/AIDS Contexts in Uganda', in *Applied Drama and Theatre as an Interdisciplinary Field in the Context of HIV/AIDS in Africa*, ed. Hazel Barnes (Amsterdam: Rodopi, 2013).
61 As above in note 6.
62 Jane Plastow, 'The Faithful Copyist or the Good Thief', in *Theatre*

Unbound: Reflections on Theatre for Development and Social Change, ed. S. A. Kafewo, T. J. Iorapuu and E. S. Dandaura (Zaria, Nigeria: Ahmadu Bello University Press, 2015).

63 Ministry of Health, 'National Malaria Control Programme, Malaria Strategic Plan 2005–2010: Scaling Up Malaria Control Interventions', Lilongwe, Malawi, 2005.
64 National Malaria Control Programme, Communities Health Sciences Unit, Ministry of Health, Lilongwe, Malawi, 2010.
65 Ministry of Health, pp. 20–33.
66 PSI is a global health organization which operates in the health sector in Malawi. PSI works in partnership with the Ministry of Health's National Malaria Control Programme, http://www.psi.org/country/malawi/#about (accessed 22 June 2015).
67 The campaign involved a number of stages: research generated key areas of malaria prevention and themes to be communicated; key message(s) were consolidated and drama groups selected and allocated towns. The drama groups created plays based on the communication briefs created by PSI (Malawi). See Zindaba Chisiza, 'When People Resist Change: Rethinking the Function of Participation in Participatory Health Communication. A Case of Malawi', unpublished MA thesis, University of Warwick, 2012.
68 Kamphiritiya Theatre Arts is a vernacular Chichewa drama group from Blantyre, situated in the southern region of Malawi.
69 J. Kuseka, Malungo Zii, Kampiritiya Theatre Arts, Namadzi, Chiladzulu, Malawi, 6 August 2011 (live performance).
70 Jane Plastow, 'Domestication or transformation'.
71 Zindaba Chisiza, 'When People Resist Change', p. 72.
72 As above in note 9.
73 World Health Organization, 'Dengue Control', http://www.who.int/denguecontrol/en/ (accessed 17 August 2015).
74 R. Jelmaye and J. T. Lewis, 'Brazil City Calls In Army to Fight Dengue', *Wall Street Journal*, 17 April 2015.
75 *Public Enemy No. 1* was directed by Johayne Hildefonso and Malu Cotrim and written by Thérèse Bellido.

Chapter 5

1. WHO. *Noncommunicable Diseases: Fact Sheet*, January 2015, http://www.who.int/mediacentre/factsheets/fs355/en/ (accessed 11 October 15).
2. WHO, *WHO Global Action Plan for the Prevention and Control of Noncommunicable Diseases 2013–2020* (Geneva: World Health Organization, 2013), p. 7.
3. Alan Mozes, 'Poverty Drains Nutrition from Family Diet', *Washington Post*, 21 February 2008, http://www.washingtonpost.com/wp-dyn/content/article/2008/02/21/AR2008022101091.html (accessed 11 October 15).
4. In their resource guide, Maria Yellow Horse Brave Heart and Tina Deschenie discuss the impact of post-colonial stress, which they describe as the 'historic and multigenerational trauma' experienced by Native people on the health of Native Americans today. 'Resource Guide: Historical Trauma and Post-Colonial Stress in American Indian Populations', *Tribal College* 17:3 (2006): 24–7.
5. WHO, *The European Health Report 2015: Targets and Beyond – Reaching New Frontiers in Evidence: Highlights* (Copenhagen: World Health Organization, 2015), pp. 6–7.
6. Mercedes de Onis, Monika Blössner and Elaine Borghi, 'Global prevalence and trends of overweight and obesity among preschool children', *American Journal of Clinical Nutrition* 92 (2010): 1257–64.
7. The term 'First Nations' refers to people registered under the Indian Act of Canada. 'Aboriginal' is the inclusive term from the Constitution Act, 1982, which refers to registered Indians, Métis and Inuit. We use the term 'Indigenous' in our work to refer to a collective of distinct cultural groups worldwide that have experienced damaging processes of colonization.
8. Augusto Boal, *Theatre of the Oppressed* (London: Pluto Press, 2008).
9. Linda Goulet and Keith Goulet, *Teaching Each Other: Nehinuw Concepts and Indigenous Pedagogies* (Vancouver: UBC Press, 2014).
10. Warren Linds and Linda Goulet, '(Un)Intentional spaces: Co-determined leadership through drama/theatre', in Warren Linds, Alison Sammel and Linda Goulet (eds.), *Emancipatory Practices: Adult/Youth Engagement for Social and Environmental Justice* (Rotterdam: Sense Publishers, 2010), pp. 221–40.

11 Linda Tuhiwai Smith, *Decolonising Methodologies: Research and Indigenous Peoples* (New York: Zed Books, 1999).
12 Russell Bishop, 'Te Kotahitanga: Kaupapa Maori in mainstream classrooms', in Norman K. Denzin, Yvonne S. Lincoln and Linda Tuhiwai Smith (eds), *Handbook of Critical and Indigenous Methodologies* (Thousand Oaks, CA: Sage Publications, 2008), pp. 439–58.
13 Manulani Aluli Meyer, 'Indigenous and authentic: Hawaiian epistemology and the triangulation of meaning', in Norman K. Denzin, Yvonne S. Lincoln and Linda Tuhiwai Smith (eds), *Handbook of Critical and Indigenous Methodologies* (Thousand Oaks, CA: Sage, 2008), pp. 217–32.
14 Augusto Boal, *Games for Actors and Non-actors*, trans. Adrian Jackson (London: Routledge, 1992), p. 49.
15 Linda Goulet, Warren Linds, Jo-Ann Episkenew and Karen Schmidt, 'A decolonizing space: Theatre and health with Indigenous youth', *Native Studies Review* 20:1 (2011): 35–61.
16 Ashley Ning and Kathi Wilson, 'A Research Review: Exploring the health of Canada's Aboriginal youth', *International Journal of Circumpolar Health* (2012): 1–10.
17 Malcolm King, Alexandra Smith and Michael Gracey, 'Indigenous health – part 2: The underlying causes of the health gap', *The Lancet* 374 (2009): 76–85.
18 See Statistics Canada, *Aboriginal Peoples in Canada 2011: Inuit, Metis and First Nations, 2011 Census Health Indicator Profile, by Aboriginal Identity, Age Group and Sex, Four Year Estimates, Canada, provinces and territories* (Ottawa: Statistics Canada Community Health Survey, 2011), Table 105 0512, http://www5.statcan.gc.ca/cansim/a26?lang=eng&retrLang=eng&id=1050512&tabMode=dataTable&srchLan=-1&p1=-1&p2=35 (accessed 3 January 2015).
19 First Nations and Inuit Health, Health Canada, 'Suicide Prevention', http://www.hc-sc.gc.ca/fniah-spnia/promotion/suicide/index-eng.php (accessed 3 January 2015).
20 Julian Robbins and Jonathan Dewar, 'Traditional Indigenous Approaches to Healing and the modern welfare of Traditional Knowledge, Spirituality and Lands: A critical reflection on practices and policies taken from the Canadian Indigenous Example', *International Indigenous*

Policy Journal 2:4 (2011), http://ir.lib.uwo.ca/iipj/vol2/iss4/2 (accessed 10 October 2014).

21. Arvol Looking Horse, 'Indigenous Philosophies and Ceremonies as a basis for Action', unpublished raw data, participant/non-presenter notes, Our People, Our Health, National Conference of the National Aboriginal Health Organization, Ottawa, 2009.
22. Royal Commission on Aboriginal Peoples, 'Appendix 3A: Traditional Health and Healing', *Report of the Royal Commission on Aboriginal Peoples*, Vol. 3, Ch. 3 (Ottawa: Royal Commission on Aboriginal Peoples, 1996).
23. These surveys were conducted by post-doctoral researcher Nuno Ribeiro.
24. Joseph Couture, 'The role of Native Elders', in Olive Patricia Dickason and David Long (eds), *Visions of the Heart: Canadian Aboriginal Issues* (Toronto: Oxford University Press, 1996), p. 26.
25. All Elders gave us permission to use their names. We do so to give credit to them for the authorship of their words and to acknowledge them as the source of this knowledge.
26. Joe O'Watch, personal interview, 7 June 2013.
27. Ron Keewatin, personal interview, 27 May 2013.
28. Keewatin, personal interview, 27 May 2013.
29. Youth interview, 21 January 2015.
30. Willie A. Ermine, 'Ethical Standards for Research Involving Traditional Healing', unpublished raw data, participant/non-presenter notes, *Our People, Our Health, National Conference of the National Aboriginal Health Organization*, Ottawa, 2009.
31. Ibid.
32. O'Watch, personal interview.
33. Ibid.
34. Youth interview, 21 January 2015.
35. Qwo-Li Driskill, 'Theatre as suture: Grassroots performance, decolonization and healing', in Renete Eigenbrod and Renée Hulan (eds), *Aboriginal Oral Traditions: Theory, Practice, Eethics* (Halifax, NS: Fernwood Publishing, 2008), p. 155.
36. Ibid.
37. Brian Fay, *Critical social science: Liberation and its Limits* (Ithaca, NY: Cornell University Press, 1987).

38 Linda Goulet, Warren Linds, Jo-Ann Episkenew and Karen Schmidt, 'A decolonizing space: Theatre and health with Indigenous youth', *Native Studies Review* 20 (2011): 35–61.
39 Robert A. Alexie, *Porcupines and China Dolls* (Toronto: Stoddart, 2002), p. 29
40 Mary Ann Hunter, 'Cultivating the art of safe space', *Research in Drama Education* 13:1 (2008), pp. 5–21, DOI:10.1080/13569780701825195).
41 Youth focus group, 30 March 2012.
42 Warren Linds and Linda Goulet, '(Un)Intentional spaces: Co-determined leadership through drama/theatre', in Warren Linds, Alison Sammel and Linda Goulet (eds.), *Emancipatory Practices: Adult/Youth Engagement for Social and Environmental Justice* (Rotterdam: Sense Publishers, 2010), pp. 221–40.
43 James Thompson, *Applied Theatre: Betwixt and Beyond* (Berne: Peter Lang, 2003).
44 Barker, Clive, *Theatre Games: A New Approach to Drama Training* (London: Eyre Methuen, 1977).
45 Felice Yuen, Alison Pedlar and Roger C. Mannell, 'Building community and social capital through children's leisure in the context of an international camp', *Journal of Leisure Research: Special Issue, Leisure and Social Capital* 37 (2005): 494–518.
46 Fyr Jean Graveline, *Circle Works: Transforming Eurocentric Consciousness* (Halifax, NS: Fernwood, 1998); Linda Tuhiwai Smith, *Decolonizing Methodologies: Research and Indigenous peoples* (New York, NY: Zed Books, 1999).
47 Youth interview, 18 March 2010.
48 Youth focus group, 30 March 2010.
49 Youth interview, 18 March 2010.
50 Boal, *Games*.
51 See more on the role of playing games in learning in M. Kangas, 'Creative and playful learning: Learning through game co-creation and games in a playful learning environment', *Thinking Skills and Creativity* 5 (2010): 1–15.
52 Youth interview, 21 January 2015.
53 Youth interview, 18 March 2010.
54 Willie Ermine, 'The ethical space of engagement', *Indigenous Law Journal* 6 (2007): 194.

55 David Turnbull, *Tricksters, Masons and Cartographers: Comparative Studies in the Sociology of Scientific and Indigenous Knowledge* (Amsterdam: Harwood Academic Publishers, 2000).
56 Linda Archibald and Jonathan Dewar, 'Creative arts, culture, and healing: Building an evidence base', *Pimatisiwin: A Journal of Aboriginal and Indigenous Community Health* 8 (2010): 1–25, http://www.pimatisiwin.com/online/?page_id=815 (accessed 28 October 2014).
57 WHO, *Preventing Chronic Disease: A Vital Investment* (Geneva: WHO, 2005).
58 Research Centre for Prevention and Health, Capital Region of Denmark, *Health Profile for Regions and Municipalities 2010, The Capital Region of Denmark* (2010).
59 Karen Wistoft, 'Health Strategies and reservoirs of knowledge among adolescents in Denmark', *Global Health Promotion* 17:2 (2010): 16–24.
60 Dan Grabowski, 'Identity, knowledge and participation: Health theatre for children', *Health Education* 113:1 (2013): 64–79.
61 http://miltonsand.dk/.
62 Anne L. Meng and John Sullivan, 'Interactive theatre: an innovation conflict resolution teaching methodology', *Journal of Nurses Staff Development* 27:2 (2011): 65–8.
63 Katja Joronen, Anne Konu, H. Sally Rankin and Päivi Åstedt-Kurki, 'An evaluation of a drama program to enhance social relationships and anti-bullying at elementary school: a controlled study', *Health Promotion International* 27:1 (2011): 5–14.
64 Carl A. Patow and Debra J. Bryan, 'Engaging physicians in CME: the power of theatre', *Minnesota Medicine* 93:11 (2010): 11–40.
65 Cheryl L. Perry, Margeurite Zauner, J. Michael Oakes, Gretchen Taylor and Donald B. Bishop, 'Evaluation of a theatre production about eating behavior in children', *Journal of School Health* 72:6 (2002): 256–61.
66 Katja Joronen, H. Sally Rankin and Päivi Astedt-Kurki, 'School-based drama interventions in health promotion for children and adolescents: systematic review', *Journal of Advanced Nursing* 63:2 (2008): 116–31.
67 Brandi S. Niemeier, Desiree L. Tande, Joyce Hwang, Sherri Stastny and Joel M. Hektner, 'Using education, exposure, and environments to increase preschool children's knowledge about fruit and vegetables', *Journal of Extension* 48:1 (2010): 1–5.

68 Bettina F. Piko and Judit Bak, 'Children's perceptions of health and illness: images and lay concepts in preadolescence', *Health Education Research* 21:5 (2006): 643–53.
69 Vasilis Grammatikopoulos, Elisavet Konstantinidou, Nikolaos Tsigilis, Evridiki Zachopoulou, Niki Tsangaridou and Jarmo Liukkonen, 'Evaluating preschool children knowledge about healthy lifestyle: preliminary examination of the healthy lifestyle evaluation instrument', *Educational Research and Review* 3:11 (2008): 351–2.
70 Dan Grabowski, 'Health-identity, participation and knowledge: A qualitative study of a computer game for health education among adolescents in Denmark', *Health Education Journal* 72:6 (2013): 761–8.
71 Louk W. H. Peters, Carin H. Wiefferink, F. Hoekstra, G. J. Buijs, G. T. M. ten Dam and Theo G. W. M. Paulussen, 'A review of similarities between domain-specific determinants of four health behaviors among adolescents', *Health Education Research* 24:2 (2009): 198–232.
72 Wistoft, 'Health Strategies', pp. 16–24.
73 Grabowski, 'Identity, knowledge and participation', pp. 64–79.
74 Dan Grabowski and Katrine K. Rasmussen, 'Adolescents' health identities: A qualitative and theoretical study of health education courses', *Social Science and Medicine* 120 (2014): 67–75.
75 Roger Hart, 'Children's Participation: From Tokenism to Citizenship', *UNICEF International* (Florence: Child Development Centre, 1992).
76 Kala Sangam Arts Centre, Bradford, UK, www.kalasangam.org (accessed 17 March 2016).
77 Kala Sukoon Arts and Wellbeing programme, 2008–10.
78 Anthony H. Barnett, A. N. Dixon, Srikanth Bellary, M. W. Hanif, J. P. O'Hare, Neil T. Raymond and Sudhesh Kumar, 'Type 2 diabetes and cardiovascular risk in the UK South Asian community', *Diabetologia* 49 (2006): 2234–46 (2241), DOI 10.1007/s00125-006-0325-1.
79 Constitution of the World Health Organization, 1948, http://www.who.int/about/mission/en/ (accessed 8 July 2015).
80 Adrian Furnham and J. Forey, 'The attitudes, behaviours and beliefs of patients of conventional vs. complementary (alternative) medicine', *Journal of Clinical Psychology* 50:3 (1994): 458–69.
81 Barnett et al., 'Type 2 diabetes'.
82 Ibid., p. 2244.

83 John Bell, 'Islamic Performance and the problem of drama', *The Drama Review* 49:4 (2005): 5–10.
84 Peter Bazalgette, 'Use the arts to boost the nation's health', *The Guardian*, 28 December 2014, http://www.theguardian.com/commentisfree/2014/dec/28/arts-boost-nations-health-nhs-funding-arts-council (accessed 30 August 2015).

Chapter 6

1 Ian Thomas, 'The History of AIDS in Africa', http://www.blackhistorymonth.org.uk/article/section/real-stories/the-history-of-aids-in-africa/ (accessed 7 October 2015).
2 UNAIDS report, 'HIV in Asia and the Pacific', 2013, http://www.unaids.org/sites/default/files/media_asset/2013_HIV-Asia-Pacific_en_0.pdf (accessed 7 October 2015).
3 UNAIDS, 'Global Report 2013.
4 Lynn Dalrymple, 'Applied Art is still art, and by any other name would smell as sweet', in H. Barnes (ed.), *Applied Drama and Theatre*, vol. 2, *Arts Activism, Education and Therapies: Transforming Communities across Africa* (Amsterdam: Rodopi, 2013).
5 Jacques Rancière, *The Emancipated Spectator* (London: Verso, 2009), p. 14.
6 Ibid., p. 17.
7 Ibid.
8 Alain de Botton, *How to Think More about Sex* (London: Macmillan, 2012), p. 3.
9 Personal discussions and communications with Dr Francis Ndowa, Coordinator for the WHO Controlling Sexually Transmitted & Reproductive Tract Infections Team, WHO, Geneva HQ, 2005.
10 Ford Hickson, 'What's the Point of HIV prevention?', conference paper, Sex, Drugs and Rock 'n' Roll: How far from the tombstone have we come? Conference, London, 24 September 2010, British Psychological Society, Division of Clinical Psychology, Faculty of HIV & Sexual Health, http://sigmaresearch.org.uk/files/Ford_Hickson_BPS_2010_HIV_prevention_(notes).pdf (accessed 7 October 2015).

11 Catherine Burns, 'Sexual Heritage', public lecture on Tedx at Wits University, 26 September 2012, http://www.youtube.com/watch?v=1qPRkmczDqY (accessed October 29 2015).
12 Sara Ahmed, *The Promise of Happiness* (London: Duke University Press, 2010), p. 120.
13 Alan Read, *Theatre, Intimacy and Engagement: The Last Human Venue* (Basingstoke: Palgrave Macmillan, 2009), p. 1.
14 I am aware that the study of semiotics has done a lot of this thinking; however, I am making an argument about feeling and affect in Applied Theatre as opposed to didacticism.
15 Hereafter known as *Four Husbands*.
16 Deborah Posel, '"Getting the nation talking about sex": reflections on the politics of sexuality and nation-building in post-apartheid South Africa', in Sylvia Tamale (ed.), *African Sexualities: A Reader* (Cape Town: Pambazuka Press, 2011), pp. 130–1.
17 Over 79% of the country is Christian, http://www.indexmundi.com/south_africa/demographics_profile.html (accessed 2 January 2016).
18 Jane Bennett, 'Subversion and Resistance: Activist Initiatives', in Sylvia Tamale (ed.), *African Sexualities: A Reader* (Cape Town: Pambazuka Press, 2011), p. 82.
19 Lydia Smith, 'Corrective rape: The homophobic fallout of post-apartheid South Africa', *The Telegraph*, 21 May 2015, http://www.telegraph.co.uk/women/womens-life/11608361/Corrective-rape-The-homophobic-fallout-of-post-apartheid-South-Africa.html (accessed 10 November 2015).
20 Rape Crisis – Cape Town Trust, http://rapecrisis.org.za/rape-in-south-africa/ (accessed 5 November 2015).
21 Africa Check, http://www.avert.org/hiv-aids-south-africa.htm (accessed 10 November 2015); https://africacheck.org/reports/will-74400-women-be-raped-this-august-in-south-africa/ (accessed 10 November 2015).
22 Esiaba Irobi, 'African Youth, Performance & the HIV/AIDS Epidemic: A Theatre of Necessity', in Michael Etherton (ed.), *African Theatre: Youth* (Oxford: James Currey, 2006), p. 34.
23 Christopher Odhiambo Joseph notes how TfD practitioners in Kenya use it to line their own pockets, while Julie Koch discusses similar practices in Tanzania. Christopher Odhiambo Joseph, 'Theatre for development in Kenya: Interrogating the ethics of practice', *Research in*

Drama Education: The Journal of Applied Theatre and Performance 10:2 (2005): 189–99; Julie Koch, *Karibuni Wananchi: Theatre for Development in Tanzania*, Bayreuth African Studies, 85 (Eckersdorf: Thielmann & Breitinger, 2008).

24 This is described in more detail by Emma Durden, 'Participatory HIV/AIDS Theatre in South Africa', in Dennis Francis (ed.), *Acting on HIV: Using Drama to Create Possibilities for Change* (Rotterdam: Sense Publishers, 2011), pp. 1–13.

25 Cf. Alexandra Sutherland, 'Dramatic Spaces in Patriarchal Contexts: Constructions and Disruptions of Gender in Theatre Interventions about HIV', in Hazel Barnes (ed.), *Applied Drama and Theatre as an Interdisciplinary Field in the Context of HIV/AIDS in Africa* (Amsterdam: Rodopi, 2013), pp. 177–85.

26 Here I am thinking of the Choices workshop which I observed as part of the Sex Actually Festival in 2014. Through the puppetry-based workshop based on HIV, relationships, and rights and responsibilities, the children were encouraged to make puppets and interact with another puppet to negotiate a safe sexual relationship. While the children clearly enjoyed creating and playing with the puppets, they appeared uncomfortable when asked to pretend the puppet was themselves while negotiating safe relationships/engagements with a classmate in a story improvised by themselves. Alongside this, when some of the mini-scenes appeared to demonstrate 'safe' relationships, the facilitator noted 'You are all playing it as it is supposed to happen [i.e. safely]. What about playing it as it sometimes happens?' There was a lack of time allocated in the workshop to carefully discuss and consider what young people's rights are and there appeared to be a particular way of negotiating sex expected by the facilitators. Similarly, *Lucky the Hero* by the Africa Centre for HIV/AIDS Management at Stellenbosch University is a mini-musical which I observed in April 2007. In this iteration of the production, the emphasis was on protection against HIV infection and included lyrics such as 'respect your life' and 'abstinence is the best policy'.

27 Gareth White, *Audience Participation in Theatre: Aesthetics of the Invitation* (Basingstoke: Palgrave Macmillan, 2013), p. 120.

28 Henceforth 'Arepp'.

29 Gordon Bilbrough, *Playing for Keeps: The Arepp: Theatre for Life*

Applied Theatre Method, South Africa: Arepp: Theatre for Life, 2010 (unpublished).
30 Gordon Bilbrough, 'After the Curtain – Reframed: Using Action Research to Reflect, Monitor, and Evaluate the Applied-Theatre Experience', in Hazel Barnes (ed.), *Applied Drama and Theatre as an Interdisciplinary Field in the Context of HIV/AIDS in Africa* (Amsterdam: Rodopi, 2013), p. 64.
31 Ibid.
32 Ibid., p. 65.
33 Josephine Machon, *Immersive Theatres: Intimacy and Immediacy in Contemporary Performance* (Basingstoke: Palgrave Macmillan, 2013), pp. 105–6.
34 Ibid. p. 106.
35 Ibid.
36 Interview with Clara Vaughan, 2 June 2015, Johannesburg, South Africa.
37 The names of the actors in *Four Husbands* have been changed.
38 Michael Warner, *The Trouble with Normal* (Cambridge, MA: Harvard University Press, 2001), pp. 35–6, cited in Jennifer Doyle, *Sex Objects: Art and the Dialectics of Desire* (Minneapolis: University Of Minnesota Press, 2006), p. xiv.
39 Interview with Namatshego Khutsoane, 27 May 2015.
40 Gareth White, *Applied Theatre: Aesthetics* (London: Bloomsbury Methuen Drama, 2015), pp. 72–3.
41 Machon, p. 73.
42 Cf. James Thompson, *Bewilderment and Beyond: Applied Theatre* (Zurich: Peter Lang, 2006).
43 Lyrics found at https://www.musixmatch.com/lyrics/Ginuwine/Pony-radio-edit (accessed 5 November 2015).
44 Hans-Thies Lehmann, *Postdramatic Theatre*, trans. and intro. Karen Jürs-Munby (Abingdon, Oxon: Routledge, 2006).
45 Chi-Chi Undie, 'The realities of "choice" in Africa: implications for sexuality, vulnerability and HIV/AIDS', in Sylvia Tamale (ed.), *African Sexualities: A Reader* (Cape Town: Pambazuka Press, 2011), p. 523.
46 Pieter Dirk Uys, *Elections and Erections: A Memoire of Fear and Fun* (Cape Town: Zebra Press, 2002).
47 Pieter Dirk Uys, *Pieter Dirk Uys CV*, 2015, http://pdu.co.za/CV.html (accessed 5 November 2015).

48 I observed Uys's work in 2003 in Port Elizabeth, South Africa.
49 Stage direction from the script of *Four Husbands for Ma Lindi* (unpublished).
50 Vaughan.
51 Robert W. Blum and Kristin Nelson Mmari, *Risk and Protective Factors Affecting Adolescent Reproductive Health in Developing Countries* (Baltimore: Johns Hopkins Bloomberg School of Public Health, 2005).
52 Douglas B. Kirby, B. A. Laris and Lori Rolleri, 'Sex and HIV Education Programs: Their Impact on Sexual Behaviors of Young People Throughout the World', *Journal of Adolescent Health* 40 (2007): 206–17.
53 Jane Kenway et al., 'Making "Hope Practical" Rather than "Despair Convincing": Feminist Post-Structuralism, Gender Reform and Educational Change', *British Journal of Sociology of Education* 15:2 (1994): 187–210.
54 Helen Cahill, 'Withholding the personal story: using theory to orient practice in applied theatre about HIV and human rights', *Research in Drama Education: The Journal of Applied Theatre and Performance* 19:1 (2014): 23–38.
55 Michael Marmot, 'Social determinants of health inequalities', *The Lancet* 365 (2005): 1099–104.
56 John B. F. de Wit et al., 'The rapidly changing paradigm of HIV prevention: time to strengthen social and behavioural approaches', *Health Education Research* 26:3 (2011): 381–92.
57 Shari L. Dworkin, Sarah Treves-Kagan and Sheri A. Lippman, 'Gender-transformative interventions to reduce HIV risks and violence with heterosexually-active men: a review of the global evidence', *AIDS and Behavior* 17:9 (2013): 2845–63.
58 Emma Fulu et al., 'Why do some men use violence against women, and how can we prevent it?', *UNDP, UNFPA, UN Women* and *UNV* (Bangkok: 2013).
59 Helen Cahill, 'Rethinking role-play for health and wellbeing: creating a pedagogy of possibilty', in K. Wright and J. McLeod (eds), *Rethinking Youth Wellbeing: Critical Perspectives* (Singapore: Springer, 2015), pp. 127–42.
60 Helen Cahill, 'Re-thinking the fiction/reality boundary: investigating the use of drama in HIV prevention projects in Vietnam', *Research in Drama*

Education: *The Journal of Applied Theatre and Performance* 15: (2010): 152–72.

Chapter 7

1 WHO, *Cancer: Fact Sheet*, February 2015, http://www.who.int/mediacentre/factsheets/fs297/en/ (accessed 1 October 2015).
2 Ibid.
3 UICC, *Galvanizing Efforts to Achieve the 2013 World Cancer Declaration Targets: An Advocacy Toolkit* (Geneva: UICC, 2013), p. 4, http://www.uicc.org/sites/main/files/private/2014_Advocacy_Toolkit.zip (accessed 11 October 2015).
4 Madhulika Sikka, 'Breast Cancer Awareness month has devolved into crass materialism', *The Guardian*, 31 October 2013, http://www.theguardian.com/commentisfree/2013/oct/31/end-of-breast-cancer-awareness (accessed 2 February 2014).
5 Steven Sutton is a recent example of this. Sutton was called 'a credit to humanity' for his 'positive' and 'inspirational' response to his own cancer diagnosis and his fundraising efforts for the Teenage Cancer Trust, http://www.bbc.co.uk/news/uk-england-27408818 (accessed 11 October 2015).
6 http://www.uicc.org/advocacy/advocacy-vision-strategy (accessed 11 October 2015).
7 http://www.cancer.gov/about-nci/organization/crchd/cancer-health-disparities-fact-sheet (accessed 11 October 2015) and in Australia http://www.ncbi.nlm.nih.gov/pmc/articles/PMC3994117/ (accessed 11 October 2015).
8 *The Fault in Our Stars*, dir. Josh Boone (Temple Hill Entertainment, 2014).
9 John Green, *The Fault in Our Stars* (London: Penguin, 2010), p. 202.
10 'After Treatment', *Teenage Cancer Trust*, 2015, https://www.teenagecancertrust.org/get-help/ive-got-cancer/treatment/after-treatment (accessed 5 February 2015).
11 Lennard J. Davis, *Bending Over Backwards: Disability, Dismodernism and Other Difficult Positions* (New York and London: New York University Press, 2002), p. 12.

12 Ibid.
13 Race for Life, http://raceforlife.cancerresearchuk.org/index.html (accessed 4 March 2015).
14 Stand Up to Cancer, http://www.standup2cancer.org/ (accessed 4 March 2015).
15 Break Through Bake Off, http://www.breakthrough.org.uk/bakeoff/ (accessed 4 March 2015).
16 Motorboating Girls for Breast Cancer Awareness, 2013, https://www.youtube.com/watch?v=AP8zXJ_xsEc (accessed 4 March 2015).
17 Sandy M. Fernandez, 'Pretty in Pink', originally printed in *MAMM Magazine* (June/July 1998) and available at *Think Before You Pink*, http://thinkbeforeyoupink.org/?page_id=26 (accessed 29 January 2012).
18 Arthur W. Frank, *The Wounded Storyteller: Body, Illness and Ethics* (Chicago: University of Chicago Press, 1996), p. 81.
19 Siddhartha Mukherjee, *The Emperor of All Maladies: A Biography of Cancer* (London: Fourth Estate, 2011), p. 319.
20 Jorge Ribalta (ed.), *Jo Spence: Beyond the Perfect Picture* (Barcelona: d'Art Contemporani de Barcelona, 2005), pp. 268–80.
21 Audre Lorde, *The Audre Lorde Compendium: Essays, Speeches and Journals* (London: Pandora, 1996), p. 290.
22 Rosemarie Garland-Thomson, *Staring: How We Look* (Oxford: Oxford University Press, 2006), p. 12.
23 Neetzan Zimmerman, 'That Legendary Tig Notaro Stand Up Set is Now Available on Louis C.K.'s Website', *Gawker* (2012), http://gawker.com/5949371/that-legendary-tig-notaro-stand-up-set-is-now-available-on-louis-cks-website (accessed 2 May 2015).
24 Tig Notaro (2012): *Live*.
25 Matuschka, 'Beauty Out of Damage', featured in Susan Ferraro, 'The Anguished Politics of Breast Cancer', *New York Times*, 15 August 1993.
26 David Jay, *The Scar Project*, http://www.thescarproject.org/david-jay/ (accessed 20 July 2015).
27 Tania Katan, *My One Night Stand With Cancer* (New York City: Alyson Books, 2005).
28 Brian Lobel, *BALL & Other Funny Stories About Cancer* (London: Oberon Books, 2012), p. 14.
29 Margaret Edson, *Wit* (New York: Faber & Faber, 1993), p. 85.

30 http://www.seslhd.health.nsw.gov.au/Multicultural_Health/ (accessed 20 July 2015).
31 Ilse Blignault, Sally Smith, Lisa Woodland, Vince Ponzio, Dushan Ristevski and Suzanna Kirov, 'Fear and Shame: Using theatre to destigmatise mental illness in an Australian Macedonian community', *Health Promotion Journal of Australia* 21:2 (2010): 121.
32 Ibid., pp. 120–6.
33 Kate Rossiter, Pia Kontos, Angela Colantonio, Julie Gilbert, Julia Gray and Michelle Keightley, 'Staging data: Theatre as a tool for analysis and knowledge transfer in health research', *Social Science and Medicine* 66 (2008): 130–46.
34 Matthew Reason, 'Asking the Audience: Audience Research and the Experience of Theatre', *About Performance* 10 (2010): 15–34, http://search.informit.com.au/documentSummary;dn=767306737561035;res=IELHSS ISSN: 1324-6089 (accessed 11 May 15).
35 Marianne F. Weber, Emily Banks, David P. Smith, Dianne O'Connell and Freddy Sitas, 'Cancer screening among migrants in an Australian cohort; Cross-sectional analyses from the 45 and Up Study', *BMC Public Health* 9 (2009): 144.
36 Ben O'Mara, Hurriyet Babacan and Helen Borland, *Sending the Right Message: ICT Access and Use for Communicating Messages of Health and Wellbeing to CALD Communities*, Footscray Park, Institute for Community, Ethnicity and Policy Alternatives (ICEPA), Victoria University and VicHealth, 2010.
37 T. Wilk, 'Social role of theatre: From antiquity to modern times', *New Educational Review* 15 (2008): 33–41.
38 Mckhlcd N. B. Al Zyoud, 'Why did the Arabs not know the theatre in the western sense until the mid-nineteenth century?', *Jordan Journal of the Arts* 2 (2009): 109–19.
39 Monica Prendergast and Juliana Saxton (eds), *Applied Theatre: International Case Studies and Challenges for Practice* (Bristol: Intellect Books, 2009).
40 http://urbantheatre.com.au/past-projects/arabic-theatre-studio/ (accessed 11 October 2015).
41 http://www.hellenicarttheatre.com.au/ (accessed 11 October 2015).
42 https://www.facebook.com/australianmacedoniantheatreofsydney (accessed 11 October 2015).

Chapter 8

1. World Health Organization, *Women's Health*, Factsheet no. 334 (September 2013), http://www.who.int/mediacentre/factsheets/fs334/en/ (accessed 23 October 2015).
2. United Nations Office on Drugs and Crime, *Global Report on Trafficking Persons*, 2009. https://www.unodc.org/documents/human-trafficking/ (accessed 11 October 2015).
3. Amrita Pande, *Wombs in Labor: Transnational Commercial Surrogacy in India* (New York: Columbia University Press, 2014).
4. *Shakti* is the Hindi word for 'strength'.
5. Amartya Sen, *Development as Freedom* (New York: Anchor Books, 2000).
6. Jocelyn Kynch and Amartya Sen, 'Indian women: wellbeing and survival', *Cambridge Journal of Economics* 7:3/4 (September/December 1983): 365–6.
7. Ibid.
8. Amartya Sen, 'Development as Capability Expansion', in S. Fukuda-Parr et al., *Readings in Human Development* (New Delhi and New York: Oxford University Press, 2003), p. 44.
9. Darpana Academy of Performing Arts, 'The Shakti Project', https://www.youtube.com/watch?v=Iwp1wffr_kY (accessed 5 January 2015).
10. Darpana Academy of Performing Arts, http://darpanaacademy.blogspot.com (accessed 5 January 2015).
11. Ibid.
12. Ibid.
13. Darpana Academy of Performing Arts, 'The "Acting Healthy" Project', https://www.youtube.com/watch?v=ExKX1VllZFQ (accessed 21 May 2015).
14. Darpana, 'The Shakti Project'.
15. Kynch and Sen, 'Indian women: wellbeing and survival', pp. 364–5.
16. Ibid.
17. Ibid.
18. Ibid.
19. Mozaffar Qizilbash, 'Dialogue: Sen on Freedom and Gender Justice', *Feminist Economics* 11:3 (November 2005): 151–2.
20. Sen, 'Development as Capability Expansion', p. 52.

21 Amartya Sen, 'When misogyny becomes a health problem: The many faces of gender inequality', *New Republic*, 17 September 2001, p. 38.
22 Ibid., p. 40.
23 Ibid.
24 Darpana, 'The Shakti Project'.
25 Ibid.
26 Ibid.
27 Ibid.
28 Ibid.
29 Ibid.
30 Ibid.
31 Ibid.
32 Ibid.
33 Ibid.
34 Ibid.
35 Sen, 'Development as Capability Expansion', p. 45.
36 www.nanzikambearts.org (accessed 20 August 2015).
37 O. O. Komolafe, J. James, M. Makoka and L. Kalongeolera, 'Epidemiology and mortality of burns at the Queen Elizabeth Central Hospital Blantyre, Malawi', *Central African Journal of Medicine* 49 (2003): 130–4.
38 Rene Albertyn, Stephen W. Bickler and H. Rode, 'Paediatric burn injuries in Sub Saharan Africa – an overview', *Burns* 32 (2006): 605–12.
39 George Virich and Chris Lavy, 'Burns in Malawi', *Annals of Burns and Fire Disasters* 19 (2006): 171–3.
40 Albertyn, Bickler and Rode, 'Paediatric burn injuries in Sub Saharan Africa', pp. 605–12.
41 A. Hyder, K. Kashyap, Steven Fishman and Salman Wali, 'Review of childhood burn injuries in sub-Saharan Africa: a forgotten public health challenge: literature review', *African Safety Promotion* 2 (2004): 43–58.
42 Charles Mock, Michael Peck, Margie Peden and Etienne Krug (eds), *A WHO Plan for Burn Prevention and Care* (Geneva: World Health Organization, 2008).
43 A. H. Outwater, Hawa Ismail, Lwidiko Mgalilwa, Justin M. Temu and Naboth A. Mbembati, 'Burns in Tanzania: morbidity and mortality, causes and risk factors: a review', *International Journal of Burns and Trauma* 3 (2013): 18–29.

44 Effie Makepeace, 'Final Report to ReBaS', *Nanzikambe Arts* (Blantyre, Malawi: ReBaS, 2010).
45 World Bank, 'Raising awareness of violence against women in the Pacific', 2012, http://www.worldbank.org/en/news/feature/2012/11/25/raising-awareness-of-violence-against-women-in-the-pacific (accessed 14 October 2014).
46 C. Taylor and S. Michael, 'Gender-based domestic violence and its big bite on small island states – Fiji, Solomon Islands and Vanuatu', paper presented at the 14th Annual Global Development Network on Inequality, Social Protection and Inclusive Growth in Manila, 19–21 June 2013, http://www.gdn.int/html/page2.php%3FMID%3D3%26SID%3D24%26SSID%3D24%26SCID%3D37%26SSCID%3D77 (accessed 14 October 2014).
47 World Health Organization, 'Violence against women in Solomon Islands: translating research into policy and action on the social determinants of health', WHO Regional Office for the Western Pacific, 2013.
48 Taylor and Michael, 'Gender-based domestic violence and its big bite on small island states – Fiji, Solomon Islands and Vanuatu'.
49 World Bank, 'Raising awareness of violence against women in the Pacific'.
50 K. Abplanalp, 'Light at the end of the tunnel', *New Zealand Herald*, 29 March 2014.
51 S. Burkey, *People First: A Guide to Self-Reliant, Participatory Rural Development* (London: Zed Books, 1993).
52 K. Worth, 'Stages of Change: unpublished interview with the Director, Nina Nawalowalo', Port Moresby, Papua New Guinea, 2014.
53 M. Hunter, 'Cultivating the art of safe space', *Research in Drama Education* 13:1 (February 2008): 5–21.
54 Worth, 'Stages of Change' interview.
55 E. Lawless, *Women Escaping Violence: Empowerment Through Narrative* (Columbia: University of Missouri Press, 2001).
56 Ibid., p. 38.
57 Ibid., p 117.
58 Ibid., p. 160.
59 Worth, 'Stages of Change interview'.

60 Secretariat of the Pacific Community, 'Solomon Islands Family Health and Support Study: A study on violence against women and children', paper presented at the 2010 Beijing +15 Conference, *Review of Progress in Implementing the Beijing Platform for Action in Pacific Island Countries and Territories* (Noumea, New Caledonia: Secretariat of the Pacific Community, 2009), http://www.spc.int/hdp/ (accessed 14 October 2014).
61 Worth, 'Stages of Change' interview.
62 Ibid.
63 Ibid.
64 Ibid.
65 Abplanalp, 'Light at the end of the tunnel'.

Chapter 9

1 American Psychiatric Association, *Diagnostic and Statistical Manual of Mental Disorders*, 5th edn (Washington, DC: American Psychiatric Association, 2013).
2 Augustine Nwoye, 'African psychology and the Africentric paradigm to clinical diagnosis and treatment', *South African Journal of Psychology* 45:3 (2015): 305–17, DOI: 10.1177/0081246315570960.
3 Ibid., p. 309.
4 Ibid., pp. 310–11.
5 Euripides/C. K. Williams, *The Bacchae* (New York: Noonday Press, 1990).
6 G. Eagle, 'Therapy at the cultural interface: Implications of African cosmology for traumatic stress intervention', *PINS* 30 (2004): 1–22.
7 M. Starkowitz, 'African traditional healers understanding of depression as a mental illness: Implications for social work practice', unpublished Master's thesis, University of Pretoria, 2013, p. 25.
8 K. Sorsdahl, D. J. Stein and C. Lund, 'Mental health services in South Africa: Scaling up and future directions', *African Journal of Psychiatry* 15:3 (2012): 168–71.
9 Ibid., p. 169.

10 Starkowitz, 'African traditional healers understanding of depression as a mental illness', p. 21.
11 K. Sorsdahl, D. J. Stein and C. Lund, 'Mental health services in South Africa: Scaling up and future directions', *African Journal of Psychiatry* 15:3 (2012): 169.
12 R. C. Bodibe, 'Traditional healing: An indigenous approach to mental health problems', in J. Uys (ed.), *Psychological Counselling in the South African Context* (Cape Town: Maskew Miller, 1992), p. 154.
13 B. Hamber, 'The burden of care: An analysis of the burden of care on caregivers of South African psychiatric outpatients', unpublished Masters research report, University of Witwatersrand, 1995, in G. Eagle, 'Therapy at the cultural interface', p. 2.
14 In Nguni languages, the prefix 'i' serves as 'the' or 'a'. Depending on the sentence, this 'i' is left out when the English 'the' is used.
15 D. Conquergood, 'Beyond the text: Towards a performative cultural politics', paper presented at The Future of Performance Studies conference, New York University, March 1995, pp. 25–36, http://www.kineticnow.com/wp-content/uploads/2014/12/conquergood-1998-beyond-the-text.pdf (accessed 29 July 2015).
16 C. Moustakas, *Phenomenological Research Methods* (Los Angeles: Sage, 1994), p. 59.
17 C. Bell, *Ritual: Perspectives and Dimensions* (New York: Oxford University Press. 1997), p. 116.
18 B. McConachie, 'An evolutionary perspective on play, performance and ritual', *Drama Review* 55 (2011): 33–50.
19 iCosilune, Richard Schechner, 'Performance Theory', 2009, http://www.icosilune.com/2009/01/richard-schechner-performance-theory (accessed 28 April 2015).
20 McConachie, 'An evolutionary perspective', p. 33.
21 Ibid., p. 38.
22 R. Landy, 'Role theory and the role method of drama therapy', in D. R. Johnson and R. Emunah, *Current Approaches in Drama Therapy* (Springfield, IL: Charles C. Thomas, 2009).
23 R. Grainger, *Drama and Healing: The Roots of Drama Therapy* (London: Jessica Kingsley, 1990).
24 D. Thomas-Williams, 'Ritual storytelling: How the Griot tradition

informs dramatherapy?', unpublished Master's thesis, New York University, 2011.
25 Ibid., pp. 9–10.
26 P. Jones, *Drama as Therapy: Theatre as Living* (London: Routledge, 1996), p. 273.
27 R. Schechner, *Performance Studies: An Introduction*, 2nd edn (New York: Routledge, 2006), p. 71.
28 Ibid., p. 83.
29 Bell, *Ritual: Perspectives and Dimensions*, p. 131.
30 J. C. Alexander, 'Cultural pragmatics: Social performance between ritual and strategy', in J. C. Alexander, B. Giesen and J. L. Mast, *Social Performance: Symbolic Action, Cultural Pragmatics and Ritual* (New York: Cambridge University Press, 2006), p. 34.
31 McConachie, 'An evolutionary perspective', p. 44.
32 Bell, *Ritual: Perspectives and Dimensions*, p. 137.
33 WHO, *Traditional Medicine Strategy 2002–2005* (Geneva: World Health Organization 2002), pp. 1–61, http://www.wpro.who.int/health_technology/book_who_traditional_medicine_strategy_2002_2005.pdf (accessed 25 April 2015).
34 Eagle, 'Therapy at the cultural interface', p. 6.
35 M. Freeman and M. Motsei, 'Planning health care in South Africa – Is there a role for traditional healers?', *Social Science and Medicine* 34 (1992): 1183–90
36 Ibid., p. 1183.
37 S. D. Edwards. 'Traditional and modern medicine in South Africa: A research study', *Social Science and Medicine* 11 (1986): 1273–6.
38 J. F. Sobiecki, 'The intersection of culture and science in South African traditional medicine', *Indo-Pacific Journal of Phenomenology* 14 (2014): 1–11.
39 Ibid., p. 2.
40 Ibid., p. 4.
41 S. Makanya, 'The missing links: A South African perspective on the theories of health in dramatherapy', *The Arts in Psychotherapy* 41 (2014): 303–6.
42 Ibid., p. 303.
43 N. Mkhize, 'Ubuntu and harmony: An African approach to morality

and ethics', in R. Nicolson, *Persons in Community: African Ethics in a Global Culture* (Scottsville: University of KwaZulu Natal Press, 2008), p. 44.
44 American Psychiatric Association, *Diagnostic and Statistical Manual of Mental Disorders*, 5th edn (Arlington, VA: American Psychiatric Association, 2013), p. 155.
45 Landy, *Drama Therapy*, p. 189.
46 C. Moret and M. Briley, 'The importance of norepinephrine in depression', *Neuropsychiatric Disease and Treatment* 7 (2011): 9–13.
47 Starkowitz, 'African traditional healers understanding of depression as a mental illness', p. 80.
48 H. Ngubane, *Body and Mind in Zulu Medicine: An Ethnography of Health and Disease in Nyuswa-Zulu Thought and Practice* (London: Academic Press, 1977).
49 G. Straker, 'Integrating African and western healing practices in South Africa', *American Journal of Psychotherapy* 48 (1994): 455–67.
50 Eagle, 'Therapy at the cultural interface'.
51 Starkowitz, 'African traditional healers understanding of depression as a mental illness'.
52 Ibid., p. 39.
53 Eagle, 'Therapy at the cultural interface', p. 7.
54 Mandla Ngwane, interview on traditional understandings of depression, 30 July 2014.
55 P. Ventevogel, M. Jordans, R. Reis and J. de Jong, 'Madness or sadness? Local concepts of mental illness in four conflict affected African communities', *Conflict and Health* (2013): 1–16.
56 Starkowitz, 'African traditional healers understanding of depression as a mental illness', p. 25.
57 Sorsdahl et al., 'Mental health services in South Africa', p. 169.
58 Mandla Ngwane, interview on traditional understandings of depression.
59 Starkowitz, 'African traditional healers understanding of depression as a mental illness', p. 97.
60 Ibid., p. 69.
61 Ibid., p. 84.
62 Ibid., p. 85.
63 Ngubane, *Body and Mind in Zulu Medicine*.

64 Sorsdahl et al., 'Mental health services in South Africa'.
65 Ibid., p. 286.
66 A. Moovanthan and L. Nivethitha, 'Scientific Evidence-Based Effects of Hydrotherapy on Various Systems of the Body', *North American Journal of Medical Sciences* 6 (2014): 199–209, DOI: 10.4103/1947-2714.132935.
67 Grainger, *Drama and Healing*, p. 50.
68 Vicki Ross, 'Narratives of my mind', *KZNSA* (2015), http://www.kznsagallery.co.za/exhibitions/ (accessed 30 April 2015).
69 Ngubane, *Body and Mind in Zulu Medicine*.
70 A. T. Bryant, *Zulu Medicine and Medicine Men* (Cape Town: C Struik, 1966)
71 A. Pienaar and I. Manaka-Mkhwanazi, *Mental Health Nursing* (Cape Town: Juta Academic, 2004), p. 131.
72 Ventevogel et al., 'Madness or sadness'.
73 Sorsdahl et al., 'Mental health services in South Africa'..
74 Psychological Association of South Africa Council Committee, *Mental Health in South Africa* (Pretoria: PASA 1989), p. 50.
75 J. T. de Jong and I. H. Komproe, 'Closing the gap between psychiatric epidemiology and mental health in post-conflict situations', *The Lancet* (2002): 1793–4.
76 L. E. Rueter and B. L. Jacobs, 'A microdialysis examination of serotonin release in the rat forebrain induced by behavioural/environmental manipulations', *Brain Research* 739 (1996): 57–69.
77 Straker, 'Integrating African and western healing practices in South Africa', p. 459.
78 Eagle, 'Therapy at the cultural interface', pp. 7–8.
79 Starkowitz, 'African traditional healers understanding of depression as a mental illness', p. 79.
80 Bobby Baker, *The Expert View: An Artist Led Symposium*, Bromley by Bow Centre, London, 8 May 2015.
81 For an extensive overview and insight into Bobby Baker's practice and critical engagement with it, see Michèle Barrett and Bobby Baker (eds), *Bobby Baker: Redeeming Features of Daily Life* (London: Routledge, 2007).
82 Bobby Baker, *The Expert View*.

83 Throughout Baker's experience in the mental health system she kept an illustrated diary, initially making a drawing a day, then a drawing a week. Over the eleven-year period before she was discharged, she compiled 711 drawings. Baker and Dora Whittuck, a clinical psychologist and Baker's daughter, curated a selection to form the exhibition *Diary Drawings*, launched at the Wellcome Collection, London, in 2009, which continues to tour nationally and internationally.
84 Bobby Baker in 'Bobby Baker Interview', in Caoimhe McAvinchey (ed.), *Performance and Community: Case Studies and Commentary* (London: Methuen, 2014), pp. 105–14 (pp. 108–9).
85 Tony Hall, *Reflections on the Cultural Olympiad and London 2012 Festival* (London: Arts Council England, 2013).
86 Bobby Baker, application to Unlimited for *Mad Gyms and Kitchens*, Daily Life Ltd, 2010.
87 Bobby Baker, *Push Me*, The Space, 2012, http://www.pushmeplease.co.uk/artists/bobby-baker/ (accessed 12 July 2015).
88 See, for example, Elaine Aston, 'Feminist Performance as Archive: Bobby Baker's "Daily Life" and *Box Story*', *Performance Research* 7:4 (2002): 78–85.
89 Daily Life Ltd, *Mad Gyms and Kitchens*, Top Tips Gallery, http://dailylifeltd.co.uk/previous-work/mad-gyms-and-kitchens/gallery/ (accessed 12 July 2015).
90 Ibid.
91 *Artful Measures* is a collaboration between Caoimhe McAvinchey and Daily Life Ltd with case studies examining the relationship between arts practices that engage with issues of mental health and the documentation and evaluation practices that evidence and account for them. The cultural labour of *Mad Gyms and Kitchens* is the focus of Case Study 1, http://artfulmeasures.dailylifeltd.co.uk (accessed 12 July 2015).
92 Bobby Baker, *The Expert View*.
93 Vitor Pordeus, 'Madness yet there's method in it', lecture at McGill University, June 2015, https://www.youtube.com/watch?v=t-ydfuFrXhw (accessed 25 September 2015).
94 William Shakespeare, *As You Like It*, Act Two, Scene Seven. 'From

Stratford to Rio: using Shakespeare to treat mental illness', BBC News, http://www.bbc.com/news/health-32241100 (accessed 16 August 2015).
95 Nise da Silveira was a Brazilian psychiatrist. She started an out-patients clinic and art centre called Casa das Palmeiras (Palms House), where she pioneered research into art as occupational therapy for the mentally ill. 'Madness and Method', *Aeon Magazine*, http://aeon.co/magazine/psychology/can-theatre-be-used-to-treat-mental-illness/ (accessed 17 August 2015).
96 Amir Haddad is the founder and director of the street theatre company Tá na Rua (It's in the Street), established in 1980.
97 The Museum of Images of the Unconscious was Nise da Silveira's exhibition space for the art works made by her patients.
98 The World of Lygia Clark, http://www.lygiaclark.org.br (accessed 27 September 2015).

Chapter 10

1 Sheila L. Macrine (ed.), *Critical Pedagogy in Uncertain Times: Hope and Possibilities* (London: Palgrave Macmillan, 2009).
2 Janet Wolff, *The Aesthetics of Uncertainty* (New York: Columbia University Press, 2008).
3 Matthew Reisz, 'University careers increasingly marked by precariousness and uncertainty, scholars hear', *Times Higher Education*, 1 December 2015, https://www.timeshighereducation.com/news/university-careers-increasingly-marked-precariousness-and-uncertainty-scholars-hear (accessed 30 December 2015).
4 Charalampos Economou, Daphne Kaitelidou et al., *The Impact of the Financial Crisis on the Health System and Health in Greece* (Geneva: WHO/European Observatory on Health Systems and Policies, 2014).
5 In October 2015, a collaboration of Hollywood and Nollywood was announced, called *93 Days*. Will Ross, 'Hollywood and Nollywood join forces to make Ebola film', http://www.bbc.com/news/world-africa-34535541 (accessed 15 October 2015).
6 United Nations Development Group, *Socio-economic impact of the Ebola Virus Disease in West African Countries: A call for national and regional*

  containment, recovery and prevention, UNDP, 2015, http://www.africa.undp.org/content/dam/rba/docs/Reports/ebola-west-africa.pdf (accessed 29 April 2016).
7 David Abram, *The Spell of the Sensuous: Perception and Language in a More-Than-Human World* (New York: Vintage Books, 1997), p. 237.
8 Violeta Luna, 'Body in Action: Cartographies for Socially Engaged Performance', keynote for the Australasian Association for Theatre Drama and Performance Studies Annual Conference, Wellington, New Zealand, 2014.
9 'Safety Assessment of Roundup Ready® Corn Event NK603', Monsanto Report, 2002, http://www.monsanto.com/products/documents/safety-summaries/corn_pss_nk603.pdf (accessed 27 January 2015).
10 Luna, 'Body in Action'.
11 *Campesino* is a Spanish word meaning 'peasant farmer'.
12 Luna, 'Body in Action'.
13 http://secosymojados.com/artists/ (accessed 13 April 2015).
14 John Holloway and Eloína Peláez (eds), *Zapatista!: Reinventing Revolution in Mexico* (London: Pluto Press, 1998).
15 Kate Rossiter, Pia Kontos, Angela Colantonio, Julie Gilbert, Julia Gray and Michelle Keightley, 'Staging Data: Theatre as a tool for analysis and knowledge transfer in health research', *Social Science and Medicine* 66:1 (2008): 130–46.
16 Jerzy Grotowski, *Towards a Poor Theatre* (New York: Simon and Schuster, 1968).
17 Susan M. Cox, 'A life of their own: Reflections on autonomy and ethics in research-based theatre', in Anna Harpin and Juliet Foster (eds), *Isolated Acts: Madness, Performance and Psychiatry* (Basingstoke: Palgrave Macmillan, 2014), pp. 65–8.
18 Ibid.
19 Rossiter *et al*. 'Staging data', p. 136.
20 IDRC, 'Executive summary: Health. An ecosystem approach', http://www.idrc.ca/EN/Resources/Publications/Pages/ArticleDetails.aspx?PublicationID=538 (accessed 27 January 2015).
21 Leslie Bank and Gary Minkley, 'Going nowhere slowly? Land, livelihoods and rural development in the Eastern Cape', *Social Dynamics* 31:1 (2005): 1–38.

22 Experience Bryon, *Integrative Performance Practice: Practice and Theory for the Interdisciplinary Performer* (London and New York: Routledge, 2014), p. 60.
23 Ibid., p. 61.
24 Ibid., p. 43.
25 Ibid., p. 212.
26 Esther Thelen and Linda B Smith, 'Dynamic Systems Theories', in William Damon and Richard M Lerner, *Handbook of Child Psychology: Volume 1 – Theoretical Models of Human Development* (Hoboken, NJ: John Wiley and Sons, 2006), p. 276.
27 Ibid., p. 258.
28 Zoe Zontou, 'Applied Theatre as an "Alternative Substance": Reflections from an Applied Theatre Project with People in Recovery from Alcohol and Drug Dependency', *Journal of Applied Arts and Health* 2:3 (2011): 303–15.
29 http://www.fallenangelsdancetheatre.co.uk (accessed 27 January 2015).
30 Williams White, *Pathways from the Culture of Addiction to the Culture of Recovery*, 2nd edn (Center City, MN: Hazelden, 1996), p. 428.
31 Betty Ford Institute Consensus Panel, 'What is Recovery? A Working Definition from The Betty Ford Institute', *Journal of Substance Abuse Treatment* 33 (2007): 221–8; Patricia Deegan, 'Recovery: The Lived Experience of Rehabilitation', *Psychosocial Rehabilitation Journal* 11 (1988): 11–19.
32 Srdjan Sremac, 'Addiction, Narrative and Spirituality: Theoretical-methodological Approaches and Overview', *Religija I Tolerancija* 8:14 (2010): 255–73.
33 Fallen Angels' participants reflective interview with the author, 11 June 2014.
34 Sally Bailey, 'Recovering Identity and Stimulating Growth Through Drama Therapy', in S. Brooke (ed.), *The Use Of Creative Therapies with Chemical Dependency Issues* (Springfield, IL: Charles C. Thomas, 2009), pp. 204–17.
35 Aline Harwick, 'The Contribution of Applied Drama to the Recovery of Adult Substance Abusers: A Qualitative Exploration', in J. Reynolds and Z. Zontou (eds), *Addiction and Performance* (Newcastle-upon-Tyne: Cambridge Scholars, 2014).

36 Odidika U. J. Umeora, Nkechi Bridget Emma-Echiegu, Maryjoanne Chinyem Umeora and Nnennaya Ajayi, 'Ebola viral disease in Nigeria: The panic and cultural threat', *African Journal of Medical and Health Sciences* 13 (2014):1–5, http://www.ajmhs.org/text.asp?2014/13/1/1/139434 (accessed 10 July 2015).

37 Tilly A. Gurman, 'Back to Basics: Improving the Conceptualization and Operationalization of Programmatic Exposure in Social and Behavior Change Communication Through Conceptual Models', *Journal of Health Communication* 20 (2015): 1–3, DOI: 10.1080/10810730.2015.1001699.

38 Jonathan Haynes, 'African cinema and Nollywood: Contradictions', *Situations* 4:1 (2007): 67–90.

39 *Ebola Doctors*, Nollywood movie, 2014, https://www.youtube.com/watch?v=s1Y3w21CiJ8 (accessed 10 July 2015).

40 *Ebola Doctors* was posted on YouTube on 18 September 2014, and a month before Nigeria was declared Ebola-free, the film had more than 300,000 viewers. Out of 751 viewers who rated the film, 571 (76 per cent) liked it, while 180 (24 per cent) did not like it.

41 '5 fake Ebola cures that are circulating online right now', 8 October 2014, http://www.rt.com/news/194200-ebola-virus-treatment-bizarre/ (accessed 10 July 2015).

42 Eric M. Leroy and Pierre Rouquet, 'Multiple Ebola virus transmission event and rapid decline in Central Africa wildlife', *Science Magazine* 303: 5656 (2004): 387–90.

Afterword

1 Jason Hickel, 'The problem with saving the world: the UN's new Sustainable Development Goals aim to save the world without changing it', *Jacobin*, 8 August 2015, https://www.jacobinmag.com/2015/08/global-poverty-climate-change-sdgs/ (accessed 13 May 2016).

2 Stephen Clift, 'Creative arts as a public health resource: Moving from practice-based research to evidence-based practice', *Perspectives in Public Health* 132: 123, cited by Eleonora Belfiore, 'The arts and healing: The power of an idea', in *Oxford Textbook of Creative Arts, Health, and Wellbeing: International perspectives on Practice, Policy and Research*,

ed. Stephen Clift and Paul M. Camic (Oxford: Oxford University Press, 2015), p. 16

3   Commission on Social Determinants of Health, *Closing the Gap in a Generation: Health Equity Through Action on the Social Determinants of Health: Commission on Social Determinants of Health Final Report* (Geneva: WHO, 2008), p. 18.

4   J. Sachs, L. Becchetti and A. Annett, *World Happiness Report 2016, Special Rome Edition, Vol. II* (New York: Sustainable Development Solutions Network, 2016).

5   http://www.actionforhappiness.org/ (accessed 11 May 2016).

6   Augusto Boal, *Legislative Theatre: Using Performance to Politics* (London: Routledge, 1998), p. 11.

7   John Ashton, 'Let's Invest in Real Health', in Arts Council England, *Create: A Journal of Perspectives on the Value of Art & Culture* (Manchester: Arts Council England, 2014), p. 95.

8   United Nations Youth Envoy, '10 things you didn't know about the world's population', April 2015, http://www.un.org/youthenvoy/2015/04/10-things-didnt-know-worlds-population/ (accessed 2 May 2016).

9   WHO, *Global Status Report On Violence Prevention* (WHO, 2014), http://www.who.int/violence_injury_prevention/violence/status_report/2014/en/ (accessed 2 May 2016).

10 Michael Balfour, Penny Bundy, Bruce Burton, Julie Dunn and Nina Woodrow, *Applied Theatre: Resettlement* (London: Methuen Bloomsbury, 2015).

11 United Nations Youth Envoy, '10 things'.

Index

adaptation 99–100, 234–8
addiction 123–35, 241–5
   and recovery 241–5
   and social stigma 241–5
aesthetics 6–7, 35, 41–71, 156–7, 235–8
   privileging western notions of 51–2
   (syn)aesthetics 153
affect 21, 23, 41, 50, 52–4, 60, 63, 71, 149
   and effect 42–4
   negative 21, 44–6
   positive 65–6
AfroReggae 34–5, 98, 114–19
Age Exchange Theatre Trust 79–80
ageing 9, 75–89
   and art 76–89
agency 33–4, 55, 58–61, 166, 191, 213, 236–7
   and imagination 130
Ahmed, Sara 148
alcohol 3, 41–2, 45, 47–51, 61–2, 101, 121, 128–9, 235, 241–5
Alive and Out There 168, 180–3
Alma Ata Declaration 26–7
anxiety 20, 90–1, 224, 229
apartheid 60–1, 101, 150, 236
Applied Theatre 4–9, 41–71, 88–9, 94–5, 107, 123–35, 145–6, 150–1, 154, 156–7, 186–8, 198–9, 249–52
   applied theatre as research (ATAR) 42
   donors 67
   ethics 54–5, 68–71,
   and globalization 56–7, 129–31
   in health 41–2, 70
   and neoliberalism 6, 19, 51–2, 54, 67, 69

Applied Theatre and Arts Processes (ATAP) 128–9
Arepp: Theatre for Life (Arepp) 152–4
arts 4–10, 12, 17–18, 21, 23–5, 40, 42, 50, 52–3, 63–4, 66–8, 77–9, 88–9, 94, 123–35, 142–4, 203–4, 206, 217–18, 249–52
   funding 67, 88
   as intervention 6, 41–4
   as medicine 12, 22–3
   as pedagogy 5, 41
   purpose 6, 42, 52
   as research 6, 40, 42, 63
Arts Council England (ACE) 21, 78
'arts for health' 5, 52, 71, 217, 249
'arts in health' 4–5, 12, 17–18, 23–6, 42, 52, 66, 71, 88–9, 142, 217, 249–52
   issues of 24–5
   value of 217–23, 249–52
Asia-Pacific region 145–6, 162–6
Australian Aboriginal People 16–17
awareness 22, 48, 62, 94–5, 98, 102, 108, 113, 147, 158, 163, 174, 180, 189, 246–8
   and social change 62, 174, 189, 202

Baker, Bobby 206, 217–23
Bandura, Albert 57–9
bereavement 89–92, 211–12
bias 162
   perception 186–9
Bilbrough, Gordon 152–3
biomedical model 249
Boal, Augusto 44, 54, 56, 69–70, 112, 114, 124, 250
body, the 14–15, 115, 112, 124, 129,

149, 153–4, 169–70, 175, 178–9, 239–40
and mind 11–12, 126–7, 152
Botton, Alain de 6–7, 53, 146–7
Brazil 34–5, 98, 114–19, 205–6, 223–7, 301 n.95
Breathe Imphefumlo 100–1
Brecht, Bertolt 45, 57, 224
British New Economics Foundation (NEF) 21–2
Brown, Jonathon D. 64
Burns, Catherine 147–8

Canada 22–3, 123–35, 235, 278 n.7
cancer 3, 13, 15, 66, 115, 167–83
    and audience 167, 168–9, 175–9
    and bodies 172, 178
    and/as disability 169, 173
    and heroism 167, 169–70
    and humour 175–8
    medical model of 169, 172–4
    narratives of 167–9, 171
    portrayals of 168–9, 171, 175–6
care 11–12, 32, 75, 78, 173, 213, 217, 221
    culture of 32, 94–5, 125, 142–3, 223–7
    residential care homes 77–89
Carina's Choice 102–11
change 25, 27, 31–2, 39, 46, 50, 56–61, 65, 69, 114, 130, 136–7, 142–4, 145, 162–3, 188, 198, 202–4, 209, 211, 222, 237, 245–8
child mortality 3, 28–9, 37
cholera 97
civil rights 175
climate change 39, 229–30, 234–8,
Climate Change Adaptation 234–8
colonization 22, 37, 122–35, 206–7, 278 n.7
    and the body 122, 123–4, 129–30
communicable diseases 3–4, 97–119
    and clinical trials 102–4, 106–7, 109–10

contagious diseases 97
increased risk of 97–8
and inequality 97–8
community 15–17, 20–2, 26–7, 42–3, 46–8, 53, 55–6, 77, 79, 109, 127–8, 133, 179
    development 46, 48–51
    and social connectedness 20–1
    temporary 92
    transformation 111–12
community arts 42, 66
community theatre 53, 181–2
community-generated (ComGen) theatre 46–8
conflict 29, 30–1, 57, 203, 236
corporeal, the 153, 233
creativity 6–7, 24, 50, 81, 142–4, 199
crisis 3, 8, 28, 39–40, 154–5, 200, 229
cultural sensitivity 142
culture 4, 18–21, 33, 44, 48–9, 93, 208–9, 231–3, 251
    and community 26–7
    and health 22–3, 122–3, 125

Daily Life Ltd. 217–22
dance 44, 118–19, 133–4, 150, 223–7, 241–5
    and symbolism 241–5
Darpana Academy of Performing Arts (Darpana) 186–99
death/dying 3–4, 35, 41–2, 70, 76, 89–95, 97, 99–100, 111, 121, 135, 167, 209
    and anxiety 90–1, 93
    and capitalism 93
    conversations about 76–90
    and economies 76
    and education 90
    and empathy 94–5
    euphemisms of 91, 272 n.42
    and humour 91
    as failure 92–3
    phobia 76, 93
    premature 3, 121

dementia 8, 75–89
  Alzheimer's 4, 78, 270 nn.2, 15
  and creativity 78, 81–2, 88–9
  and economies 75–6, 78
  and improvization 77–8, 80–9
Democratic Republic Of The Congo (DRC) 37–8, 212
Dengue Fever 97–8, 114–19
Denmark 122, 135–41
depression 206–17 *see also* mental health
  as a continuum 208, 212–13
  localized understandings of 211–12
  and social withdrawal 211, 215
desire 64, 147–8, 150, 155–6, 164–5
development 7–8, 28–32, 48–50, 55–6, 62–3, 111–14, 121, 167, 188–9
  deficit model 62
  international narratives of 7–8, 23, 28–32, 110
diabetes 3, 121–7, 135–44
diagnosis 78, 82, 170, 174, 205, 210
Diagnostic and Statistical Manual of Mental Disorders (DSM) 205–6
disability 34, 169–80, 219, 238–41, 261 n.105, 262–3 n.122
  medical model of 169, 172–4
  social models of 169, 172–3, 175, 179
Disability Adjusted Life Years (DALYs) 36–7, 41–2, 261 n.105
disease 3–5, 27–9, 36–7, 42, 52, 65, 97–120, 172–3, 207, 211, 245–8
  communicable diseases 4
  and inequality 3–4, 8, 25–6, 31, 97–8
  lack of 13–16, 125
  lifestyle-related 42, 121–2, 136–41
  Non-Communicable Diseases (NCDS) 27–8, 36, 121–44

parasitic 29, 97–111
pathological 27
perception of 99–100
  as political 12, 27
  and poverty 3–4, 36, 116–18
diversity 19, 44, 156–207
  biodiversity 230–5
domestic violence 62, 186, 201–4, 251
  by intimate partners 202
  and silence 203
drama, form/subject of 43, 104, 123, 143, 162, 165, 188–9, 199, 208, 263–4 n.9
dramatherapy 79, 205, 207–8
dramaturgy 225, 230, 238–41
drugs 126–9, 164, 174, 241–5

Ebola Doctors 230, 245–8
Ebola Virus Disease (EVD) 71, 229–30, 245–8
education 5–6, 25–8, 41–4, 54–9, 71, 90, 104, 112, 123–35, 162–6, 185–6, 192–201
  and entertainment 57–9
  and humour 90, 135–41
  knowledge economy 54
  peer 62, 107
  and the academy 54
emancipation 43, 113, 152
embodiment 106, 123–4, 130–4, 149, 153, 208, 214–17, 234–8, 242
emotion 7, 12, 21, 42–4, 56, 58, 60, 71, 127, 143, 146–54, 170–2, 203, 206–17
  and cognition 7, 42–6, 71
  emotional engagement 44–6
empowerment 53, 55–6, 62–3, 189, 203
Entertainment-Education (EE) 57–9
epidemic 27–9, 100–11, 162–6
ethnicity 34, 75, 142, 168

facilitation 48, 68–71, 84–9, 107
failure 30, 58–9, 65, 76–7, 92–3, 163

Fallen Angels Dance Theatre
  Company 230, 241–5
family 65–6, 91, 143–4, 182, 193,
  195–7
Farmer, Paul 33–4, 55
feedback 71, 90–1, 182, 194–5
feelings 12, 16, 20, 149–61, 211–16
  see also emotion
  structures of 16, 23
feminism 20–1, 178, 219
film 100–1, 147, 168–71, 229
  comedy 245–8
First Nations (Canada) 22, 123–35,
  278 n.7
food 27, 49, 110, 125–7, 135–41,
  229–38 *see also* healthy eating
For Facts' Sake 159–60
form 1, 47, 67, 77–8, 80–2, 115,
  157–9, 230–1, 235, 243
  and content 53, 107, 218
  and function 43, 57
Four Husbands 149, 154–61
Freire, Paulo 112
fundraising 167, 171, 174, 178, 289
  n.5
  and consumerism 167, 174
funerals 90

geographies 8, 34, 35–7
gender 8, 147, 149–61, 163–4, 171
  inequality 8–9, 28–9, 32–5,
  185–204
genetically modified (GM) crops
  229–38
Gilroy, Andrea 88
GINI index 8
Global Burden Of Disease Study
  (GBD) 3, 36, 261 n.102
global community 3
Global North 5–8, 37, 52, 75, 78, 249
global political economy 8
Global South 3, 5–8, 27–9, 36–7, 41,
  52, 57, 75, 100, 111, 121–2,
  145, 185, 249–50

Gramsci, Antonio 48–9
Greece 12
  Ancient 27
Guatemala 62–3

Haiti 33, 97
healing 11–2, 56–7, 130, 203, 205–6,
  224–5
  and prayer 180, 216
  as performative 205–17
  traditional practices of 125–8,
  206–17
health
  and communication 14, 26, 38,
    47–8, 59, 131, 136, 140, 149,
    151, 245
  and community 16–7, 22, 42,
    103, 142
  and confidence 63–5, 131, 134,
    144, 180, 204
  definition of 11–16
  ecological 32, 230–4
  and economies 8, 19, 27–8,
    32–40, 48, 55–6, 75–8,
    110–11, 202, 229–30, 249–50
  education 5–6, 25–8, 41–6, 52, 54,
    57–9, 104, 107, 110–11, 137,
    140–1, 162–5, 245–8
  and happiness 16, 18–19, 21, 250
  and human rights 16, 33, 50
  and humour 70, 91, 115–16, 154,
    159–61, 164–5, 177, 217
  and indigenous populations
    123–35
  inequality and 32–40, 75–6, 97–8,
    163, 174
  and intermediality 238–41
  and language 39, 126, 167, 173,
    211–12
  and location 33, 36–7, 75–6 *see
    also* geographies
  maternal 28–9, 189, 194, 251
  and normativity 13–18, 31, 147
  poverty and 4, 27, 28–31, 33,

37–42, 48, 54–5, 101, 107, 109, 116–17, 125, 163, 185, 212, 249
promotion 16, 25–8, 40, 59, 122, 135–6, 139, 146, 162, 180–3, 213
and religion 15, 99–100, 64, 208–10
social 11, 15, 17, 27–8, 79
spiritual 16, 126–7, 205, 209–17, 242–3, 250
transnational 26
and utopia 16
women's *see* women's health
and youth 22, 122–35, 148, 251
healthcare 11, 16, 41, 75–6, 125, 169, 180–3, 187, 222, 250
disproportionate access to 26–7, 32, 37, 52, 75
healthy 13–16, 22, 49, 123–35, 147, 171, 191, 210–3, 236, 261 n.105 *see also* unhealthy
healthy eating 121, 125–7, 135–41
Heathcote, Edwin 11–12
Heddon, Deidre 24
helplessness 59–60, 64–5
Hickson, Ford 147
Hildefonso, Johayne 98, 114–19
history 24–5, 30, 33, 129–30, 206–7
HIV/AIDS 8, 14, 28–30, 36, 42, 54–5, 59, 62, 70, 97, 145–62, 170, 229–30, 235, 257
and fear 145–7, 151, 163
and homophobia 147, 174
and morality 146–7, 163
relationship to TB 30, 101–2, 106, 111
and shame 146–7, 151, 163
hope 36, 148, 186, 204
and theatre 163, 186
homosexuality 145, 150
homophobia 163–4
Hughes, Jenny 88–9
hybrid practices of 207

identity 122, 136–41, 170–1, 176–7, 225, 231–3, 245
impact 3–4, 6–7, 21, 24–5, 42–4, 50–3, 66–8, 88–9, 123, 143, 168, 182, 186–8, 206, 208, 245–8, 249–50
and evaluation 42–4, 67–8, 88–9
and value 24
improvization 77–89, 104, 137, 225–6,
as a facilitation strategy 77, 80, 85–7
and 'saying yes' 77, 83, 85
In Your Circle 149–50, 154–9
India 145, 186, 188–99
Indigenous 22, 49, 71, 122–35, 225–6, 230–4
populations 101, 122–35
youth 122–35
inequality 8, 25–8, 31–40, 66, 75, 97–8, 124–5, 163, 171, 185, 192
infection 4, 8, 36, 61, 97–8, 99–111, 145, 199, 207, 245–6
parasitic 98
injury 4, 36, 42, 200
instrumentalism 6, 25–6, 41–71, 146
interaction 23, 107, 123–4, 130, 147–8, 157, 226, 238–40
intergenerational 5, 79, 126, 166
International Health Regulations 27–8
intervention 6, 34, 41–4, 46–52, 54–6, 61–2, 66, 70, 131, 135, 170–2, 207
intimacy 148–61, 240
and belonging 149
collective 149, 154, 160

Jones, Phil 208
Joseph, Christopher Odhiambo 68–9, 285 n.23

Kala Sangam 123, 142–4

Kellehear, Allan 76
Kenya 48, 68–9
Khutsoane, Namatshego 150, 156, 161
Kicking the Bucket 89–95

La Bohème 99–100
Latin America 229, 231–2
Lawlor, Clark 99–100
leadership 49–50, 111, 132–4
   collaborative 111, 132
   resistance to 132–3
learning 22, 42, 45, 50, 54, 57–9, 64, 70, 104, 112, 131, 136, 149, 153–4, 207
   arts-based 134
   experiential 152
Liberia 245–6
life expectancy 3–4, 36, 38, 75, 187, 262–3 n.122
lifestyle 16, 62, 121, 123–35, 139–40, 142–4, 242
   'choices' 121, 123–35
   diseases 121, 136
Lorde, Audre 169, 174–5, 179
Luna, Violeta 229, 230–4

Machon, Josephine 149, 153–4, 157
Mad Gyms and Kitchens 206, 217–23, 300 n.91
Madness Hotel, The 206, 223–7
malaria 3, 28–9, 36, 55, 97–8, 111–14, 277 n.67
Malaria Ebola 246–7
Malawi 49, 98, 111–14, 186, 199–201
McAvinchey, Caoimhe 77–8, 80, 89
Mda, Zakes 46–9,
medicine 11–12, 24, 27, 93, 102, 223–7
   and the medical event 239
   traditional 127, 207, 209–10, 213–17
Memory Ensemble 82–3
mental health 23–4, 37, 180–3, 205–28
   and agency 59–60, 130, 213, 236
   biopsychosocial (BPS) model 205
   care 207
   and counselling 210
   cultural understandings of 205, 211–13
   and emotional resilience 205
   and strategies for wellness 221–3
Mexico 230–4
Millennium Development Goals (MDGs) 27–32, 167, 249
Milton-Sand & Søn 122, 135–41
multiple health conditions 75

Nanzikambe Arts Development Organisation 199–201
narrative 30, 56, 80, 82, 152–3, 179, 187, 203–4, 243
   personal 240–2
National Health Service (NHS) (UK) 142, 222, 262–3 n.122
neoliberalism 6, 19–20, 22, 31, 51, 54, 67, 100, 234, 250
Nicholson, Helen 81
Nigeria 226, 245–8
NK603: Action for Performer & e-Maiz 230–4
Non-Governmental Organizations (NGOs) 4, 61, 112–14, 199, 245
non-participatory methodologies 46, 106–7
Notaro, Tig 168–9, 175–7, 179
nutrition 101, 106–10, 142, 187, 219

obesity 121–2, 135–42
oppression 47, 54–6, 69, 131, 234
Osnes, Beth 62–3

Papua New Guinea 16, 202–4
participation 6, 17, 23, 46–8, 50, 65–7, 77–89, 94, 107, 113, 137–8, 141, 149, 151–2
   and development 42

in schools 107–8
in theatre and performance 66–7, 77–8, 133, 181, 245
Participatory Agit-Prop 46–7, 49
pedagogy 5–6, 41–2, 44, 52, 54, 134, 140–1, 145–6, 224
non-formal learning 42
performance 4–5, 15, 31–2, 38, 42–4, 46, 53, 65, 70, 77–8, 88, 145–6, 151, 153, 169, 171, 177, 208–9, 225, 245–8, 250–2
cultural 44, 49, 53, 158, 204, 209
non-Eurocentric 49, 71, 207–8
and ritual 206–17
techniques of 49, 104, 165, 203
training 104, 189
performance research 6
performativity 131, 207–9, 216–17
pharmaceuticals 109–10, 226–7
and expense 109–10
phenomenology 238–41
Plastow, Jane 112
Pordeus, Vitor 206, 223–7
positive psychology 42, 64–5
Post-Colonial Stress Disorder 22, 123–35, 278 n.4
post-colonialism 22, 122, 123–35, 278 n.4
power 26, 33–4, 39, 48–9, 51–2, 57, 123–4, 146–7, 160–1, 203
Practice as Research (PaR) 238–41
praxis 41, 50, 67
precarity 229–30
Prentki, Tim 41, 43, 48
prevention 4, 16, 98, 102–8, 111–14, 162–6, 199–201
and fear 102, 162–3
issues with 136
rather than cure 4
psychiatry 180, 206, 218, 223–7
and pharmaceuticals 226–7
psychologism 56–7
public health 7, 24, 26, 34–5, 38, 121, 135, 147, 162, 166

quality of life 17, 25, 82
quantitative evidence 24, 67–8, 122
issues with 24, 31, 67–8

Ranciere, Jacques 43–4, 145–6
rape 44–6, 150, 185
Read, Alan 148–9
rehearsal 48, 56, 65, 80, 104–5, 209
relationships, 18, 22, 26, 57, 61, 64–6, 127–8, 130, 131, 147–61, 172, 210, 286 n.26
representation 99–100, 143, 175, 208, 218, 226, 245
Research and Intervention into Sexual Health: Theory to Action (RISHTA) 61–2
resilience 42, 59, 63–6, 205, 208, 212–13, 216, 234, 236
risk 15, 25–6, 31, 61, 67, 70–1, 97, 108, 130–1, 149, 155, 159–63, 199–200, 248
ritual 12, 90, 189, 206, 208–17, 223–7, 231
performance of 12, 208–17
Rogoff, Irit 54
role models 125–8
role play 63, 84, 87, 204
Rothschild, Liz 76, 89–95

Sayre's law 52, 265 n.35
self-esteem 17, 64–5, 119, 213
and dignity 17
Sen, Amartya 34, 62, 187–8, 190–9
sense-making 149–50, 152–4, 157
sex 106, 146–66
and morality 146–8, 151
pathologisation of 147, 155
and playfulness 148–9, 157–8
and rationality 162–3
sex work 61, 164
sexual health 61–2, 145–66
and communication 148–9
discussions of 148, 159–60
and positivity 147, 151, 154–5

and stigma 147, 151, 163–4, 166
sexuality 146–61
sexually transmitted infections (STIs) 61, 147, 108, 124–5
Shakti 186–99, 292 n.4
shame 76, 111, 129, 146, 148, 163, 180–3, 187, 203
Shaughnessy, Nicola 94–5
Sierra Leone 245
sickness 13, 127, 155, 168–80, 205–6
and 'the sick role' 167, 174–5, 179
Singapore 16
Social Cognitive Learning Theory 57–9
social exclusion 38, 53, 243
social justice 34, 41, 50–2, 69
social traditions 21
socioeconomics 32–3, 41–2, 55–6, 64–6, 110–11, 202, 215, 229, 249–50
Solomon Islands 186, 201–4
Sontag, Susan 12
South Africa 8, 16, 45, 60–1, 66, 70, 98–111, 145, 147–61, 206–17, 229–30, 234–8
Spence, Jo 169, 174–5, 179
Sri Lanka 50–1, 56
Stages of Change 186, 201–4
Staging Addiction Recovery (SAR) 241–5
Stander, Genevieve 60–1
stigma 100, 109, 111, 143, 147, 163–6, 180–3, 218, 242–3, 248
Storybox 83–9
storytelling 80–9, 203
issues with 81
street theatre 61–2, 224
sustainability 16–17, 55–6, 62, 68, 202, 237
Sustainable Development Goals (SDGs) 249
Sweden 37, 66–7

Tanzania 55
Taylor, Shelley E. 64–5

teacher-centred learning 107
theatre
affective properties 43–4, 60
application of 41, 145–6
cognitive potential 43, 46, 71
as collective tradition 224
and communication 38, 47–8, 61, 112, 149
and dementia care 75–89
dialogical 68–9, 70, 111–14, 176–7, 222
Documentary Theatre 79
games 123, 127–35, 281 n.42
interactive 143, 151, 181
interventionist 6, 41–63, 131, 207–8
pedagogical 41–54, 141
and the postdramatic 158
Reminiscence Theatre 79–81
research-based 235
responses to health 32
strategies of 55, 136, 162
theatre of necessity 1502
theatre-making 4–7, 57, 65, 148, 150–1, 157
Theatre For Development (TFD) 41, 98, 111–14, 199
and behaviour change 55, 111–14
funding 51–2, 68–9, 112
socialist ideologies of 43
therapy 6–7, 88, 223–7, 242
Thompson, James 43, 56–7
Timeslips 81–3
transformation 44, 57, 111–12, 114, 130, 152, 162, 203–4, 216
transgender 164
treatment 27, 70, 88, 101–2, 121, 127–31, 170–4, 178, 182, 199, 205–17, 238–41
holistic 11–12
Tselikas, Elektra 57
tuberculosis 3–4, 42, 97–111
cultural associations of 99–101

history of 99–101
multi-drug resistant (MDR-TB) 98, 102
relationship to HIV/AIDS 30, 101–2, 106, 111
representation in literature and performance 99–101
typhoid 27

Uganda 145
Underwood-Lee, Emily 169, 175–80
Undie, Chi-Chi 158–9
unhealthy 14, 121, 135–42 see also *healthy*
United Kingdom (UK) 4, 8, 37, 40, 64, 66–8, 75, 78, 89–95, 123, 142–4, 147, 169, 171–4, 217–23
United States of America (USA) 8, 20, 82, 171–4
Universal Declaration Of Human Rights 50
universal health care 3, 28, 169 see also healthcare

vaccines 102, 104–11
Van Erven, Eugene 53
violence 42, 62, 147–8, 150, 163–4, 185–6, 193, 203–8
domestic *see* domestic violence
interpersonal 251
structural 33–6
Virchow, Rudolf 27
Vukani! 234–8
vulnerability 158, 212, 240

well-being 4, 11–25, 29, 34, 42, 50, 59, 63–8, 88, 123–35, 186–99, 205–6, 209, 213, 217–23, 242, 244–5, 249–52
and ecologies 231–4
and gender 185–99, 202
and happiness 16, 19
holistic understanding of 17, 126–7
mental 15, 17
and neoliberalism 18–25
physical 15, 17
and safety 20
social 15, 17, 51
and social connectedness 20–1
as a social construct 11
subjective 19, 21, 23
and wellness 190, 221–2
White, Gareth 151–2, 154, 156–8
White, Mike 17, 23–4, 26, 52–3
women's health 28, 32, 102, 150, 171, 174, 178, 185–204, 251
access to healthcare 187 *see also* healthcare
and capability 186–8, 191, 199
and education 185, 192–3, 198
and marriage 185, 189, 193–7
and representations of victimhood 45, 187, 194
and reproduction 185, 195–6, 251
and trust 192–4
understandings of 185, 190–1
and unemployment 185
and violence 185, 193, 202–4
World Health Organization (WHO) 15, 41–2, 102, 142, 146, 185, 250

www.ingramcontent.com/pod-product-compliance
Lightning Source LLC
Chambersburg PA
CBHW050135240426
43673CB00043B/1671